# Aflatoxins - Occurrence, Detoxification, Determination and Health Risks

*Edited by Lukman Bola Abdulra'uf*

Published in London, United Kingdom

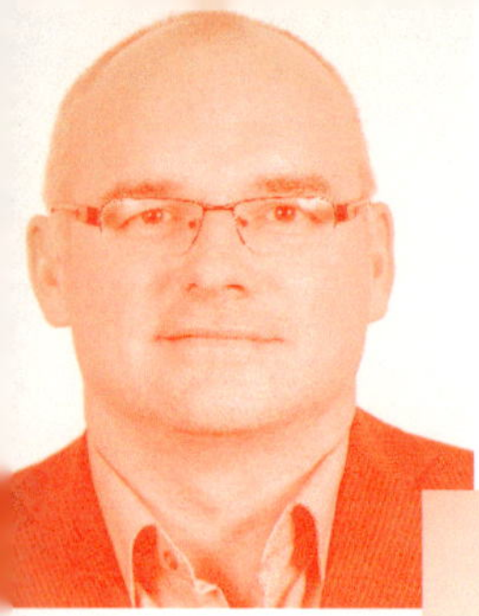
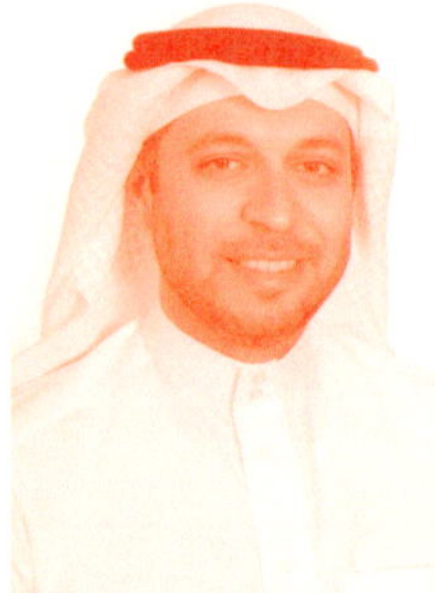
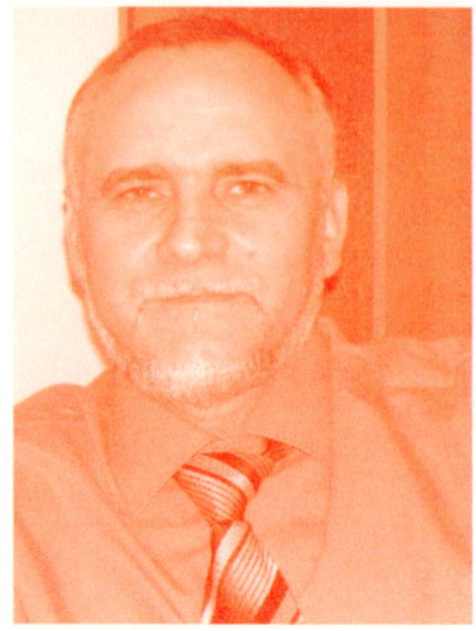
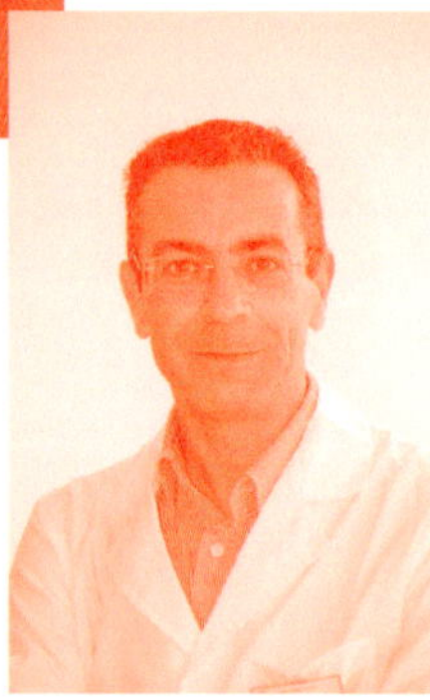
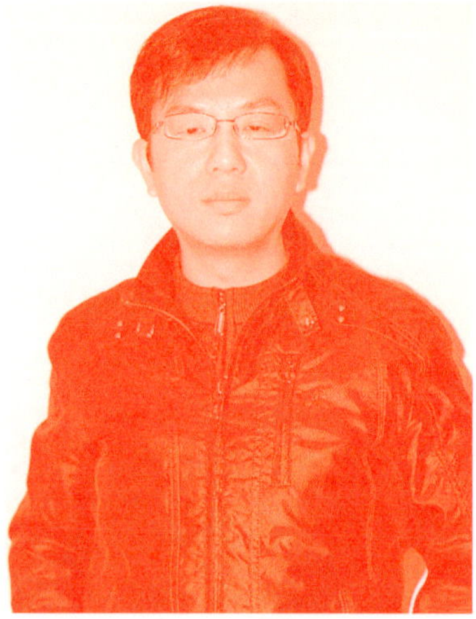
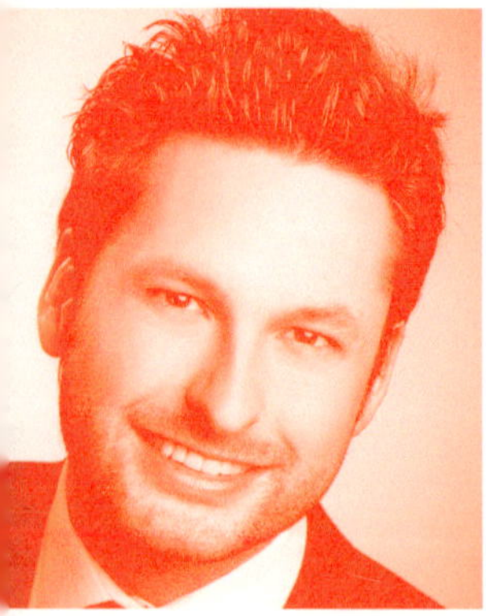
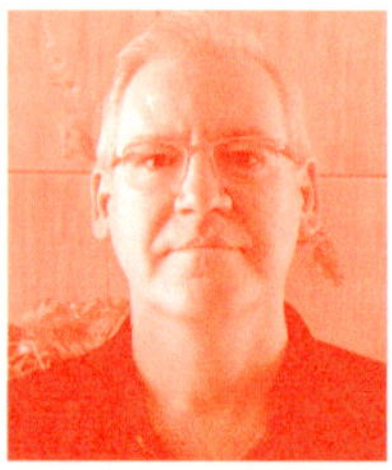

IntechOpen

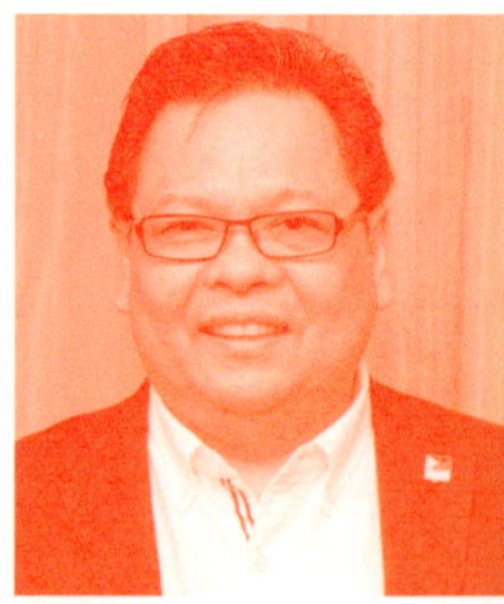
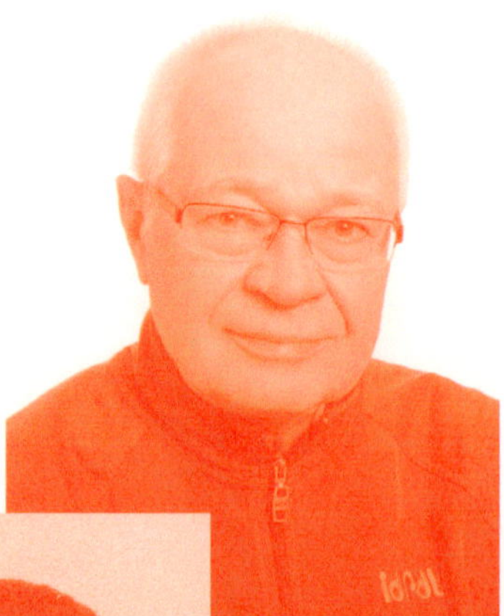
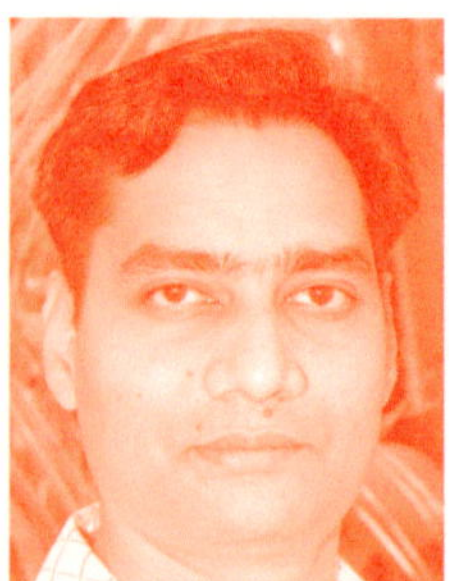
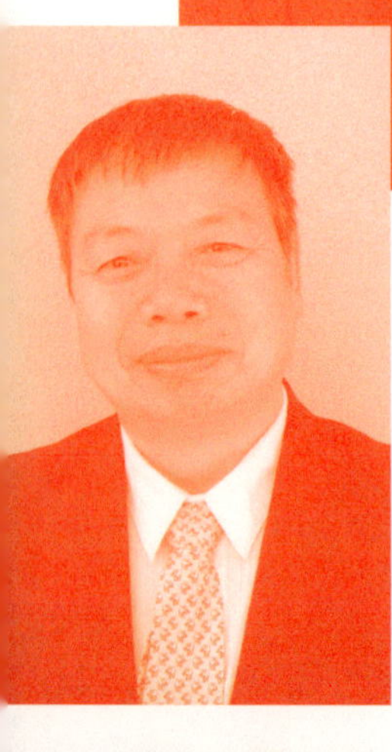
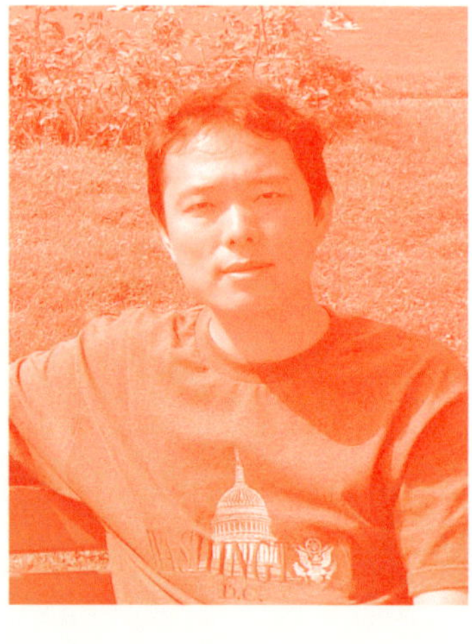
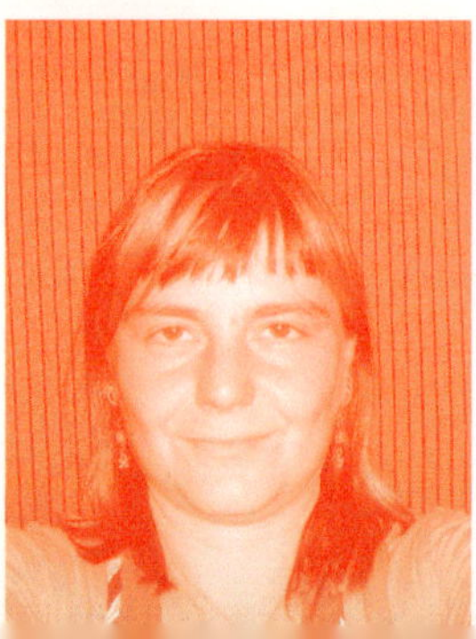

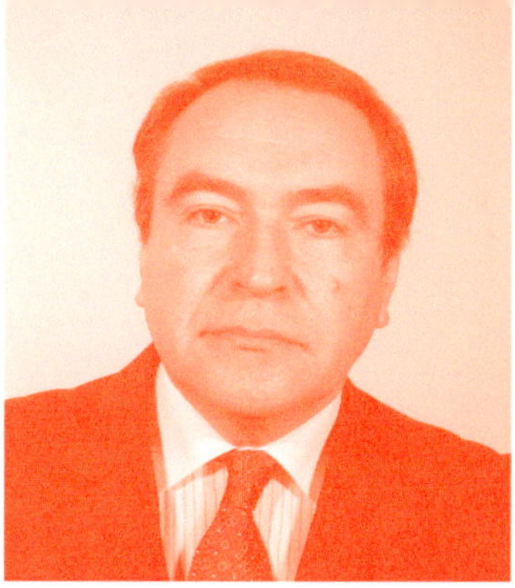
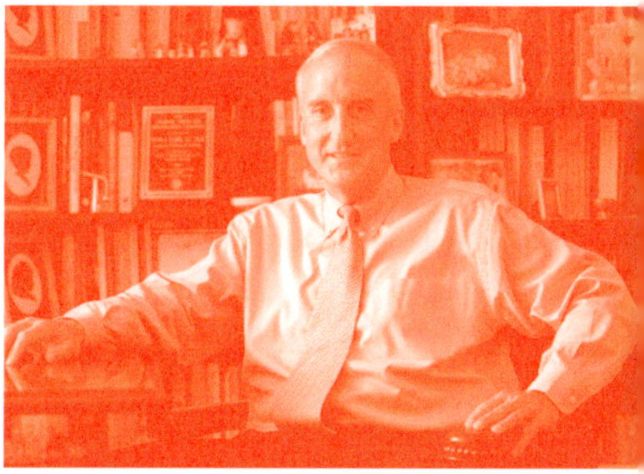
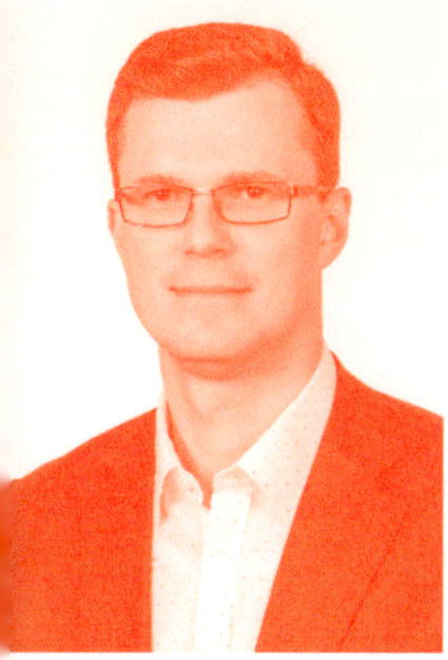
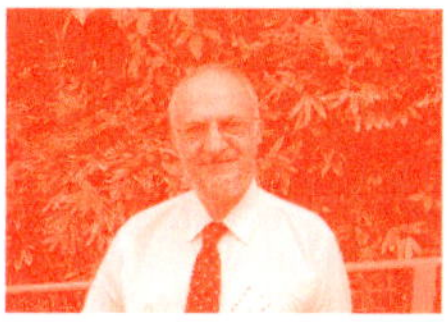
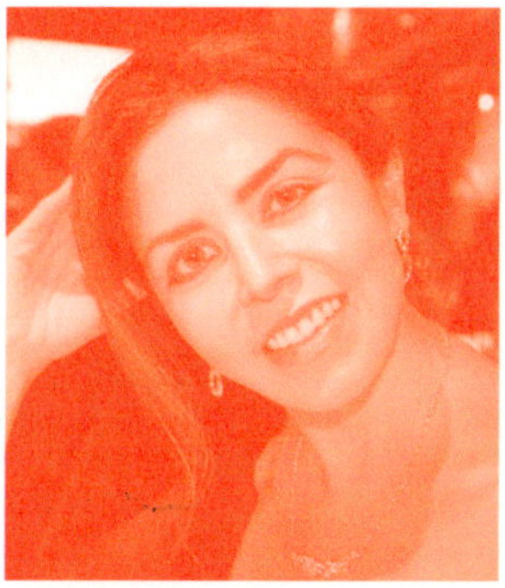

*Supporting open minds since 2005*

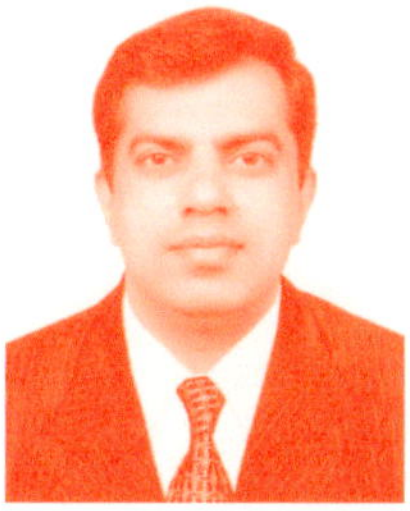
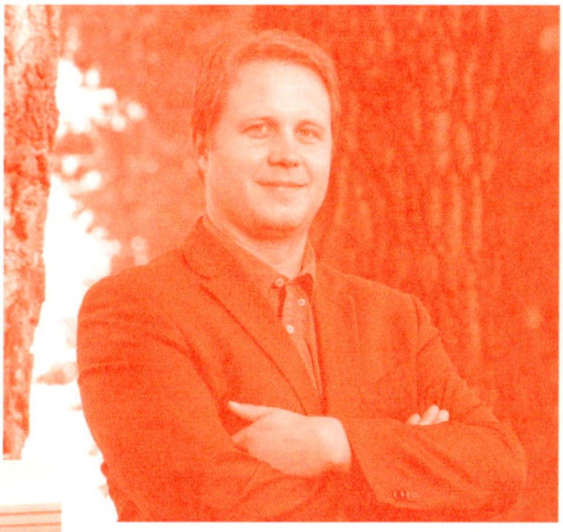
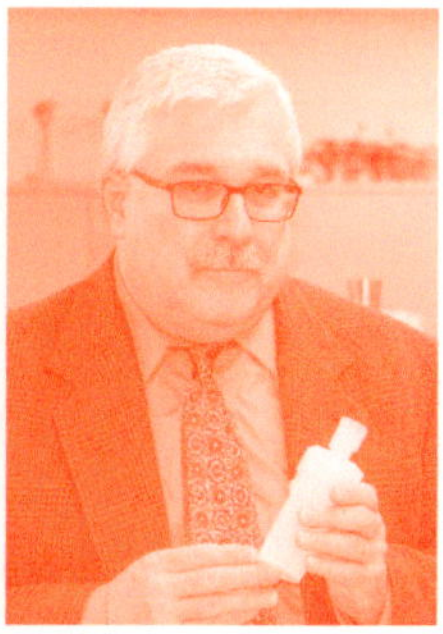
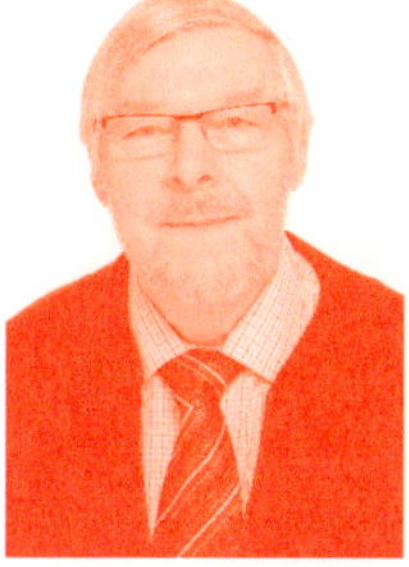
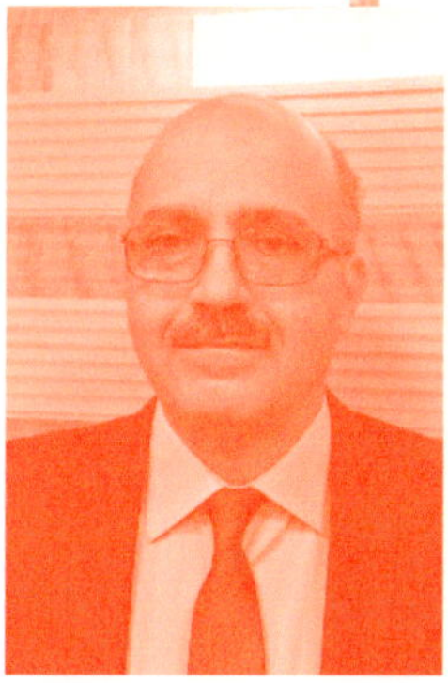
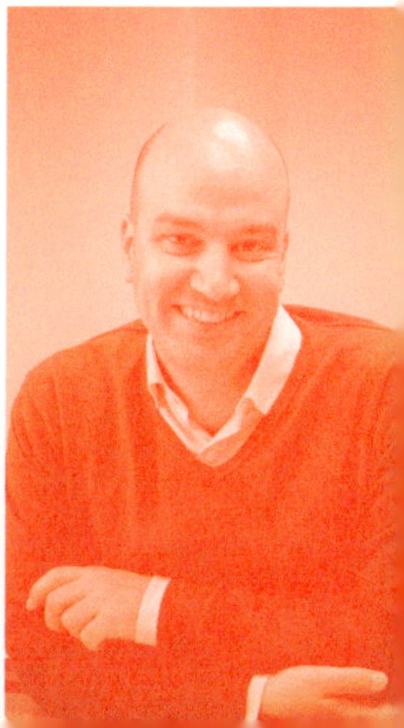
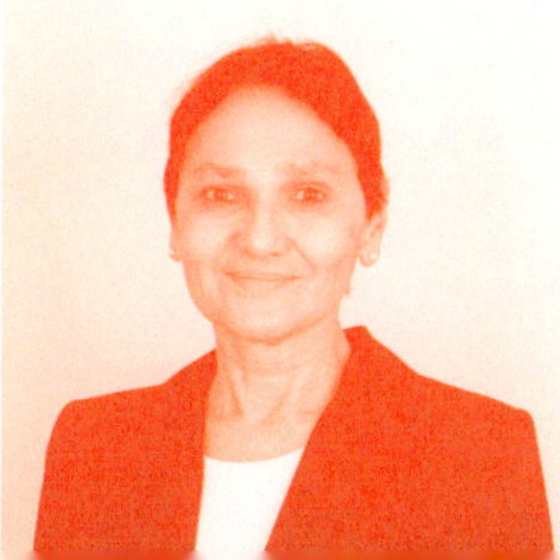

Aflatoxins - Occurrence, Detoxification, Determination and Health Risks
http://dx.doi.org/10.5772/intechopen.92518
Edited by Lukman Bola Abdulra'uf

Contributors
Esiegbuya Daniel Daniel Ofeoritse, Ojieabu Amarachi, Abdul Rashid Hudu, Mahunu Gustav Komla, Nelson Opoku, Nadeem A. Ramadan, Hadeel A. Al-Ameri, Muralidharan Velappan, Deecaraman Munusamy, Vishakha Pandey, Prem Chandra, Enespa, Adewale Segun Segun James, Emmanuel Ifeanyichukwu Ugwor, Victoria Ayomide Adebiyi, Emmanuel Obinna Ezenandu, Victory Chukwudalu Chukwudalu Ugbaja, Farman Ahmed, Muhammad Asif Asghar, Mateen Abbas, Pilar Viòas, Natalia Arroyo-Manzanares, Natalia Campillo, Ignacio Lûpez-Garcìa, Edgar Manuel Cambaza, Alberto Sineque, Edson Mongo, Aline Gatambire, Edirsse Mateonane, Raquel Chissumba



First published in London, United Kingdom, 2022 by IntechOpen
IntechOpen is the global imprint of INTECHOPEN LIMITED, registered in England and Wales, registration number: 11086078, 5 Princes Gate Court, London, SW7 2QJ, United Kingdom
Printed in Croatia

British Library Cataloguing-in-Publication Data
A catalogue record for this book is available from the British Library

Additional hard and PDF copies can be obtained from orders@intechopen.com

Aflatoxins - Occurrence, Detoxification, Determination and Health Risks
Edited by Lukman Bola Abdulra'uf
p. cm.
Print ISBN 978-1-83969-303-8
Online ISBN 978-1-83969-304-5
eBook (PDF) ISBN 978-1-83969-305-2

For EU product safety concerns:
IN TECH d.o.o., Prolaz Marije Krucifikse Kozulić 3, 51000 Rijeka, Croatia, info@intechopen.com or visit our website at intechopen.com.

# Meet the editor

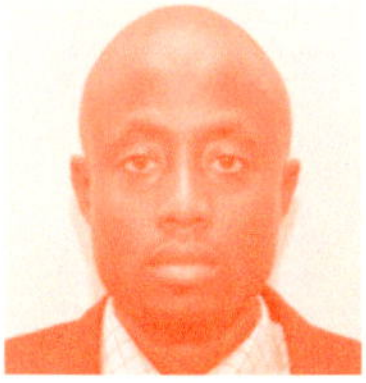

Dr. Lukman Bola Abdulra'uf is a senior lecturer at the Kwara State University, Malete, Ilorin, Nigeria. He started his teaching career at the Kwara State College of Education, Ilorin in 2006. He had his Ph.D. in analytical chemistry at the University of Malaya, Kuala Lumpur, Malaysia, MSc at the University of Ilorin, Nigeria, and BSc at the Bayero University, Kano, Nigeria. He was a TWAS postdoctoral research fellow at the COMSATS University, Islamabad, Pakistan. His research focuses on the analysis of contaminants, such as pesticide residues, mycotoxins, food additives, and veterinary drug residues in food samples using microextraction techniques. His current research interests are focused on the synthesis of carbon nanomaterials, ionic liquids, and solgel for analytical applications and the use of graphene nanomaterial as electrochemical biosensors.

# Contents

# Preface

The book *Aflatoxins - Occurrence, Detoxification, Determination and Health Risks* comprises 11 chapters organized in 2 sections and is a collection of original research and review articles. The topics discussed in this volume as related to aflatoxins include food safety and health hazards, role of and knowledge on socioeconomic factors, information dissemination, food processing, and analysis.

The first section of the book comprises five chapters (Chapters 1–5) and provides a general review on aflatoxins. Chapter 1 provided a review on fungi *Aspergillus flavus*: methods of identification, control, and effects on health and productivity. Chapter 2 is dedicated to food safety, human health hazards, and prevention of aflatoxin contamination in foods. Chapter 3 discussed the roles of socioeconomic factors (such as, level of education; methods of skill acquisition, food vending, and handling, especially in the hygienic practices; storage methods; and poor water supply) on food contamination. Chapter 4 discussed the occurrence of aflatoxins as result of indigenous food processing methods, such as, fermentation, roasting, and cooking. Chapter 5 emphasized the role of press or mass media in creating awareness and increasing media coverage on aflatoxin research development activities and the role to be played by research institutions in translating technical information published in scientific journals to assist reporters in understanding the research implications.

The second section (Chapters 6–11) is devoted to the techniques and approaches in the detoxification of food and the determination of aflatoxins using chromatographic analysis. Chapter 6 discussed the numerous methods for detoxification of aflatoxins in food to ensure food security. Chapter 7 reviewed the presence of mycotoxins in freshwater fish species and their effects on human health. Chapter 8 described the occurrence of aflatoxins in spices. Chapter 9 described disruption of metabolic activities through inhibition of ATP generation, carbohydrate, and lipid metabolism. Chapters 10 and 11 reviewed the chromatographic analysis of aflatoxins in food samples; it also described various extractions and cleanup methods prior to chromatographic analysis.

The book reviews up-to-date literature of leading experts in aflatoxins, and the references at the end of each chapter provide a starting point in acquiring a deeper knowledge on occurrence, detoxification, and analysis of aflatoxins in food samples. I hope this will serve as reference book for researchers and students.

I gratefully acknowledge the efforts and expertise of the contributing authors for their time and effort in preparing the chapters and for their interest in the book project.

I am indebted to the Vice-Chancellor Prof. Muhammed Mustapha Akanbi of Kwara State University, Malete, Nigeria, my colleagues in the Department of Chemistry and Industrial Chemistry, and also my former colleagues in the School of Basic and Remedial Studies of Kwara State College of Education, Ilorin, Kwara State for their support and encouragement. I also acknowledge my wife Mrs. Rihanat B. Abdulrauf and my children Haleemah, Habeebah, Hameedah, Abdulrauf, Abdulrahman, and Hameemah for their patience, understanding, and support during the chapter review process.

My special appreciation goes to the editorial team and publishing manager of *IntechOpen* for their promptness, encouragement, understanding, and patience during the review and publication processes.

**Dr. Lukman Bola Abdulra'uf**
Department of Chemistry and Industrial Chemistry,
Kwara State University,
Malete, Ilorin, Nigeria

Section 1

# Aflatoxin Occurrences and Food Safety

Chapter 1

# Aflatoxins

*Nadeem A. Ramadan and Hadeel A. Al-Ameri*

## Abstract

The aflatoxin producing fungi Aspergillus flavus, *A. parasiticus*, and A. nomius, although they are also produced by other species of Aspergillus as well as by Emericella spp.(Telemorph). There are many types of aflatoxins, but the four main ones are aflatoxin B1 (AFB1), aflatoxin B2 (AFB2), aflatoxin G1 (AFG1), and aflatoxin G2 (AFG2, while aflatoxin M1 (AFM1) and M2 (AFM2) are the hydroxylated metabolites of AFB1 and AFB2. Aflatoxin B1, which is a genotoxic hepatocarcinogen, which presumptively causes cancer by inducing DNA, adducts leading to genetic changes in target liver cells. Cytochrome-P450 enzymes to the reactive intermediate AFB1–8, 9 epoxide (AFBO) which binds to liver cell DNA, resulting in DNA adducts, metabolize AFB1 Ingestion of contaminated food is the main source of exposure to aflatoxins, which adversely affect the health of both humans and animals. The compounds can cause acute or chronic toxic effects of a teratogenic, mutagenic, carcinogenic, immunotoxic or hepatotoxic character. You can reduce your aflatoxin exposure by buying only major commercial brands of food and by discarding that look moldy, discolored, or shriveled.

**Keywords:** flatoxin, *Aspergillus flavus*

## 1. Introduction

Aflatoxins are a type of toxins produced by *Aspergillus* species, including *A. flavus* Link, *A. parasiticus* Speare, and *A. nomius* Kurtzman, Horn and Hesseltine. These toxins are responsible for harming 25 percent of the food crops in the world. The fungi produce both pre- and post-harvest contaminant toxins. Aflatoxin is responsible for major economic losses to agriculture in the United States and other developed countries, but aflatoxins also cause human and animal disease in developing countries where the use of contaminated grain cannot always be avoided. Aflatoxin exposure leads to the production of liver cancer in areas of the world where it is endemic, making it a major contributor to a serious public health epidemic. The presence in field samples of other mycotoxins, in particular fumonisins, along with aflatoxin, poses additional questions about the safety of food and feed supplies.

Until the 1980s, reviews and numerous studies on the effect of aflatoxin on livestock were available. To today from the 1990s, A number of clinical reports have been published on the toxicological issues caused by aflatoxins, concentrating mainly on the molecular biology of aflatoxin in both host and fungus, aflatoxin control by traditional breeding, and genetic engineering to develop resistant aflatoxin.

## 2. *Aspergillus* infection and aflatoxins development

A large family of fungi occupying very diverse ecological niches is the genus *Aspergillus*. Although there is a worldwide distribution of members, *Aspergillus* spp. Between latitudes north or south of the equator, 26° to 35°, the most abundant appear [1]. In subtropical and warm temperate climates, these fungi are thus more common. Aspergillus spp., generally known as saprophytes, In nutrient cycling, they grow on a large number of substrates and are very important. They are well suited to colonizing a number of grain and nut crops due to their ability to thrive in high temperatures and with relatively low. Some species have limited parasitic abilities under favorable conditions and can colonize crops in the field.

Some of the most significant fermentation fungi, e.g. *A. niger*, *A. sojae*, *A. oryzae* are grown for their ability to generate industrial enzymes and metabolites and to provide food with flavor. However, other members are infamous for the mycotoxins created by them. *Aspergillus* species-associated mycotoxins include aflatoxins, ochratoxins, versicolorins, sterigmatocystin, gliotoxin,

## 3. *Aspergillus flavus*

The major class of mycotoxins formed by Aspergillus spp. are aflatoxins. Aflatoxins are produced by only four species of fungi and each belongs to *Aspergillus* section Flavi [2, 3]. These species are *A. parasiticus, A. flavus*, *A. pseudotamarii* and *A.nomius.* But only *A. flavus* and *A. parasiticus* are economically important. These two fungi have overlapping niches in the production of maize, peanut, cotton, almond, and pistachio seeds and may produce aflatoxin. Other tree nuts are also affected, such as walnuts and Brazilian nuts. It is also possible to infect figs, but the occurrence is poor. These fungi may also develop aflatoxin on much of the substrate that is poorly preserved. The predominant species for all commodities is *Aspergillus flavus*, while *A. parasiticus* is prevalent in peanuts [4].

As early as 1920, *Aspergillus flavus* cause an ear mold of maize, but until the 1960s, when it was shown to produce the factor (later recognized as aflatoxin) associated with Turkey X disease, the fungus was of little concern. The meaning of *Aspergillus flavus* preharvest corn infection. Prior to 1971, was largely discounted as aflatoxin contamination was thought to be just a storage problem. In the Southern and Midwestern United States in the 1970s, the study of aflatoxin contamination awakened the scientific community to the importance of preharvest contamination [5, 6].

The occurrence of aflatoxin contamination is sporadic and highly dependent on environmental conditions. Contamination with aflatoxin is intermittent and highly dependent on environmental factors. Each year in the southern United States, large populations of *A. flavus* and aflatoxin infection occur, but significant outbreaks are related to above-average temperatures and below-average rainfall. In the United States' corn belt between 1983 and 1988, these two environmental factors were related to a high incidence of aflatoxin pollution. Aflatoxin has been found in high concentrations in southern China, Southeast Asia, and Africa [7].

In corn, the infection process of *A. flavus* is better represented [5]. It is reproduces through asexual conidia, inhabiting the soil. Shortly after pollination, conidia carried to the corn silks by wind or insects may expand into the ear and colonize kernel surfaces. The fungus can directly invade seeds and cobs if environmental conditions are favorable, or it may enter through wounds caused by insects. Major infection and aflatoxin contamination do not happen in either case until the moisture of the kernel is below 32 percent. In kernels, Aflatoxin will continue to be produced until the moisture reaches 15%. While insects are not necessary to contaminate with aflatoxin, their presence raises the level of contamination and high levels of aflatoxin are almost always associated with injury to insects, in particular *Ostrinia nubilalis*, the European corn borer [6].

There is proof that peanut flowers can be contaminated with *A. flavus* when compared to infection of the pods, this route of infection seems minor. It is not known the exact route of infection in pods, but insects tend to play a major role. Established vectors of the fungus are both mites and lesser stalk borer larvae (*Elsmopalpus lingosellus*). And microscopic damage to the pods increases fungus infection [8].

Even though there is evidence for direct infection of cotton by *A. flavus* [9, 10], A high level of aflatoxin in the environment is often associated with insects. The entry point for the fungus tends to be the exit holes created by the Pink Boll Worm Larvae (Pectinophora gossypiella Saunders). Pistachios infection by *A. flavus* Early splits are associated with a disorder in which the hull splits before maturation of the nut. High aflatoxin contamination is associated with the damage of navel orange worm larvae in both pistachios and almonds [11, 12].

Temperature and moisture are the two major factors causing aflatoxin contamination [5, 6]. High temperatures and drought stress lead to high levels of aflatoxin contamination in maize and peanuts. Under field conditions where soil humidity and temperature have been regulated, [13] showed that neither by itself is sufficient. The researchers discovered that there was no aflatoxin in peanuts grown with sufficient moisture. Similarly, peanuts grown under prolonged drought were aflatoxin free at temperatures lower than 25°C or higher than 320°C. Colonization by *A. flavus* and aflatoxin contamination at 30.5°C was maximized. The airborne inoculum of the fungus is increased by high temperatures and drought conditions [14]. Increased growth and reproduction at higher temperatures of the fungus is probably linked to its relatively high optimum temperature of growth. Over a wide range of temperatures (12 to 48°C), the fungus can grow, but its optimum for growth is 37°C. Higher temperatures and conditions of drought can also favor *A. flavus* over other fungi due to its capacity to thrive on low water activity substrates. The fungus can grow at an aW as low as −35 Megapascals (MPa). Interestingly, the optimal temperature is 25 to 30°C for the processing of aflatoxin. The plant is also likely to be predisposed to increased infection by temperature and drought stress, but little is known about the mechanisms [1].

The effects of temperature on cottonseed aflatoxin contamination appear more nuanced and poorly understood [5]. While cottonseed aflatoxin contamination is rarely a problem in the southern United States, western-grown cotton can be a serious problem. High night temperatures are important, they have argued. Higher aflatoxin levels in almonds have also been related to high day and night temperatures [15].

Source of Inoculum for *A. flavus* is the soil, but there is no known prevailing survival structure. In the southern United States in society and in cornfields, the fungus produces sclerotia; in the Midwest, however, sclerotia has not been identified. The fungus is likely to survive as mycelium and, to some degree, as sclerotia and conidia [5]. The temperature and humidity of the soil significantly affect the amount of conidia in the soil and air [14].

## 4. Types of aflatoxins

While aflatoxins are of global concern, in developing countries located in the tropical and sub-tropical regions, their negative effect on health, the economy and social life is greater. Agricultural products from SSA countries, e.g. Uganda, Gambia Tanzania, Kenya, and SEA countries, e.g. Thailand, China, Indonesia, Vietnam, have historically been associated with the highest incidence of aflatoxin, which has been associated with the highest incidence of hepatocellular carcinoma and the frequency of episodes of acute aflatoxicosis in the region [16]. In fact, these regions were the primary destination for scientists to perform epidemiological studies on the relationship between dietary exposure to aflatoxins and liver cancer, which was a major contributor to the production of aflatoxins as an etiological factor in human disease. Among more than 18 different forms and metabolites currently recognized, four major aflatoxin types [aflatoxin B1, aflatoxin B2 (AFB1), aflatoxin G1 (AFG1), and aflatoxin G2 (AFG2)] are the best known and the most studied [17].

The production of aflatoxins has been reported in members of three sections of *Aspergillus* genus; section Flavi (B- and G-type aflatoxins), section Ochraceorosei (aflatoxins B1 and B2), and section Nidulantes (formerly Emericella genus; aflatoxin B1) [18, 19]. However, the most widespread and potent aflatoxin-producing moulds are species of Section Flavi, with *A. flavus* and *A. parasiticus* Due to their widespread distribution in the agricultural environment and their versatility to grow and produce aflatoxins under different ecological conditions, *A. parasiticus* is the most commonly found in agricultural products [17]. A recent polyphase-based classification revealed that 18 of the 33 species in the Flavi segment are aflatoxigenic and each of the 16 species is capable of producing four major aflatoxins (AFB1, AFB2, AFG1 and AFG2), while the other two species produce either AFB1 alone (*A. togoensis*) or AFB1 and AFB2 respectively (*A. pseudotamarii*) [20] (**Table 1**). The latter writers observed that *A. flavus* Contrary to the prevalent view that this species exclusively generates B aflatoxins strains of Korean origin generate G aflatoxins [21]. Currently, the production of G aflatoxin by *A. flavus* was mentioned when these aflatoxins were first identified [20, 22, 23].

But when G-aflatoxin-producing strains NRRL 2999, 3000, and 3145 were originally classified as *A. flavus* a dispute was raised, re-classified as *A. parasiticus* [19]. Subsequently, Wicklow and Shotwell confirmed the production of aflatoxins G and B by other *A. flavus* strains; NRRL strains 3357, 6412, 6554, 6555, and 13003. However, *A. flavus* inability to produce G aflatoxins was later confirmed and validated by genetic research connecting indel genes to aflatoxins. (short insertions or deletions) mutations in the cyp A/nor B region in *A. flavus* to the impairment of the expression of genes coding for P450 monooxygenase enzyme required for the biosynthesis of G aflatoxins [24, 25]. It has been argued, however, that this mutation does not occur in all strains, and some *A. flavus* Depending on the morphotype (S or L) and phylogenetic group (I or II) to which they belong, the strains may still produce B or G aflatoxins. The morphotypes are described by the strain-formed sclerotia size; 'S' for small sclerotia (diameter $< 400$ μ) and 'L' for large sclerotia (diameter $> 400$ μ). In this regard, it was revealed that phylogenetic group I contains both S- and L-morphotype strains that only produce B aflatoxins, while group II only contains S-morphotype strains that produce aflatoxins G and B [26]. However, it was later shown that, irrespective of the morphotype, the phylogenetic group I strains develop both B and G aflatoxins, and that the phylogenetic group II is not limited to the S-morphotype strains, but also includes the 'L' morphotype strains [27, 28]. In addition, some S-trains (SBG) have been shown to produce both B and G aflatoxins, while others (SB) only produce B aflatoxins [29]. Latest studies in taxonomy using a blend of advanced analytical methods have verified that *A. flavus* can Indeed produce B and G aflatoxins regardless of the morphotype [20, 28]. However, it is well known that S-morphotype strains are more aflatoxigenic than their counterparts of the L-morphotype and accumulate greater quantities of aflatoxins regardless of the type of aflatoxin [28, 29]. This has been clarified by the fact

| Aflatoxin | Source | Frequently Contaminated Products |
|---|---|---|
| Difurocoumarocyclopentenone | | |
| Aflatoxin B1 | *Section Flavi: A. flavus, A. togoensis, A. pseudotamarii, A. austwickii, A. aflatoxiformans, A. arachidicola, A. cerealis, A. mottae, A. minisclerotigenes, A. luteovirescens (formerly A. bombycis), A. novoparasiticus, A. parasiticus, A. nomius, A. pipericola, A. pseudonomius, A. pseudocaelatus, A. transmontanensis, A. sergii, Section Ochraceorosei: A. ochraceoroseus,A. rambellii Section Nidulantes: A. miraensis, A. astellatus A. venezuelensis,, A. olivicola* | Cereals (like, rice, sorghum, wheat, barely, maize), oil seeds (like., cotton seeds, rape seeds, seeds of sunflower), seeds of nuts (like, pistachio, groundnut, peanuts), spices (like, black and red pepper, turmeric, allspices, ginger), dairy products, meats, dried fruits, fruit juices, eggs, foods derived from these products |
| Aflatoxin B2 | *Section Flavi: A. flavus, A. aflatoxiformans, A. pseudotamarii, A. cerealis, A. austwickii, A. minisclerotigenes, A. arachidicola, A. luteovirescens, A. mottae, A. novoparasiticus, A. nomius, A. pipericola, A. parasiticus, A. pseudonomius, A. pseudocaelatus, A. transmontanensis, A. sergii Section Ochraceorosei: A. ochraceoroseus and A. rambellii* | Cereals (like, rice, sorghum, barely, wheat, corn,), seeds oil (like, sunflower seed, oilseed rape cotton seed,), nuts (like, groundnut, pistachio, peanuts), Spices (like, black and red pepper, ginger, turmeric), milk products, meats, dried fruit, eggs, fruit juices, and foodstuffs derived from such products. |
| Aflatoxin B2a | Aflatoxin B1 hydroxylated metabolite obtained by water addition to the terminal furan double bond under acidic conditions in the liver, stomach or soil (no evidence of the involvement of particular enzymes) produced naturally by *A. Parasiticus A. flavus*. | NA |
| Aflatoxin M1 | Hepatic microsomal mixed-function oxidase (MFO) system (mainly cytochrome) hydroxylated aflatoxin B1 metabolite in mammalian liver Formed in vitro by liver homogenates from aflatoxin B1 produced naturally by *A. Parasiticus A. flavus.* | Milk (human milk included) and dairy products Meat products (liver, kidney) Groundnut and corn moulds |
| Aflatoxin M2 | Hydroxylated B2 metabolite by mammalian hepatic microsomal MFO produced naturally by *A. parasiticus* | Idem as aflatoxin M1 |
| Aflatoxin M2a | Hydration of the dilute acid terminal furan ring of aflatoxin M1 to yield the hemicetal derivative Homogenates in the liver in vitro | dairy products and Milk |
| Aflatoxin P1 | Demethylated aflatoxin B1 metabolite by O-demethylase-catalyzed liver microsomal oxidase | Dairy products, Mainly excreted in the humans urine and urine animals. |
| Aflatoxin Q1 | Hydroxylated metabolite of aflatoxin B1 by microsomal enzymes in higher vertebrate and poultry liver (main monkey metabolite of aflatoxin B1) | Assumed to be in edible parts of bovine fed on aflatoxin B1-contaminated feed |
| Aflatoxin Q2a | Acid hydration of aflatoxin Q1 | NA |
| Aflatoxicol (R0) | In vitro biotransformation of aflatoxin B1 by a soluble cytoplasm reductase system in fish, rats and human liver preparations In vitro biotransformation of aflatoxin B1 in fish, rodents, and human liver preparations by a soluble cytoplasm reductase system A naturally occurring hybrid of *A. parasiticus* and *A. flavus.* | Predominantly avian goods (primary metabolite in B1-contaminated feed fed to avian species). Dairy products Does not accumulate in edible parts of aflatoxin B1-infected bovine and pig feed. |

| Aflatoxin | Source | Frequently Contaminated Products |
|---|---|---|
| Aflatoxicol M1 | Reduced metabolites of liver-catalyzed aflatoxin B1, aflatoxin R0 or aflatoxin M1 by soluble NADPH-dependent reductases | Dairy products and milk |
| Aflatoxicol H1 | Reduced metabolites of soluble NADPH-dependent reductases catalyzed by aflatoxin B1 and aflatoxin Q1 in the liver | Dairy products and milk |
| Difurocoumarolactone | | |
| Aflatoxin G1 | *A. aflatoxiformans, A. flavus, A. cerealis, A. austwickii, A. minisclerotigenes, A. arachidicola, A. luteovirescens, A. mottae, A. novoparasiticus, A. nomius, A. pipericola, A. parasiticus, A. pseudonomius, A. pseudocaelatus, A. transmontanensis, A. sergii.* | Cereals (like, rice, sorghum, wheat, barely, maize), oily seeds (like, cotton seeds, rape seeds, sunflower seeds), nuts (like, peanuts, groundnuts, pistachio nuts), spices (like, ginger, black and red pepper, turmeric), milk products, meats, dried fruits, fruit juices, poultry, and feed and foods extracted from such products. |
| Aflatoxin G2 | *A. flavus*[1], *A. austwickii, A. aflatoxiformans, A. arachidicola, A. cerealis, A. mottae, A. minisclerotigenes, A. nomius, A. luteovirescens, A. transmontanensis, A. parasiticus, A. novoparasiticus, A. pseudocaelatus, A. pipericola, A. sergii, A. pseudonomius* | Same as aflatoxin G1 |
| Aflatoxin G2a | A hydroxylated aflatoxin G1 metabolite obtained by catalytic addition of water to the terminal furan double bond in the presence of acidic conditions in the liver, intestine, or soil (no evidence of unique enzyme involvement). Manufactured naturally by *A. flavus* | NA |
| Aflatoxin GM1 | MFO produces a hydroxylated metabolite of aflatoxin G1 in the liver of mammals. *A. parasiticus* fed aspertoxin as a precursor produced it in vitro. *A. flavus* creates it naturally. | Dairy products and milk |
| Aflatoxin GM2 | Hydroxylated mammalian liver derivative of aflatoxin G2 by MFO In vitro, developed by A. Dihydro-O-methylsterigmatocystin-parasiticus (DHOMST) | Dairy products and milk |
| Aflatoxin GM2a | Metabolite of aflatoxin GM1 in the mammalian liver<br>Hydration of the dilute acid terminal furan ring of aflatoxin M1 to generate hemicetal in vitro in liver homogenates | Dairy products and milk |
| Parasiticol (aflatoxin B3) | An aflatoxin G1 metabolite from biodegradation (hydrolysis and decarboxylation reactions) in *Rhizopus stolonifer, A. flavus, Rhizopus oryzae, Rhizopus arrhizus,* | such as aflatoxins G1 and B1 |
| Others | | |
| Parasiticol (aflatoxin B3) | An aflatoxin G1 metabolite from biodegradation (hydrolysis and decarboxylation reactions)in *Rhizopus stolonifer, A. flavus, Rhizopus oryzae Rhizopus arrhizus,* produced naturally by *A. flavus, A. parasiticus, A. nomius, A. novoparasiticus, A. mottae.* | Aflatoxin B1 and G1 are the same |

| Aflatoxin | Source | Frequently Contaminated Products |
|---|---|---|
| Aspertoxin b | *A. parasiticus* and *A. flavus* | Mainly plant products that are vulnerable to contamination with *A. parasiticus* and *A. flavus*; Food products of animal origin are not considered to be important. |

[a]*It is not a standard G-type producer of aflatoxins, but some strains have been reported to produce aflatoxins in addition to B1 and B2. [20].*
[b]*Typically regarded as an* A. flavus *produced sperate mycotoxin. Because of structural variations between aflatoxins and the difurocoumarin structure that characterizes them. Abbreviations: NA: Not available.*

**Table 1.**
*Origins of aflatoxins and the products most exposed to contamination.*

that aflatoxin production increases as the size of sclerotia decreases during its development [20, 30]. Indeed, in the low-elevation regions in Kenya where the S-morphotype is predominating (>90%), the concentration of aflatoxin B1 in maize was reported to exceed 1000 μg/kg [26, 31]. This was practically illustrated by the higher incidence of deadly acute aflatoxicosis in these regions compared with those where the S-morphotype strains are less common [32].

## 5. Physical, chemical, and toxicological properties of aflatoxins

More than 18 different forms of aflatoxin are currently known to occur naturally or as a result of feed and food carryover phenomena (**Table 1**). There are about 13 forms of aflatoxins that are naturally produced by toxic fungi, some of which can be metabolized to produce toxicity-retaining derivatives by humans, animals, or other microorganisms, Compared to the parent molecules, but typically with a lower potency. AFB1, AFB2, AFG1, and AFG2, especially AFB1. has high incidence and toxicities, they are of the greatest concern to the economy and public health, Aflatoxin M1 (AFM1), on the other hand, is of particular concern for the safety of dairy products because it is commonly found in the milk of lactating animals feeding on aflatoxin B1-contaminated feed, in addition to its high toxicity and possible carcinogenicity in humans [33, 34]. Other aflatoxins, however, should not be underestimated because of their inherent toxicity, which may not be negligible, or because the most active AFB1 can readily be inverted. They may also be intermediates for the more toxic mycotoxin biosynthesis [35, 36]. The physicochemical and toxicological properties of major aflatoxins are summarized in **Table 2**.

## 6. Structural diversity of aflatoxins

Structurally, aflatoxins are difuranocournarins/difurocoumarins synthesized through the polyketide pathway and consist of a coumarin nucleus (**Figure 1A, B**, center green) to which one side of the difuran moiety (**Figure 1A**, left blue) and one side of the pentene ring (**Figure 1A**, left red) or the other side of the six-sided lactone ring (**Figure 1A**, left blue) are linked (**Figure 1B**, red on the right). On this basis, aflatoxins fall into two main groups: (i) difurocoumarocyclopentenones comprised typically of aflatoxin B series and derivatives (**Table 1** and **Figure 1A**), and (ii) difurocoumarolactones with the aflatoxin G series as the main representatives, typically including AFG1, AFG2, AFGM1, AFGM2, and AFG2a

| Aflatoxin | MW (g/mol) | Formula | Melting Point (°C)[a] | Toxicity | | | Adverse Health Effects[b] |
|---|---|---|---|---|---|---|---|
| | | | | LD50 (mg/kg bw) | Test Organism | Route | |
| Aflatoxin B1 | 312.063 | C17H12O6 | 268.5 | 0.24–60 3.0 | Various human chick embryo and species of animals and | In vitro experiments of injection in chick embryo,Oral intraperitoneal | Genotoxicity, carcinogenicity, hepatotoxicity, teratogenicity, immuno-toxicity |
| Aflatoxin B2 | 314.079 | C17H14O6 | 286–289 | 1.7 | Duck | Orally | Carcinogenicity,hepatotoxicity, Week mutagenicity |
| Aflatoxin B2a | 330.074 | C17H14O7 | 240 | >400 μg showed a weak toxicity | Ducklings | Orally | Low toxicity (200-fold less than B1) |
| Aflatoxin M1 | 328.058 | C17H12O7 | 297–299 | 0.32<br>1.5 | Duck Rat | Unreported Oral | Carcinogenicity, nephrotoxicity, Hepatotoxicity |
| Aflatoxin G2 | 330.074 | C17H14O7 | 237–240<br>226–229 | 2.5<br>Weekly mutagenic | Duckling<br>S. typhimurium | test of oral Ames' | Low toxicity, no evidence in animals for carcinogenicity |
| Aflatoxin G2a c | 346.069 | C17H14O8 | 243.13 (Predicted) | NA | NA | NA | Low toxicity to inactive (a detoxified form of G1) |

*Data compiled from PubChem of the National Center for Biotechnology Information (Pubchem. Explore Chemistry. 2020 https://pubchem.ncbi.nlm.nih.gov) and ChemSpider of the Royal Society of Chemistry (Chemspider. Search and Share Chemistry. 2020. http://www.chemspider.com) databases, unless references are indicated beside the data.*
*[a]Details collected on the ChemSpider website (http://www.chemspider.com) The IARC claimed in the most recent classification of mycotoxins that 'sufficient evidence' exists for the carcinogenicity of aflatoxins B1, G1 and M1 in laboratory animals, unless indicated by an imbedded citation.*
*[b]But there is "limited evidence" or "insufficient evidence" for the carcinogenicity of aflatoxin B2 and G2 respectively, respectively, in laboratory animals.; However, in the light of mechanistic studies showing the ability of major aflatoxins (B1, G1, B2, G2, M1) as a first step in genotoxicity to form DNA adducts, They were listed as carcinogens in group 1 [IARC (International Organization for Cancer Research.; c Salmonella typhimurium-induced mutagenicity is <1 percent of aflatoxin B1 taken as a guide [37]. Abbreviations: NA: Not available.*

**Table 2.**
*Key properties of aflatoxins and their metabolites.*

*DOI: http://dx.doi.org/10.5772/intechopen.97292*

(**Table 1** and **Figure 1B**). Parasiticol (also designated as aflatoxin B3) despite the absence of the characteristic six-membered lactone ring, it is generally categorized as a member of the latter group (**Figure 1C**, right). There is also a doubt as to whether or not aspertoxin is an aflatoxin that is not linked to members of any of the difurocoumarin groups due to its bifuroxhanthone structure (**Figure 1C**, left). This mycotoxin, which is associated with sterigmatocystin structurally (an intermediate metabolite of aflatoxins B1 and G1) [38] A precursor of aflatoxin GM1 may also be [39], Which may explain why it is regarded by some writers as a member of the category of difurocoumarolactones. Aspertoxin has earned the

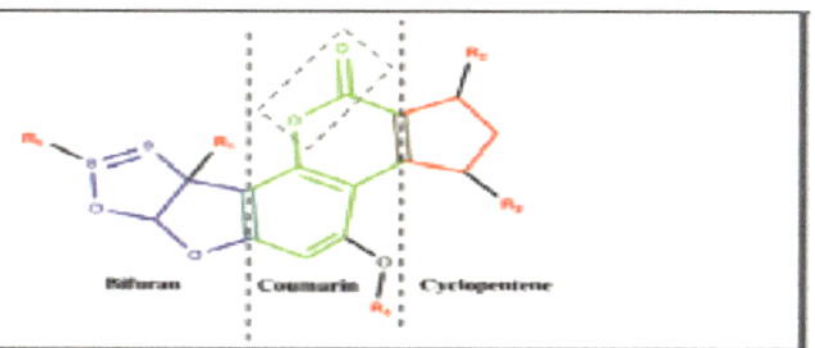


| Aflatoxin | $R_1$ | $R_2$ | $R_3$ | $R_4$ | $R_5$ | $C_8$-$C_9$ bond |
|---|---|---|---|---|---|---|
| B1 | H | =O | H | $CH_3$ | H | Unsaturated |
| B2 | H | =O | H | $CH_3$ | H | Saturated |
| $B2_a$ | H | =O | H | $CH_3$ | OH | Saturated |
| M1 | OH | =O | H | $CH_3$ | H | Unsaturated |
| M2 | OH | =O | H | $CH_3$ | H | Saturated |
| $M2_a$ | OH | =O | H | $CH_3$ | OH | Saturated |
| P1 | H | =O | H | H | H | unsaturated |
| Q1 | H | =O | OH | $CH_3$ | H | Unsaturated |
| $Q2_a$ | H | =O | OH | CH3 | OH | Saturated |
| Aflatoxicol B | H | OH | H | $CH_3$ | H | Unsaturated |
| Aflatoxicol M1 | OH | OH | H | $CH_3$ | H | Unsaturated |
| Aflatoxicol H1 | H | OH | OH | $CH_3$ | H | Unsaturated |

**(A)** Difurocoumarocyclopentenone aflatoxins

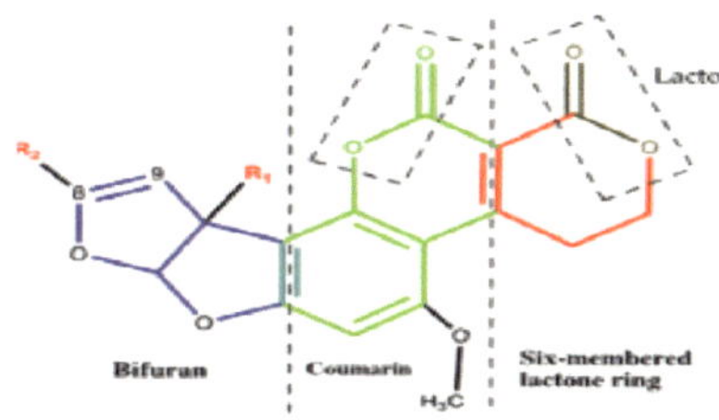


| Aflatoxin | $R_1$ | $R_2$ | $C_8$-$C_9$ bond |
|---|---|---|---|
| G1 | H | H | Unsaturated |
| G2 | H | H | Saturated |
| $G2_a$ | H | OH | Saturated |
| GM1 | OH | H | Unsaturated |
| GM2 | OH | H | Saturated |
| $GM2_a$ | H | OH | Saturated |

**(B)** Difurocoumarolactone aflatoxins

**(C) Structure of aflatoxins B1, B2, G1, G2 and M1**

**AflatoxinB$_1$** **Aflatoxin B$_2$**

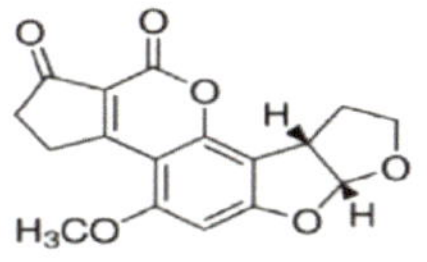

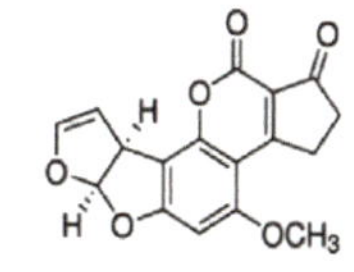

**Aflatoxin G1** **Aflatoxin G2** **Aflatoxin M1**

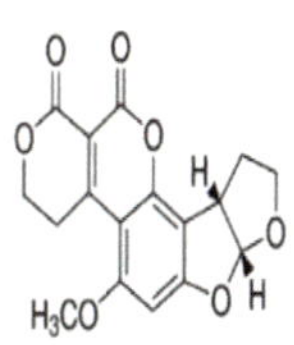

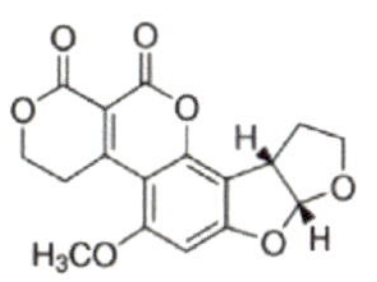

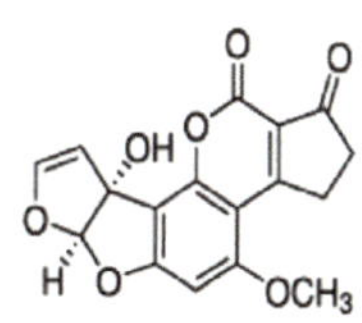

**(D) Other aflatoxins**

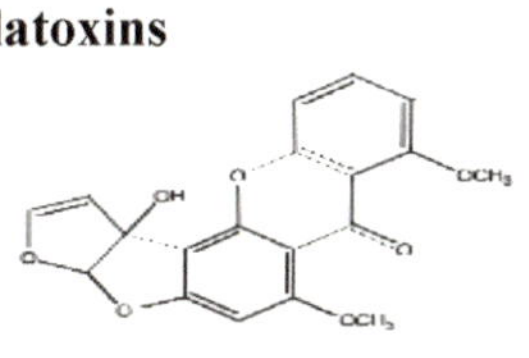

Aspertoxin

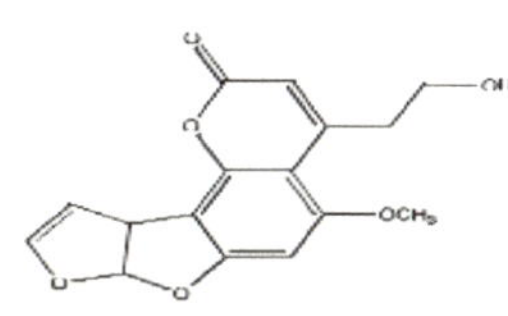

Parasiticol

**Figure 1.**

*Diversity of aflatoxin chemical structures in difurocoumarocyclopentenone (A) and in difurocoumarolactone (B) Structure of aflatoxins B1, B2, G1, G2 and M1 (C). groups. a difuranoxanthane, Aspertoxin,, parasiticol, lacking the lactone ring of its parent aflatoxin G1, are occasionally considered as standalone mycotoxins (D).*

least publicity, unlike other aflatoxins, considering its demonstrated toxicity in chicken embryos where it causes malformations, generalized oedema, muscle tone loss, and umbilical vessel haemorrhage leading to death. It should be noted that saturated (AFG2, AFGM2, and AFM2) or hydrated (AFB2a, AFG2a, AFM2a, AFQ2a, AFG2a, AFGM2a) terminal furan ring aflatoxins are the least toxic, suggesting that the C8 = C9 double bond of this furan moiety plays a crucial role in aflatoxin toxicity [40].

## 7. Preharvest control strategies

To optimize plant output and minimize plant tension, any management activity can reduce aflatoxin contamination [5, 6, 13]. This involves planting adapted varieties, proper fertilization, control of weeds, and irrigation required. In years favorable for disease growth, even the best management methods can not eradicate aflatoxin contamination. It has been shown that previous cropping history affects soil fungus populations [4]. However, the meaning of the initial inoculum has not been established. In addition, *Aspergillus* molds grow from pistachio trees on litter, but it is not known whether infection and aflatoxin contamination can be minimized by practices to minimize this litter. Decreasing damage to the navel orange worm could decrease the contamination of aflatoxin. Cropping history and plant debris potentially play a minor role in aflatoxin contamination relative to plant stress [11, 12].

Breeding projects for all major crops affected by aflatoxin contamination are underway, but no genotypes with sufficient resistance to aflatoxin accumulation are commercially available. Inbred corn lines [6] And peanut genotypes with some resistance to the accumulation of aflatoxin have been reported. There is evidence of tolerance in maize and peanuts to the production of perse aflatoxin. In almonds, breeding for resistance to aflatoxin contamination is also ongoing.

Because chemical control procedures for contaminating mycotoxins are not economically feasible for most grain crops, there is an interest in developing effective biocontrol agents to reduce the contamination of mycotoxins. Recent research shows the potential for a biocontrol agent to minimize cotton, peanuts, aflatoxin contamination [41, 42], and corn. These crops were treated by researchers with nonaflatoxigenic isolates Either *A. flavus* or *A. parasiticus*. The reason for using nonaflatoxigenic isolates of the two fungi is that they are possibly the better biocompetitors, since they occupy the same or similar ecological niche as the aflatoxigenic strains, So far, there is no evidence that the ability to produce aflatoxin confers a competitive advantage to *A. flavus* or *A. parasiticus*.

Bock and Cotty carried out the most rigorous trials of a biocontrol agent for the prevention of aflatoxin contamination (1999). They received a U.S. permit. Environmental Protection Agency (EPA) for the treatment of wheat seed colonized by a naturally occurring nonaflatoxigenic strain (AF36) of *A. flavus* in Arizona cotton fields.This procedure has increased the AF36 population and decreased the cottonseed toxin strain and aflatoxin concentrations.

### 7.1 Aflatoxins: human and animal health; economic impact

The biologically active secondary metabolites produced by certain strains of *Aspergillus parasiticus* are aflatoxins (*Aspergillus flavus* toxins). These ubiquitous fungi are capable of infecting a large variety of crops that can be infected with this powerful mycotoxin under certain conditions. Acute toxicity, including hepatotoxicity, teratogenicity, immunotoxicity and even death, can result from ingestion of food or feed that is highly contaminated with aflatoxin. The most abundant and toxic chemical form of Aflatoxin B1 (AFBl) is highly mutagenic and is one of the most active carcinogens ever tested in rats [43], suggesting that chronic exposure to very low levels of aflatoxin is cause for concern.

In humans, hepatot-oxicity is correlated with ingestion of aflatoxin. Epidemiological studies have also shown that areas with elevated aflatoxin levels in the world are associated with a high incidence of liver cancer. The prevalence of the hepatitis B virus in these areas makes it difficult to create a clear cause-effect relationship. However, the International Agency for Research on Cancer has, on the basis of the available evidence, designated AFBl as a possible human carcinogen. The US Food and Drug Administration developed action levels of 20 p.p.b. for food for human consumption (except milk, where the level is 0–5 p.p.b.) and 20–300 p.p.b. for most animal feeds because of this high level of concern regarding aflatoxin [44]. In the world, other countries have set even lower standards of intervention.

From an economic point of view, mycotoxins impact approximately 25 of the world's crops annually [44, 45]. This is equivalent to a direct expense of billions of dollars due to the loss of crops and livestock, plus the secret indirect costs of tracking crop aflatoxin levels and the reduced output of farm animals that eat aflatoxin and other mycotoxins. In the US and in many other regions of the world, the removal of aflatoxin is a critical economic and health issue.

In recent years, aflatoxins have been the subject of multiple reviews covering ecology as a testimony of their significance [46], Incidence [47], identification [48, 49], human health consequences (toxicity, carcinogenicity) [43, 50–52], genetics [53], biosynthesis [54, 55] biosynthesis [54, 55] and substances that interfere with biosynthesis [56], as well as the avoidance of aflatoxin contamination [57–59]; (for general reviews see [44, 60, 61]). Recent efforts in several laboratories have centered on developing an in-depth understanding of the molecular biology of the aflatoxin biosynthetic pathway due to the difficulties of effectively and economically regulating aflatoxin contamination of food and feed by conventional agricultural methods (see below). The purpose of this analysis is to provide current knowledge on the molecular biology of aflatoxin biosynthesis and how this information is used to: (1) extract toxin from the food chain; (2) understand aflatoxin pathway regulation and evolution; (3) to comprehend aflatoxin's biological significance to the fungus that creates it. This analysis is timely because it provides a summary of several major breakthroughs that have resulted from intensive research activity over the past 2 years - knowledge not available in previously published articles on the molecular biology of aflatoxin biosynthesis [62–64]. Since aspergilli contains opportunistic mammalian, insect and plant pathogens, promoting our understanding of gene expression regulation, production and secondary metabolism in this diverse genus may provide important clues to their ecology and biology, leading not only to efficient aflatoxin management, but also to more general means of controlling this whole community of pathogens.

### 7.2 Biological significance of aflatoxins: a role in fungal development

The size of the cluster of aflatoxins and the striking serving of genes and organization of the cluster clearly imply that aflatoxins play a key role in the fungi' life cycle or survival. Are there any hints as to what that feature might be? The two key origins of inoculum for the survival or dissemination of these filamentous fungi are conidia (asexual spores of aspergilli) and sclerotia (resting/survival structures).

There is no direct correlation between sclerotia development and aflatoxin (if any). Bennett and Horowitz [65] found no association between sclerotia production and aflatoxin production in toxigenic and atoxigenic strains of *A. flavus*. Other study, on the other hand, has found that the regulation of aflatoxin synthesis in toxigenic strains has an effect on sclerotia growth. (reviewed in [46]). Mutations have been shown to cause cancer in preliminary experiments using molecular biology methods (UV or gene disruption) that result in the accumulation of certain intermediate aflatoxin pathways also result in the inhibition of sclerotic growth. Genetic blocks that remove AFBl and intermediate synthesis result in improved development of sclerotia. Restoration of function by complementation often restores normal growth of sclerotia. These findings indicate that the synthesis of aflatoxin and fungal growth may be related. The existence and value of such a relation can be revealed by the continuation of these studies [66, 67].

### 7.3 Aflatoxicosis

The association of aflatoxins with animal diseases has been extensively studied [68]. The relationship of aflatoxins to hepatocellular carcinoma and other human diseases is still being studied, while acute aflatoxicosis is well known in humans. In Africa, the Philippines, and China, multiple epidemiological studies have implicated aflatoxins in the increased occurrence of human gastrointestinal (GI) and hepatic neoplasms. In human liver cell carcinoma, aflatoxin B1 was also involved [69].

### 7.4 Acute aflatoxicosis

In humans, acute disease due to ingestion of aflatoxin has been manifested as acute hepatitis, typically associated with highly contaminated foodstuffs, in particular corn. Exposure to aflatoxins in selected tissues was acceptable in some cases, and histopathological evidence was convincingly adequate to allow for the diagnosis of aflatoxicosis. Jaundice, low-grade fever, depression, anorexia, and diarrhea are common but nonspecific changes in patients with acute aflatoxicosis, with fatty degenerative changes in the liver apparent upon histopathological examination, such as Centro lobular necrosis and fatty infiltration. In patients with acute, aflatoxin-caused hepatitis in Kenya, tenderness was evident near the liver; ascites can develop. In outbreaks in India, mortality reached 25%. The liver samples collected from patients who died contained detectable aflatoxin B1 levels [70].

The ingestion of aflatoxin-contaminated foods was associated with two human diseases of undefined etiology: kwashiorkor and Reye's syndrome. The seasonal occurrence and distribution of aflatoxin in food has been geographically correlated with Kwashiorkor. Some of the same attributes of kwashiorkor, namely, hypoalbuminemia, fatty liver, and immunosuppression, were present in animals given dietary aflatoxin. Aflatoxins have been found in liver tissue by autopsy in 36 children with kwashiorkor, contributing to the reputation of aflatoxin as the cause of this human disease without any other known etiology. In some patients with kwashiorkor, malnutrition may change the metabolism of dietary aflatoxin, resulting in its detection [71].

However, the etiology of Reye's syndrome is more troublesome. Aflatoxin has been associated with this condition, which includes acute encephalopathy with viscera fat degeneration, since this mycotoxin was detected in patients with Reye's syndrome in Thailand, New Zealand, the former Czechoslovakia and the United States. In addition, aflatoxin B1 in macaque monkeys developed a disease similar to Reye's syndrome in [71].

Nelson, *et al.* [72], however, found no substantial variations in serum and urine between matched controls and patients with Reye's syndrome compared to aflatoxins. Similar differences were noticed concerning the incidence in patients of aflatoxins in tissues and Reye's syndrome. The U.S. cases often seem to lack any geographical relationship to the exposure to aflatoxin. Again, in some patients, Reye's syndrome, which involves the liver, can alter dietary aflatoxin metabolism [71].

### 7.5 Chronic aflatoxicosis

The association of this mycotoxin with hepatocellular carcinoma typically suggests chronic aflatoxicosis in humans. Several epidemiological studies have investigated the importance of dietary aflatoxin and other factors associated with this disease in countries or localities with a high incidence of liver cancer. Most of the research, which occurred predominantly prior to 1980, attempted to determine and compare dietary levels of aflatoxin B1 with the existence of hepatocellular carcinoma.

Some earlier studies have been criticized for not understanding the hepatitis B virus exposure of the studied populations (HBV). In relation to the incidence of hepatocellular carcinoma, most post-1980 studies investigated hepatitis B surface antigen (HBsAg) as well as aflatoxin exposure. Most of them considered an aflatoxin effect independent of the prevalence of HBsAg [73]. No aflatoxin effect on liver cancer was observed when all racial, social, and cultural groups were included, but a positive association was found by an independent assessment of the Bantu people.

The consequence is that aflatoxin has been related to unique p53 mutations where codon 249 has a G $\rightarrow$ T trans-version in the third position. These particular tumor mutations may provide substantial evidence as to their origin. Epidemiological research on the relationship between aflatoxins and human hepatocellular carcinoma greatly benefit from the armament of biomarkers. Epidemiological research on the relationship between aflatoxins and human hepatocellular carcinoma greatly benefit from the armament of biomarkers. The findings showed that human liver cancer is associated with a particular biomarker for aflatoxin and that HBV and aflatoxin B1 interact as risk factors for liver cancer [74].

## 8. General effects of aflatoxins on health and productivity

Aflatoxins are powerful toxins in the liver. In animals, their effects differ with dosage, period of exposure, species, race, and diet or nutritional status (**Figure 2**). When ingested in large doses, these toxins can be lethal. Sublethal doses cause chronic toxicity, and low levels of chronic exposure in some species can lead to cancer, mainly liver cancer [75]. In general, young animals are more sensitive to the toxic effects of aflatoxin than older animals. Due to their widespread occurrence in many dietary staples, such as peanuts, tree nuts, milk, maize, dried fruits, and their potential as human carcinogens, aflatoxins have created the greatest public health concern.

In the early tests of aflatoxicosis, one of the experimental species used was trout. The LD50 was estimated to be equal to 0.5 to 1.0 mg/kg of crystalline aflatoxins B1 and G1 in the same amounts, and they seem to be very sensitive to the effects of the aflatoxins. Eighty components per billion total dietary aflatoxins produced a very high incidence of hepatomas in the trout. Rainbow trout are very susceptible to hepatogenicity in the early stages of development. Nine months later, immersion of fry or embryo in 0.5 ppm aflatoxin B1 for 0.5 h resulted in a 30 to 40% incidence of hepatocellular carcinoma. Aflatoxicosis epizootics also occur in fish and were possibly the cause of epizootic trout liver cancer that occurred in hatcheries in California from 1939 to 1942. In this outbreak, aflatoxin-contaminated cottonseed meal was implicated as the causative agent.

Aflatoxin fed trout grow hepatic cancer. In suckling piglets, rising and finishing swine, and breeder stock, aflatoxin toxicity has been reported. Decreased weight gain rates, decreased feed conversion performance, toxic hepatitis, nephrosis, and

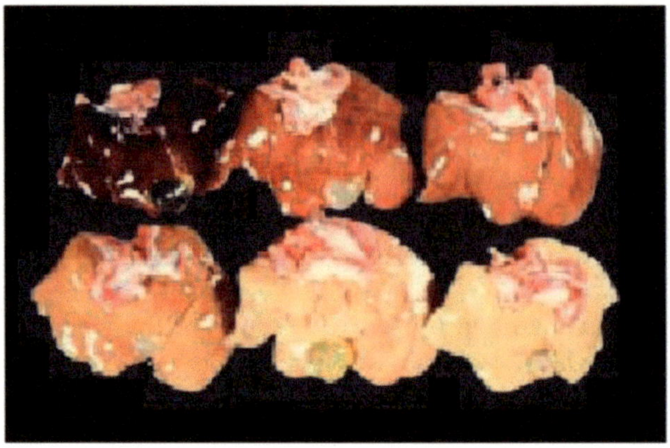

**Figure 2.**
*Guinea pig livers are given increasing doses of aflatoxin for the same period of time. From left to right, starting with the liver of a guinea pig given no aflatoxin in the upper left corner, and the liver of a guinea pig given the maximum dose of aflatoxin in the lower right corner. With increasing doses of aflatoxin, remember the increasingly pale livers. With increasing doses of aflatoxin, remember the increasingly pale livers. Picture courtesy of John L. Richard, USDA, ARS, Ames, Iowa, National Animal Disease Center; now at Romer Labs, Inc., Missouri, Union.*

systemic hemorrhages are clinical and pathological symptoms. Depending on age, diet, concentration, and duration of exposure, the effects of aflatoxin in pigs differ. Swines tend to be immune to dietary aflatoxin levels of up to 300 ppb from weaning to marketing [76].

Acute aflatoxicosis has been comprehensively identified in cattle. Decreased feed intake, dramatic declines in milk production, weight loss, and liver damage are clinical symptoms. However, due to reduced feed quality, immunosuppression, and lower reproductivity, chronic exposure of dairy and beef cattle to naturally occurring aflatoxin levels may have an even greater economic effect. Aflatoxins affect the function of the rumen in vitro and in vivo by reducing the digestion of cellulose, volatile fatty acids and proteolysis [77, 78] showed reduced motility of the rumen in steers given a single aflatoxin dose.

Significant health concerns resulting from prolonged exposure of a dairy herd to aflatoxin-contaminated corn (120 ppb). In addition, breeding performance decreased by 2 percent for a five-month period after exposure, while milk production increased by 28 percent after the diet was removed from aflatoxin-contaminated corn. The birth of smaller and unhealthy calves, diarrhea, acute mastitis, respiratory disorders, prolapsed rectum, hair loss, and reduced feeding intake are other concerns.

The conversion of aflatoxin B1 to the hydroxylated metabolite, aflatoxin M1, which is excreted in milk, is another feature of aflatoxin exposure in dairy cattle. Aflatoxin M1 is present in milk from Holstein cows given aflatoxin B1 for seven days, while aflatoxin M1 is not detected in milk for four days after the end of aflatoxin B1 administration [68]. As a percentage of aflatoxin B1, the excreted quantities of aflatoxin M1 average 1 to 2 percent, but values as high as 6 percent have been recorded at kg of aflatoxin B1 daily intake levels. In the poultry industry, Aflatoxicoses have caused significant economic losses affecting ducklings, broilers, layers, turkeys, and quail. Anorexia, reduced weight gain, decreased egg development, bleeding, embryotoxicity, and increased vulnerability to environmental and microbial stressors are clinical symptoms of intoxication [79].

In chickens given a high level (1.5 ppm) of dietary aflatoxins, histopathologic changes, including fatty liver, necrosis, and bile duct hyperplasia, are observed. Clinical responses include hypoproteinemia; decreased hemoglobin; and decreased serum triglycerides, phospholipids, and cholesterol in chickens provided half of this dose. Aflatoxins can reduce the activity of several enzymes in broiler chickens that are essential for the digestion of starches, proteins, lipids and nucleic acids. The decreased activity of the enzymes pancreatic amylase, trypsin, lipase, ribonucleic acid (RNA) and DNAse could lead to the malabsorption of aflatoxicosis-associated nutrients [80].

Hamilton [81] reported a decrease in egg production to 5% of normal in laying hens given near- LD50 aflatoxin levels in naturally contaminated maize. Egg production and size are decreased by aflatoxin-contaminated feed (up to 10 ppm) ingested by layers for 4 weeks. As a percentage of total egg weight, total yolk and yolk weight decreased, followed by higher yolk and plasma carotenoid concentrations [82].

## 9. Immunologic effects

While they are mainly referred to as hepatotoxins and hepatocarcinogens, aflatoxins tend to have been implicated in domesticated animal outbreaks of infectious diseases. Salmonellosis, a bacterial infection, and candidiasis, a yeast infection, were related to outbreaks of aflatoxin-induced Turkey X disease in 1960. Following the discovery of high levels of aflatoxins in the regional corn crop in 1977, outbreaks of salmonellosis in swine occurred in the southeastern United States [83]. Several animal species' resistance to bacterial, fungal, and parasitic infections has been shown to be lowered by aflatoxins, according to comprehensive experimental evidence [84].

**Table 3** summarizes the general characteristics of aflatoxin immunosuppression. Special care is required to interpret the findings of the aflatoxin and immunity studies, since some used aflatoxin mixtures, while others used purified aflatoxin B1. In this regard, differences were seen between aflatoxin B1 and its metabolites [85].

Data from experimental models generally supports the argument that aflatoxin B1 suppresses the cell-mediated immune response in particular. Several reviews have addressed Aflatoxin-induced immune modulation [86, 87].

Since aflatoxin poses an economic threat to the poultry industry, there has been comprehensive analysis of its effects on avian immunity. As reflected by decreased thymus weight and lower peripheral T lymphocyte numbers in chickens fed aflatoxin B11, cell-mediated responses are especially responsive [88, 89]. Graft versus host response in chickens given 300 ppm of aflatoxin B11 is suppressed [90]. In broiler

| **Cellular responses Effects** |
|---|
| Macrophage phagocytosis was reduced. |
| Cutaneous hypersensitivity Reduced with a delay |
| Reduced Lymphoblastogenesis (response to mitogens) |
| Graft versus host response reduced |
| **Humorous factors' impact** |
| Concentrations of Immunoglobulins (lgA and lgG) in serum |
| may be reduced |
| Complementary activity has declined. |
| Reduced of Bactericidal activity of serum |

**Table 3.**
*Aflatoxin's effect on immunity.*

chicks given 1 ppm of aflatoxin B1 feed, the delayed hypersensitivity response to dinitro-fluorobenzene is decreased [88]. Oral administration of aflatoxin B1 to chicks at 0.1 and 0.5 mg/kg body weight decreases the proliferation of peripheral blood lymphocyte responses to mitogenic T cell concanavalin A (Con A) [91].

Aflatoxin B1 is reliably inhibited by the phagocytic functions of macrophages and of the reticuloendothelial system. In chickens, aflatoxin B1 (0.3 to 1.0 ppm) depresses the percentage of nitroblue tetrazolium positive cells in spleen tissue, suggesting depressed macrophage activity [88]. In rats, oral administration of aflatoxin B1 (0.35 to 0.7 mg/kg bw) depresses both the amount and function of macrophages [92]. In chicks given aflatoxin B1 (0.3 mg/kg feed), the clearance of circulating colloidal carbon is reduced, indicating a decreased phagocytic status of the reticuloendothelial system. In vitro results suggest in vivo phagocytic activity suppression in chickens and rats as well. In rat peritoneal macrophages exposed to aflatoxins in vitro, phagocytosis, intracellular killing of *Candida albicans* and spontaneous superoxide anion (O2-) development are suppressed [93]. For macrophage toxicity, activation of aflatoxin B1 by mixed-function oxidases is apparently needed [94, 95].

Aflatoxins inhibit the activity of the mononuclear phagocyte system of more than one cell type. This decrease in activity appears to be linked to effects on phagocyte cells (**Figure 3**) but, perhaps more importantly, to the serum heat-stable substance needed for phagocyte activity [91].

In many immune reactions, complement, a serum constituent formed by the liver, plays an important role. The deficiency of this operation indicates a reduction in the immunological capacity of an essential part of the host. In pigs given feed containing 500 ppm aflatoxin B1, serum complement activity is decreased; in pigs given 300 ppm aflatoxin B1 in feed and in rabbits given 95 ppm aflatoxin B1 in feed, complement activity is not affected [96]. Aflatoxins decrease the activity of a hemolytic complement in guinea pigs [97] and other species [98].

Aflatoxin B1 modulatory effects on humoral immunity are less clear than those on cell-mediated immunity, particularly in cross-species comparisons. There is no substantial difference in antibody titers in swine fed up to 500 ppm aflatoxin B1 and inoculated with Erysipelothrix rhusiopathiae bacteria compared to inoculated swine fed uncontaminated feed [99]. Aflatoxin (0.045 mg/kg bw) administered orally is not impaired by the ability of guinea pigs to develop *Brucella abortus* antibodies [100]. The antibody-forming response to sheep red blood cells (SR-BCs), a T cell-dependent

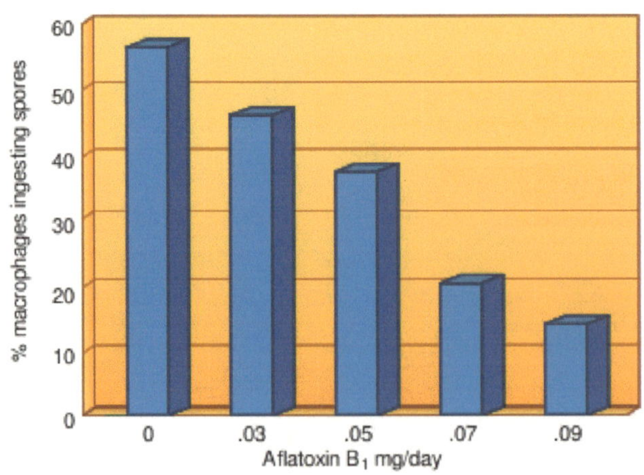


**Figure 3.**
*Decreased macrophage phagocytosis with increased doses of rabbit aflatoxin [84].*

antigen, is unchanged in rabbits given aflatoxin (approx. 24 ppm feed) relative to animals given aflatoxin B1-free diets [96].

To sum up, aflatoxin B1 suppresses immunity that is mediated by cells to a greater degree than humoral immunity. Aflatoxin B1 also inhibits some aspects of innate immunity, especially phagocytic responses. It is clear that aflatoxins are immunomodulatory in the low ppm range.

## 10. Hematopoietic effects of aflatoxins

The presence of aflatoxin-producing fungi has been associated with hemorrhagic anemia syndrome, caused by the ingestion of poultry moldy feed. Large hemorrhagic lesions in the main organs and musculature are typical of the condition. In broiler chicks that ingested aflatoxin, a suspected hemolytic anemia with bone marrow hyperplasia and a rise in bone marrow nucleic acid occurred. Hemoglobin, packed cell length, and erythrocytes circulating decreased significantly [101]. In broiler chicks fed aflatoxins for 3 weeks, Aflatoxins have triggered substantial period increases in whole blood clotting, recalcification, and pro-thrombin [102]. However, aflatoxins in the feed (20 ppm) of mature broilers induced only mild anemia for 4 weeks without raising erythrocyte fragility [103]. Lanza, *et al.* [104] provided evidence indicating that a secondary result of extreme hypoproteinemia was the production of anemia in aflatoxin-treated animals. As mentioned in the following section, these effects can be secondary to primary liver damage. Exposure to aflatoxins may also affect haemostasis in embryo development. Hatched chicks had substantially reduced cell counts, hematocrite, and hemoglobin concentrations following embryonic exposure to aflatoxin B1 [105]. However, no variations were observed between erythrocytes in the treated and control groups.

### 10.1 Aflatoxin biosynthetic pathway

*A. flavus, A. nomius* and *A. parasiticus* are the only fungal species known to produce aflatoxins [46]. Nevertheless, as many as 20 various Aspergilli, including A. Sterigmatocystin (ST) [106], a highly toxic intermediate in the biosynthetic pathway of AFBl, is produced by nidulans and species of Bipolaris, Chaetomium, Farrowia and Monocillium. Even though the AFBl biosynthetic pathway in *A. flavus* and *A. parasiticus* and the ST biosynthetic pathway in *A. nidulans* are believed to be similar, In order to recognize any key differences that may occur in biosynthesis or regulation and to shed light on the evolution and acquisition of the Aspergilli pathway and other genera, cooperative studies using all three species are being pursued.

Primary contributions in elucidating the biochemistry and molecular biology of the aflatoxin pathway have been the isolation and characterization of many mutants blocked in aflatoxin biosynthesis. Our current understanding of the order and mechanism of reactions in this complex biosynthetic pathway, which includes approximately 17 different enzymes, was developed by bioconversion experiments using these aflatoxin-blocked mutants, metabolic inhibitors and stable radio-isotopeor isotopelabelled precursors or pathway intermediates [55].

Polymerization of acetate and nine malonate units (with CO loss) by polyketide synthetase (PKS) in a manner analogous to fatty acid biosynthesis is proposed as the initial step in the generation of the polyketide backbone of AFBl [54, 55]. The synthesis of a 6-carbon hexanoate starter unit by a fatty acid synthase (FAS), which is then expanded by a PKS (without further ketoreduction) to produce a 20-carbon decaketide, noranthrone, is an alternative and maybe more probable hypothesis

[107]. Noranthrone is then oxidized by a hypothesized oxidase into anthraquinone norsolorinic acid (NA) in either scheme. The rest of the proposed pathway is summarized in **Figure 4** [54, 55, 57, 108]. Versicolorin A (VA) is important because it is the first molecule containing a double bond in the difuran moiety at the 2.3 position in the AFBl pathway. This double bond is the target of microsomal cytochrome P450 enzymes that produce a highly reactive epoxide resulting in DNA and protein activation and adduct formation. (reviewed in [52]). In contrast, aflatoxin B2 (AFB2), which lacks this double bond, is hundreds of times less carcinogenic [52].

It is stated that many enzymes involved in the aflatoxin pathway have been purified for homogeneity. Two distinct 0-methyltransferases include them [109, 110].

NA reductase (or probably two different enzymes) is involved in the conversion of ST to 0-methylsterigmatocystin [111, 112]. NA to averantin (AVN), which is involved in the conversion of versicon to versicolorin B, is transformed by cyclase reversible conversion [107, 113].

NA reductase, which is involved in the conversion of ST to 0-methylsterigmatocystin (or possibly two separate enzymes) [111, 112]. Involved in the cyclase reversible conversion of NA to averantin (AVN), which is involved in the conversion of versicon to versicolorin B [107, 113] The reaction between versiconal hemiacetal acetate and versiconol acetate is catalyzed by two versiconal hemiacetal acetate reductases (VHA reductase I and 11; possibly isozymes). (VHA reductase I and 11; probably isozymes) [114]. Such purified enzymes have provided essential tools for gene cloning.

## 10.2 Gene cloning strategied/structure and function of cloned genes

The secret to understanding the molecular biology of the pathway is the cloning of genes involved in aflatoxin biosynthesis. Cloned genes are useful probes to elucidate the molecular mechanisms that govern these genes' timing and level of expression. In the cloning of aflatoxin biosynthetic genes, two separate methods have been successfully used.

The isolation of genes encoding three enzymes in the pathway was achieved using a genetic complementation method, *nor-1*, *ver-1* and *uvm*8, and aflR, a

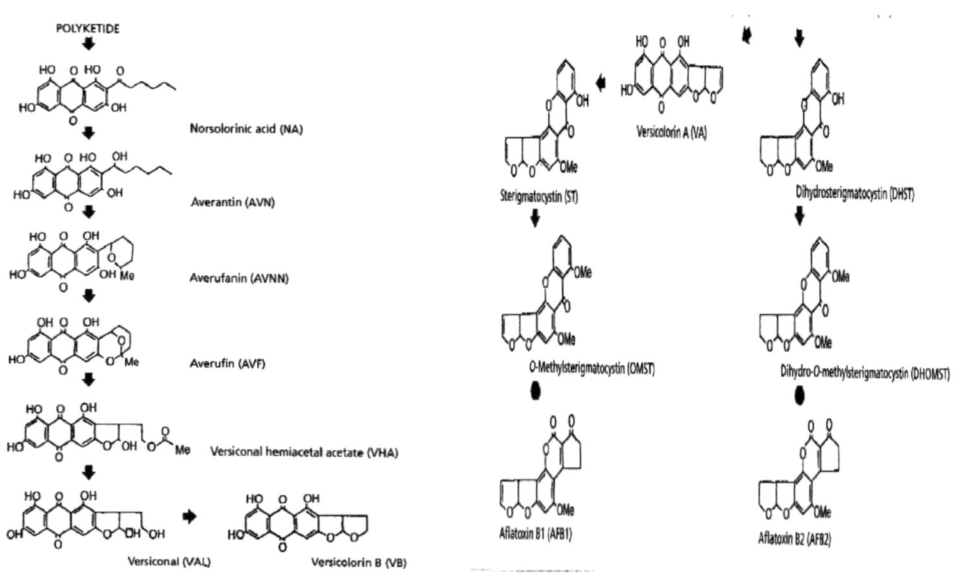


**Figure 4.**
*Aflatoxin B1 and 62 biosynthetic pathway.*

regulatory gene. Transformation systems for *A. parasiticus* were established to incorporate DNA into the fungus [115, 116] and *A. flavus* [117].

The *nor-1* (nar-*1* was developed for NA-related problems [118] and *ver-1* genes [66] By complementing aflatoxin-resistant mutants B62, they were cloned (an niaD mutant derived from *A. parasiticus* ATCC 24690, nor-7, bm-7, [119] and CSlO (an niaD mutant derived from *A. parasiticus* ATCC 36537, ver-7, wh-7, NA (brick-red) and VA (yellow) are two brightly colored pathway intermediates. The addition of a cosmid DNA library derived from genomic DNA from a wild type aflatoxin-producing *A. parasiticus* strain produced complementation (SU-1). By hybridizing *ver-1* to an *A. nidulans* genomic DNA library, the functionally homologous *ver-1* gene of *A. nidulans* was isolated. *Ver-1* and *ver-1* gene products have almost identical predicted amino acid sequences [120], demonstrating the high degree of similarity among these *Aspergillus* species' aflatoxin biosynthetic genes The predicted amino acid sequences of *nor-1*, *ver-1*, and verA show significant identity and contain a NAD(P)H binding motif near the amino terminus (ver-1/verA 33%; *nor-1* 23%) Several NADPH and NADH-dependent reductase/dehydrogenase enzymes are involved. A short-chain alcohol dehydrogenase motif occurs in each sequence [121].

Recombination inactivation (gene disruption) was performed in the toxigenic strains of *A. parasiticus* to confirm the function of these genes in aflatoxin biosynthesis (*nor- 1*, [121]; *ver-1*, [122]) and *A. nidulans* verA, [120]. *A. nidulans* lost measurable ST and accumulated VA after the verA gene was disrupted, confirming its role in the conversion of VA to ST. Likewise, As a result of the disruption of ver-1, the aflatoxin pathway was blocked, resulting in VA accumulation. The disruption of nor-1 resulted in a significant accumulation of NA. The ability of disrupted strains to generate low levels of aflatoxin was maintained, suggesting that the aflatoxin pathway has one or more alternative routes (or enzymic activities) for synthesizing averufin from NA [108]. In *E. coli*, a nor-1/maltose-binding protein (MBP) fusion protein was recently expressed [123]. Crude *E. coli* cell extracts containing the fusion protein transformed NA to AVN only when NADPH was present, supporting the prediction that nor-1 encodes a NA-to-AVN reductase.

Complementation of an aflatoxin-blocking mutant, avm8, derived from UV mutagenesis of A. parasiticus mutant strain B62, was used to clone the gene avm8 (niaD, brn-1, *nor- 1*) [124]. Metabolite conversion studies showed that avm8 has two AFBl pathway blocks, one at nor-1 and the other prior to nor-1. The P-subunit of FASs (FAS1) from *Saccharomyces cerevisiae* and Yarrowia lipobtica had a high degree of similarity (67%) and identity (48%) to the predicted peptide sequence of extensive regions of the avm8 gene product [125]. As a result, it was proposed that uvm8 encodes a FAS activity required for the synthesis of the proposed hexanoate starter. Due to the complete reduction of two keto groups in hexanoate to hydrocarbon, a FAS involved in its synthesis would be expected to contain three main enzyme activities, ketoreductase, dehydratase, and enoyl reductase, in addition to a P-ketoacyl- synthase. Limited nucleotide sequencing revealed an enoyl reductase domain in zivm8 (based on similarity to *S. cerevisiae* FAS1), which is not needed for aflatoxin PKS in theory.

In *A. parasiticus* the zivm8 gene has been disrupted. No detectable AFBl or pathway intermediates consistent with a functional role in polyketide backbone synthesis were accumulated by the disrupted strains.

A second approach to gene isolation, reverse genetics, was based on the enzymes of the purified pathway described above. Where purification was necessary, the generation of enzyme antibodies and the isolation of the gene from the library of cDNA expression in *E. coli*, it can be done.

The omt-1 gene from *A. flavus*, which encodes the 0-methyltransferase activity responsible for the conversion of ST to 0-methylsterigmato- cystin, was cloned using this process [126]. Antibodies raised against the native methyltransferase were used to screen an *A. parasitica* scDNA library made from RNA from an aflatoxin-induced culture. A motif found in other S-adenosylmethionine-dependent methyl-transferases was found in the predicted amino acid sequence derived from the cloned cDNA. Both the purified native protein and a fusion protein produced in *E. coli* from the cDNA showed substrate-specific methyltransferase activity. Omt-I is the only pathway gene that has been cloned using a reverse genetics approach to date. However, cloning several other genes encoding purified pathway enzymes should be possible using this process.

Feng, *et al.* [127] have used another molecular genetic method for gene cloning, subtractive hybridization, to isolate many genes whose expression pattern coincides with the development of aflatoxin in *A. parasiticus*. As in the two previous approaches, this approach is not dependent on precise knowledge of the role of the gene product and can therefore be beneficial when the timing of gene expression induction is understood, but pure enzymes or blocked pathway mutants are not usable. To date, no clear identification has been recorded of the activities of genes isolated by this process.

### 10.3 Regulation of aflatoxin gene expression

Polyketides are a wide and diverse family of secondary metabolites that are mainly formed by actino-mycetides, fungi, and higher plants, but are also synthesized in animals, including other species. The regulation of synthesis of these secondary metabolites is different from the regulation of primary metabolism, since secondary metabolism relies on energy, enzyme cofactors and building blocks of primary metabolism (i.e. acetate). Luchese and Harrigan [128] have reviewed the impact of primary metabolism on aflatoxin biosynthesis.

during idiophase, *A. parasiticus* and *A. flavus* produce aflatoxins, In culture, When it has slowed or stopped exponential growth and secondary metabolites are produced. Buchanan, *et al.* [129] demonstrated, using transcription and translation inhibitors, that de novo protein synthesis is necessary for the development of aflatoxin. Other studies have shown that the activity of at least four of the enzymes involved in the pathway is not detected before idiophase is formed [130–132]. During fermentation of batches of *A. parasiticus* During the transition between active growth and stationary phase, the *ver-1* and *nor-I* RNA transcripts accumulated most quickly [133]. A similar pattern was shown to follow the accumulation of RNA transcripts from the *afl*R gene, proposed to encode a key regulatory protein (see later) [134]. Coordinate transcription of these genes indicated that they are partly regulated at the transcription level, possibly by a common regulatory factor. A gene suggested to encode one significant regulatory factor, the afE-2 gene, was cloned using a wildtype genomic DNA library from *A. flavas* by complementing an aflatoxin-nonproducing mutant [134]. Afl-2 is involved in aflatoxin biosynthesis before NA, according to genetic evidence and metabolite feeding studies. *A. flavus* mutant strain, missing afE-2 was unable to convert a number of exogenously supplied pathway intermediates to aflatoxin, suggesting the absence of main pathway enzymes. Complementation of mutant strains with the wild-type afl-2 gene restored expression of several aflatoxin pathway enzyme activities in crude cell extracts, which is a requirement for a trans-acting regulatory factor encoding gene.

In *A. parasiticus* After transformation, apa-2 was cloned with a single cosmid clone (NorA) containing both the aflatoxin genes nor-1 and ver-1 on the basis of overproduction of aflatoxin pathway intermediates [118]. The apa-2 was replaced by an A. The Favas afE-2 mutant strain shows that apa-2 and 4–2 are functional homologues for the development of aflatoxin. The genetic data was confirmed by nucleotide sequence analysis, which revealed that these genes share more than 95% nucleotide sequence identity [118]. In the predicted amino acid sequences of apa-2 and aj-2, a cysteine-rich zinc cluster motif, Cys-Xaa2-Cys-Xaab-Cys-XaaG-Cys-Xaa2-Cys-Xaa6-Cys, was discovered [118, 135]. This zinc cluster motif is found in a family of fungal transcriptional activators, the most well-studied of which is *S. cerevisiae* GAL4. GAL4 controls the expression of genes involved in galactose utilization in yeast. The homologues apa-2 and a/−2 have been renamed aflR because the overwhelming evidence indicates that they are positive regulators of aflatoxin synthesis [134].

### 10.4 The gene cluster for aflatoxin

Since there is no known perfect (sexual) stage for *A. parasiticus* and *A. flavus*, Classical genetic experiments using the parasexual cycle have been performed. Parasexual study of eight blocked mutants with aflatoxin in *A. flavus* reported that they were all genetically related to linkage group VIII markers [136]. However, attempts to demonstrate parasexual studies to connect *nor-1* and *ver-1* were confounding due to problems inherent in analyzing segregant ploid levels and the non-random segregation of certain genes during haploidization (re viewed by [53]).

Many of the genes involved in aflatoxin biosynthesis in *A. parasiticus* and *A. flavus* are physically clustered on one chromosome, according to molecular genetic studies. One cosmid, Nor A, was discovered during the cloning and characterization of the *nor- 1* and *ver- 1* genes from *A. parasiticus*, and it hybridized to probes of both genes. Physical mapping of the corresponding area in the fungal genome in *A. parasiticus* later supported this preliminary evidence for linkage [67]. Later, the genes aftR, uvm8, and omt-1 were found to belong to this cluster, as well as a cluster of aflatoxin genes in *A. flavus* [67, 137]. The physical order of genes in the cluster tends to be identical to the order of enzyme reactions catalyzed by their gene products, which is an interesting finding. It's unclear if this feature has any practical meaning.

Since 17 enzyme activities are thought to be needed for complete aflatoxin synthesis, it was hypothesized that several other pathway enzymes were encoded by the cosmid Nor A (and the corresponding region in *A. flavus*). In order to determine the size, Several more pathway enzymes were encoded. A transcriptional map of the genomic DNA insertion in cosmid Nor A was completed to determine the size, location and pattern of expression of other genes in the cluster. This cluster was localized to twelve separate RNA transcripts. They were tentatively known as aflatoxin genes because the timing of their expression was close to that observed for *nor-1* and *ver-1*. In a VA-accumulating mutation, CS10, and OMST development in an OMST-accumulating strain, genetic disruption of a gene (encoding a 7–0 kb transcript) located adjacent to nor-1 in the gene cluster blocked VA production. Predicted amino acid sequence data from an extensive region of this gene showed a high degree of identity to the β- ketoacyl-synthase (Identity 67%.) and the acyltransferase (Identity 32%) functional domains [67]. In *A. nidulans*, the V A gene product encodes a PKS involved in conidial pigment development. P.-K. Chang and others (personal communication) found high homology between the acyl carrier protein domain of the w A gene product and the acyl carrier protein domain of the w A gene product. It's likely that this putative aflatoxin PKS is involved in extending the tlvm8-produced hexanoate starter cell [138].

A nucleotide sequence approach combined with biochemical studies of genetically disrupted strains can similarly classify the unique function of other genes in the cluster located by transcript mapping. Feeding interrupted strains with intermediates of the pathway of aflatoxin and analyzing their ability to transform. These substrates to subsequent intermediates can aid in determining the stage of gene disruption. This approach to function of gene recognition is extended to another interesting gene adjacent to *nor-1* (encodes a 6.5 kb transcript).

A limited portion of this gene in nucleotide sequence analysis showed that The predicted protein has a high degree of similarity to the real thing (51% over 150 amino acid residues) with the enoyl-reductase domain in the same yeast FASl products as observed in the uvm88 analysis [67]. It's probable that the hexanoate starter requires two FAS subunits (and; encoded by separate genes) that are similar to those found in yeast. This hypothesis will be tested by combining gene disruption with feeding experiments. A common phenomenon is the clustering of genes involved in secondary metabolism. For example, a number of polyketide-derived antibiotics, including erythromycin, tetracenomycin, actinorhodin, griseusin and granaticin, are produced by different species of Streptomyes (reviewed in [139, 140]). Several genes contained in their biosynthetic pathways display a high degree of identity in comparable pathways with genes and are clustered on the chromosome in identical patterns.

There have also been studies of the clustering of fungal genes involved in the synthesis of secondary metabolites. The genes that encode penicillin and cephalosporin enzymes (members of the antibiotic β-lactam class) in the *Penicillium chrysogenum* and *Cephalosporium acremonium* pathways (reviewed in [141]), *A. nidulans* [142], *Fursarium sporotrichioides* genes involved in the trichothecene process (toxic sesquiterpenes) [143], Gene clusters can be found. However, recent studies indicate that the clustering of fungal genes is not limited to secondary metabolite synthesis. Some of the genes involved in melanin biosynthesis (a dark-brown polyketide-derived pigment) are clustered within a 30 kb stretch of genomic DNA in the filamentous fungus *Alternaria alternata* [144].

The role of gene clustering in the aflatoxin biosynthetic pathway's significance (if any), regulation or evolution has not yet been elucidated. However, with growing evidence that the structure of chromatin is involved in gene regulation [145–147], A role in cluster expression can be played by the chromosome structure. This is an unexplored area that can benefit from molecular biology techniques.

### 10.5 Aflatoxin gene duplication

The presence of at least two copies of the ver- 1 gene, Per- IA and ver- IB, in different regions of the *A. parasiticus* genome was discovered during physical mapping studies of the cosmid NorA. [122]. It was established that the gene originally cloned was ver- IA by comparing the restriction enzyme polymorphisms present in these two chromosomal copies with the cloned ver-1 gene. Subsequently, ver- IB was cloned and its nucleotide sequence was calculated. These genes were found to share 93% of the identity of the nucleotide series. Near the center of the predicted ver-IB gene transcript, a stop codon was found, indicating that it may encode a truncated polypeptide that has little to no role. A duplicate chromosomal region extending from ver-IA and ver-IB approximately 12 kb upstream was found, which also includes an additional copy of aflR [122]. The higher stability of toxin production in *A. parasiticus* compared to *A. flavus*, which does not have such a duplication, may be explained by duplication of the ver-1 and aflR genes. More than 90% of *A. parasitictrs* isolates contain aflatoxin, while only 50% of A. flavus isolates are toxigenic (50 YO or less) [53].

### 10.6 Aflatoxin genes chromosomal organization

Keller et al. [148] successfully used pulsed field gel electrophoresis as a tool for genetic analysis of aflatoxigenic fungi. Genetic karyotyping and Southern blot analysis using many different gene probes revealed similarities and differences between the genomes of *A. parasiticus* and *A. flavus*, as well as those of *A. niger* and *A. nidulans*.

Under identical electrophoretic conditions, *A. flavus* (5 to 8 chromosomal visible bands), A. *parasiticus* (5 to 6 bands of chromosomes) and *A. versicolor*, a related species reported to produce precursors (six chromosomal bands) in pathway of aflatoxin, showed chromosome numbers that were identical but varied.

The total size of the genome of these fungi was close to that of the size recorded for *A. nidulans*, as well as *A. niger* (31–38.5 Mb). These studies have yielded an additional, potentially significant finding. The karyotype patterns in 19 different *A. flavus* isolates were all different, suggesting that genetic diversity in this species is widespread [53].

An indicator of chromosomal rearrangement via gross translocation leading to specific karyotype patterns may be the size variation. Imperfect fungi can tolerate such rearrangements because, unlike sexual reproduction, Asexual reproduction (via mitosis) necessitates only the separation of similar chromatids, which necessitates the pairing of identical chromosomes and is strictly regulated genetically. The heterogeneity in the genomes of different isolates of *A. flavus* can be linked to the apparent instability in the ability to generate aflatoxins, which is of practical importance. Keller et al. [120] recently demonstrated that the verA gene of *A. nidulans* hybridizes strongly to chromosome IV in a similar sample (2.9 Mb in size). It should now be possible to identify the positions of duplicated aflatoxin gene clusters on the same or different chromosomes in *A. parasiticus* using identical procedures.

### 10.7 Ongoing studies

The molecular biology of aflatoxin synthesis is currently being studied in two areas: (1) The genes structure, role, organization, and comparative mapping and gene clusters of aflatoxin (or ST) in *A. parasiticus, A. flavus* and *A. nidtrlans*; and (2) the discovery of pathway genes controlling molecular pathways (Aflatoxin promoter structure and function; regulatory genes).

### 10.8 Structure and function of genelcluster

Analysis of the nucleotide transcript mapping and sequence of most of genes in *A. parasiticus* and *A. nidulans* should be finished in the immediate future while studies of disruption continue as candidate genes are identified. The function and localization of enzymes pathway is being pursued in related work. For instance, maltose-binding protein fusion products *nor-1* and *ver-1* were expressed in *E. coli* It has developed and polyclonal antibodies (pAb) that seem to recognize the native fungal proteins [122, 123]. These antibodies will be used to locate these proteins in the cell, along with the available antibodies to the $nor - 1$ protein, and to decide if proteins function individually or in enzyme complexes. Preliminary results using the polyclonal antibody *ver-1* indicate that *ver-1* proteins are primarily localized in the fungal cell membrane fraction [122]. For studies on plant resistance mechanisms against the development of aflatoxin, immunolabelling will also be helpful in exploring the kinetics and level of expression of aflatoxin enzymes in host plant tissues.

### 10.9 Pathway genes regulated molecular mechanisms

Afl- 1, a second putative regulatory locus (besides aflR), was discovered by Leaich and Papa [149] in *A. flavus* by use UV mutagenesis and determination to be linked to *nor- 1* by parasexual analysis (reviewed by [53]). In diploids, afl I mutants are functionally dominant, resulting in aflatoxin development loss. The afl- I mutation suppresses transcription of the three structural genes studied, according to recent research [150] (nor- 1, ver- 1 and omt-I). In these strains, aflR transcription was natural. Cloning afl-1 and determining its position in regulation will be the subject of future research.

Following the cloning of aflR and the discovery of a$-I, the next logical step is to investigate the mechanisms of influence exerted by the genes' products. Identifying the cis-acting sites and trans-acting proteins that control aflatoxin gene function is the latest strategy for conducting these studies. The nor- 1, ver- 1, and aflR promoters have been fused to the *E. coli* gene encoding/3-glucuronidase (zcidA), also known as the GUS gene, whose gene product can be easily detected using colorimetric or fluorometric assays [151, 152]. This reporter construct is now being used in fungal strains: (1) to monitor fungi in plants under various conditions and to detect the induction of aflatoxin genes in fungi grown under various crop conditions; (2) classify, by deletion or site-directed mutation analysis, the cis regulatory regions related to the control of these promoters. By mobility shift assays, promoter regions are also being studied. It is then possible to identify and purify proteins which bind specifically. Preliminary data indicate that in the *nor-1* promoter, there are at least two distinct DNA/protein interactions [151]. To be demon strated, the practical importance of these relationships remains. The study of aflatoxin biosynthesis in culture offers a model framework for understanding the biosynthesis of aflatoxin on natural substrates. Applications of molecular biology to the reduction, evolution and biological significance of the aflatoxin pathway. Factors that are essential for the regulation of aflatoxin biosynthesis in the host plant, however, can differ from those that work in the culture. More studies of the fungus in the host plant must require future work. In turn, these studies can lead to new toxin control techniques and increased understanding of the aflatoxin pathway's evolution and biological function.

### 10.10 Elimination of aflatoxins from food and feed

**Figure** 5 shows how the molecular biology contributions mentioned above can be extended to the removal of aflatoxin from food and feed. They will quickly summarize each of these applications.

Several methods (grouped into pre-harvest and post-harvest strategies) are currently being used or have been suggested for use in the food chain reduction or elimination of aflatoxin. Preharvest strategies are designed to block the host plant (crop) from fungal infection or to block the fungal pathogen's ability to grow or synthesize aflatoxins on the plant and are likely to have the greatest effect on human and animal health in the future. In reversing aflatoxin screening/detection, removal/adsorption, decontamination or altered aflatoxin metabolism/DNA adduct formation, expensive and/or inadequate post-harvest elimination strategies would not need to be relied on as vital treatment measures, but can provide a safety net to eliminate low levels of aflatoxins that can escape pre-harvest monitoring. Existing approaches to pre-harvesting, including irrigation, the use of fungicides or insecticides and the use of resistant or regionally adapted crop varieties, lack successful control. It is also psychologically inappropriate or too expensive to use pesticides or irrigation, though genetically stable, highly resistant crops have not been successfully obtained using traditional breeding methods. However, for potential use, several promising preharvest techniques have been suggested for aflatoxin regulation. These strategies concentrate on two main areas: (1) genetically modified crops to minimize the growth of fungi or inhibit biosynthesis of aflatoxin (long-term

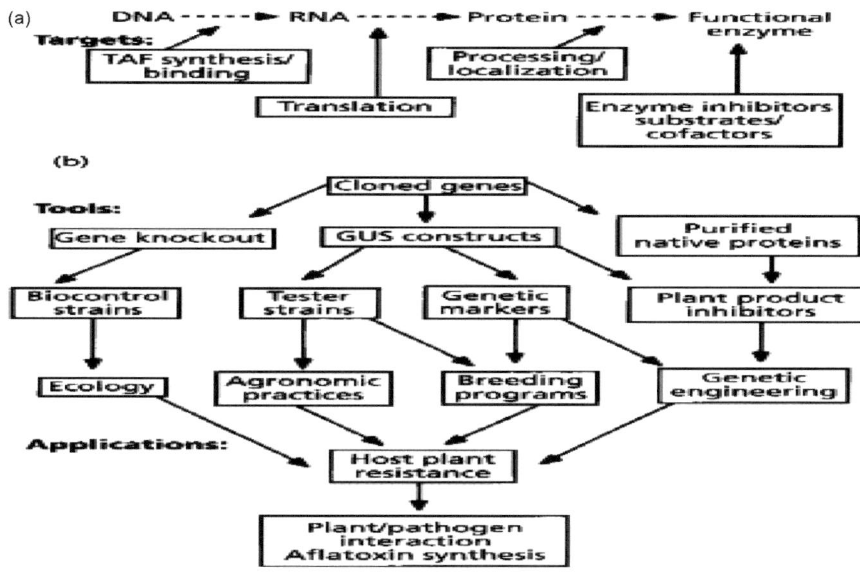


**Figure 5.**
*Elimination of aflatoxin by applications of molecular biology. (a) Targets for inhibiting aflatoxin gene expression. Natural plant products or other agents that can be identified using GUS reporter constructs or polyclonal antibodies for each gene mentioned in the text can theoretically inhibit each step in gene expression, transcription, RNA transport and processing, translation, protein processing, and localization. TAF stands for trans-acting component. (regulatory protein). (b) The potential application of tools derived from cloned aflatoxin genes to increase host plant resistance to fungal growth, infection, or toxin biosynthesis. Biocontrol strains, fungal strains with GUS reporter constructs (i.e. tester strains), and polyclonal antibodies raised to pure native proteins or proteins expressed in* E. coli *are the main tools in development.*

approach); and (2) the use of biological control species to exclude the toxigenic fungus from infecting the crop competitively (short-term approach). These other possible applications of molecular biology for the removal of aflatoxin have recently been studied in detail [57]. However, they are briefly outlined here to provide a basis for the discussion of aflatoxin synthesis molecular biology crop genetic engineering. This method employs molecular genetics to increase the expression of genes that control natural (endogenous) resistance and/or to introduce resistance genes from other sources into susceptible plants. *A. parasiticus* and *A. flavus* are weak pathogens of the plant's reproductive organs that are particularly aggressive in mature seeds with high oil concentrations [46]. Successful genetic manipulation of crops should be aided by the identification of the signals exchanged between host and pathogen that stimulate aflatoxin production in susceptible plants under host stress or that inhibit toxin formation in 'naturally resistant' crops. There is still a lot of work to be done in this field; however, the approach is promising because it may be reasonably easy to increase natural or endogenous resistance by modulating gene expression that is a common part of the plant genome.

In principle, resistance genes from other sources can be obtained by finding naturally occurring plant compounds that inhibit *A. flavus* and *A. parasiticus.* Growth and/or aflatoxin production. Crude botanical extracts that display these characteristics have been recognized (reviewed by [56]). By genetic engineering, genes that encode the synthesis of these novel compounds can be inserted into crops. Clearly, if one or two genes enable the biosynthesis of the compound, success will be more easily obtained and will only be obtained if the compound is non-toxic to humans, animals and engineered plants. In addition, at the correct time, the additional genes must be expressed in the engineered plant in the right organ. For the identification of plant compounds (or other agents) that promote or inhibit fungal invasion, growth or toxin biosynthesis, the aflatoxin gene/GUS reporter con structures are extremely useful tools.

### 10.11 Biological control

Strains of *A. flavus* and *A. parasiticus* showed potential to reduce the level of the resident fungal population and showed a substantial reduction in aflatoxin contamination (80–90%) in greenhouse and field studies. ([42]; reviewed in [46]). Since this strategy depends on the survival and successful occupation by the biocontrol strain of an ecological niche, identification of environmental factors that benefit certain isolates of *A. flavus* and *A. parasiticus* must be recognized by others. The strains of *A. flavus* are an interesting aspect of this strategy, which must be considered for its successful execution. *A. flavus* appears to be a replacement for other strains of more successfully than *A. parasiticus*. Therefore, combinations of strains of both species are likely to be needed [153]. Recent studies have suggested that nontoxigenic isolates of *A. flavus* occur naturally. In as yet undetermined environmental conditions, weaknesses may have the genetic capacity to synthesize AFBl [154]. Under as yet undetermined conditions of the environment. Using a molecular genetics approach, genetically stable *Aspergillus* toxigenic biocontrol strains that are known to compete well can be produced once these genes have been identified by specific deletions of key genes in the biosynthetic pathway. Using a molecular genetics approach, genetically stable *Aspergillus* toxigenic biocontrol strains that are known to compete well can be produced once these genes have been identified by specific deletions of key genes in the biosynthetic pathway. A minimum of one genetically engineered fungal biocontrol strain (tlvm8 disruption strain - Dis3) has been made available for field research using this gene disruption technology [124].

### 10.12 Evolution

A high degree of sequence identity between the genes of aflatoxin (*ver-1*, aflR, omt-1) in *A. parasiticus*, *A. nidulans* and *A.flavus*. The organization of the gene cluster also is well conserved. Interestingly, the *nor-1* and *ver-1* genes are present in *A. sajae, A. oryzae* and nontoxigenic *A. flavus* strains [154]. These data indicate that the AFBl or ST pathway was also included in the progenitor *Aspergillus* strain that gave rise to the present species under analysis (it will be interesting to determine if *A. nidulans* has the genetic capacity to produce AFB1; i.e. genes for the 0-methyltransferase and oxido reductase required to convert ST to AFB1). Physical clustering can also mean that the progenitor strain has acquired the intact pathway from some other organism by horizontal transfer (i.e. *Streptomyes* spp. produce anthraquinone polyketide antibiotics, structurally related to inter mediates in AFBl synthesis). Alternatively, cluster organization preservation can indicate that an intact structural organization relies on the role or control of aflatoxin synthesis. The aflatoxin pathway formed from a pre-existing pathway for the synthesis of a fungal polyketide, perhaps a mycelial or spore pigment, is another possibility that should receive further research. The putative aflatoxin PKS demonstrates a high degree of sequence identity to the PKS involved in conidial pigment synthesis in *A. nidulans* in support of this notion. Interestingly, the chemical intermediate structure in the synthesis of conidial pigment in *A. Parasiticus* (a polyketide called naphthapyranone) also has a good resemblance to NA [155]. A similar study determined that an ascospore pigment (ascoquinone A) in *A. nidulans* is a dimer of an anthraquinone and is likely to be polyketide in origin [156]. Recent studies on melanin biosynthesis in Magnaportbegriseaa have provided additional data that may support a correlation between pigment synthesis and aflatoxin synthesis [157].

*A. Parasiticus* 56% identity of the *ver-1* gene product in A was reported to share the predicted amino acid sequence of the gene encoding a polyhydroxynaphthalene reductase involved in melanin biosynthesis. This may indicate that a common ancestral polyketide pathway is used to derive these biosynthetic pathways (or parts of the pathways).

## Author details

Nadeem A. Ramadan and Hadeel A. Al-Ameri*
Department of Biology, College of Sciences, University of Mosul, Republic of Iraq

*Address all correspondence to: hadeelahmed.um@gmail.com

## References

[1] Klich, M. A., L. H. Tiffany, and G. Knaphus. (1994). Ecology of the aspergilli of soils and litter. Pp. 329–353. In M. A. Klich and J. W. Bennett (Eds.). Aspergillus Biology and Industrial Applications. Butterworth-Heineman, Boston.

[2] Ito, Y., S. W. Peterson, D. T. Wicklow, and T. Goto. (2001). Aspergillus pseudotamarii, a new aflatoxin producing species in Aspergillus section flavi. Mycological Res 105:233–239.

[3] Kurtzman, C. P., B. W. Horn, and C. W. Hesseltine. (1987). Aspergil-lus nomius, a new aflatoxin-producing species related to Aspergillus flavus and Aspergillus tamarii. Antonie van Leeuwen-hoek 53:147–158.

[4] Horn, B. W., R. L. Greene, and J. W. Dorner. (1994). Effect of corn and peanut cultivation on soil populations of Aspergillus flavus and A. parasiticus in southwestern Georgia. Appl Environ Mi-crobiol 61:2472.(19940.

[5] Payne, G. A. (1998). Process of contamination by aflatoxin-producing fungi and their impact on crops. Pp. 279–306. In K. K. S. Sinha and D. Bhatnagar (Eds.). Mycotoxins in Agriculture and Food Safety. Marcel Dekker, Inc., New York.

[6] Widstrom, N. W. (1996). The aflatoxin problem with corn grain. Pp 219–280. In D. Sparks (Ed.). Advances in Agronomy. Academic Press, New York.

[7] Hall, A. J. and C. P. Wild. (1994). Epidemiology of aflatoxin-related disease. Pp. 233–258. In D. L. Eaton and J. D. Groopman (Eds.). The Toxicology of Aflatoxins: Human Health, Veterinary, and Agricultural Significance. Academic Press, San Diego, California.

[8] Lynch, R. E. and D. M. Wilson. (1991). Enhanced infecion of peanut, *Arachis hypogaea* L., seeds with Aspergillus flavus group due to external scarification of peanut pods by lesser cornstalk borer, Elasmophalpus lignosellus (Zeller). Peanut Sci 18: 110–116.

[9] Klich, M. A. and M. A. Chmielewski. (1985). Nectaries as entry sites for Aspergillus flavus in developing cotton bolls. Appl Environ Microbiol 50: 602–604.

[10] Klich, M. A., S. H. Thomas, and J. E. Mellon. (1984). Field studies on the mode of entry of Aspergillus flavus into cotton seeds. Mycopathologia 76: 665–669.

[11] Doster, M. A. and T. J. Michailides. (1994a). Aspergillus molds and aflatoxins in pistachio nuts in California. Phytopathology 84:583–590.

[12] Doster, M. A. and T. J. Michailides. (1994b). Development of Aspergillus molds in litter from pistachio trees. Plant Dis 78:393–397.

[13] Cole, R. J., J. W. Dorner, and C. C. Holbrook. (1995). Advances in Mycotoxin Elimination and Resistance. Pp. 456–474. In H. E. Pattee and H. T. Stalker (Eds.). Advances in Peanut Science. American Peanut Research and Education Society, Stillwater, Oklahoma.

[14] McGee, D. C., O. M. Olanya, and G. M. Hoyos. (1996). Populations of Aspergillus flavus in the Iowa cornfield ecosystems in years not favorable for aflatoxin contamination of corn grain. Plant Dis 80:742–746.

[15] Doster,M.A.and T.J.Michailides. (1995).The relationship between date of hull splitting and decay of pistachio nuts by Aspergillus species. Plant Dis 79: 766–769.

[16] Liu, Y.; Wu, F. Global burden of aflatoxin-induced hepatocellular carcinoma: a risk assessment. Environ. Health Perspect. 2010, 118, 818–824. [CrossRef].

[17] Okoth, S.; De Boevre, M.; Vidal, A.; Diana Di Mavungu, J.; Landschoot, S.; Kyallo, M.; Njuguna, J.; Harvey, J.; De Saeger, S. (2018). Genetic and toxigenic variability within Aspergillus flavus population isolated from maize in two diverse environments in Kenya. Front. Microbiol., 9, 57.

[18] Linz, W.J. E., Woloshuk C. P., and Payne, G. A. (1993). Cloning of the Aspergillus parasiticus apa-2 gene associated with the regulation of aflatoxin biosynthesis. Appl Environ Microbiol59, 3273–3279.

[19] Pildain, M.B.; Frisvad, J.C.; Vaamonde, G.; Cabral, D.; Varga, J.; Samson, R.A. (2008). Two novel aflatoxin-producing Aspergillus species from Argentinean peanuts. Int. J. Syst. Evol. Microbiol., 58, 725–735.

[20] Frisvad, J.C.; Hubka, V.; Ezekiel, C. N.; Hong, S.B.; Nováková, A.; Chen, A. J.; Arzanlou, M.; Larsen, T.O.; Sklenár, F.; Mahakarnchanakul, W.; *et al.* (2019). Taxonomy of Aspergillus section Flavi and their production of aflatoxins, ochratoxins and other mycotoxins. Stud. Mycol., 93, 1–63.

[21] Abdin, M.Z.; Ahmad, M.M.; Javed, S. (2010). Advances in molecular detection of Aspergillus: An update. Arch. Microbiol., 192, 409–425.

[22] Bennett, J. W. and Goldblatt, L. A. (1973). The isolation of mutants of Aspergillus flavus and Aspergillus parasiticus with altered aflatoxin producing ability. Sabouraudia 11, 235–241.

[23] Richard, J. L., J. R. Thurston, E. B. Lillehoj, S. J. Cysewski, and Robens, J. F. and J. L. Richard. (1992). Aflatoxins in Animal and Human Health. Pp. 69–94. In G. W. Ware (Ed.). Reviews of Environmental Contamination and Toxicology. Vol. 127. Springer-Verlag, New York.

[24] Ehrlich, K.C.; Chang, P.K.; Yu, J.; Cotty, P.J.(2004). Aflatoxin biosynthesis cluster gene cypA is required for G aflatoxin formation. Appl. Environ. Microbiol., 70, 6518–6524.

[25] Probst, C.; Callicott, K.A.; Cotty, P.J. (2012). Deadly strains of Kenyan Aspergillus are distinct from other aflatoxin producers. Eur. J. Plant Pathol., 132, 419–429.

[26] Mutegi, C.K.; Cotty, P.J.; Bandyopadhyay, R.(2018). Prevalence and mitigation of aflatoxins in Kenya (1960-to date). World Mycotoxin J., 11, 341–357.

[27] Cole, R. J. and COX, R. H. (1981). Sterigmatocystins. In Handbook of Toxic Fungal Metabolites, pp. 67–93. Edited by R. J. Cole and R. H. Cox. New York: Academic Press.

[28] Gilbert, M.K.; Mack, B.M.; Moore, G.G.; Downey, D.L.; Lebar, M.D.; Joardar, V.; Losada, L.; Yu, J.; Nierman, W.C.; Bhatnagar, D. (2018). Whole genome comparison of Aspergillus flavus L-morphotype strain NRRL 3357 (type) and S-morphotype strain AF70. PLoS ONE, 13, e0199169.

[29] Kachapulula, P.W.; Akello, J.; Bandyopadhyay, R.; Cotty, P.J. (2017). Aflatoxin contamination of groundnut and maize in Zambia: observed and potential concentrations. J. Appl. Microbiol., 122, 1471–1482.

[30] Whelan, J., Chichester, J., Wiley., S., Horn, B., Dorner, J., Greene, R., Blankenship, P. and Cole, R. (1994). Effect of Aspergillus parasiticus soil inoculum on invasion of peanut seeds. Mycopatbologia 125, 179–191.

[31] Pier, A. C., J. L. Richard, and J. R. Thurston. (1980a). Effects of mycotoxins on immunity and resistance of animals. Pp. 691–699. In D. Eaker and T. Wadstrom (Eds.). Natural Toxins. Pergamon Press, New York.

[32] Probst, C.; Schulthess, F.; Cotty, P.J. (2010). Impact of Aspergillus section Flavi community structure on the development of lethal levels of aflatoxins in Kenyan maize (*Zea mays*). J. Appl. Microbiol., 108, 600–610.

[33] Benkerroum, N. (2019). Retrospective and prospective look at aflatoxin research and development from a practical standpoint. Int. J. Environ. Res. Public Health, 16, 3633.

[34] Eaton, D. L. and Groopman, J. D. (Eds.) (1994). The Toxicology of Aflatoxins: Human Health, Veterinary and Agricultural Significance. Academic Press, New York.

[35] Theumer, M.G.; Henneb, Y.; Khoury, L.; Snini, S.P.; Tadrist, S.; Canlet, C.; Puel, O.; Oswald, I.P.; Audebert, M. (2018). Genotoxicity of aflatoxins and their precursors in human cells. Toxicol. Lett., 287, 100–107.

[36] Townsend, C.A.(2014). Aflatoxin and deconstruction of type I, iterative polyketide synthase function. Nat. Prod. Rep., 31, 1260–1265.

[37] Wong, J.J.; Hsieh, D.P. (1976) Mutagenicity of aflatoxins related to their metabolism and carcinogenic potential. Proc. Natl. Acad. Sci. USA, 73, 2241–2244.

[38] Yu, J.; Chang, P.-K.; Ehrlich, K.C.; Cary, J.W.; Bhatnagar, D.; Cleveland, T. E.; Payne, G.A.; Linz, J.E.; Woloshuk, C. P.; Bennett, J.W. (2004). Clustered pathway genes in aflatoxin biosynthesis. Appl. Environ. Microbiol., 70, 1253.

[39] Yabe, K., Chihaya, N.; Hatabayashi, H.; Kito, M.; Hoshino, S.; Zeng, H.; Cai, J.; Nakajima, H.(2012). Production of M−/GM-group aflatoxins catalyzed by the OrdA enzyme in aflatoxin biosynthesis. Fungal Genet. Biol., 49, 744–754.

[40] Bbosa, G.; Kitya, D.; Odda, J.; Ogwal-Okeng, J.(2013). Aflatoxins metabolism, effects on epigenetic mechanisms and their role in carcinogenesis. Health (N. Y.), 5, 14–34.

[41] Chemspider. Search and Share Chemistry. 2020. Available online: h ttp://www.chemspider.com (accessed on11 February 2020).

[42] Dorner, J. W., Cole, R. J. and Blankenship, P. D. (1992). Use of a biocompetitive agent to control preharvest aflatoxin in drought stressed peanuts. J Food Prot 55, 888–892.

[43] Eaton, D. L. and Gallagher, E. P. (1994). Mechanisms of aflatoxin carcinogenesis. Annu Rev. Pbarmacol Toxicol34, 135–1 72.

[44] CAST (1989). Council for Agricultural Science and Technology. Mycotoxins: Economic and Health Risks. Report 11 6.

[45] Pubchem. Explore Chemistry. 2020. Available online: https://pubchem. ncbi. nlm.nih.gov (accessed on 11 February 2020).

[46] Cotty, P. J., Bayman, P., Egel, D. S. and Elias, D. 5. (1994). Agricul ture, aflatoxins, and Aspergillus. In The Genus Aspergillus, pp. 1–27. Edited by K. A. Powell, A. Fenwick and J. F. Peberdy. New York: Plenum Press.

[47] Jelinek, C. F., Pohland, A. E. and Wood, G. E. (1989). Review of mycotoxin in food and feeds - an update. J Assoc of Anal Cbem 72,

[48] Pestka, J. 1. (1988). Enhanced surveillance of foodborne mycotoxins

by immunochemical assay. J Assoc Of Anal Chem 71,

[49] Pestka, J. J. (1986). Fungi and Mycotoxins in Meats. In Advances in Meat Research, vol. 11, pp. 277–309. Westport, CT: AVI Publishing.

[50] Bray, G. A. & Ryan, D. H. (1991). Mycotoxins, Cancer, and Health. Penington Center Nutrition Series, vol. I. Baton Rouge: Louisiana State University.

[51] Chu, F. S. (1991). Mycotoxins: food contamination, mechanism, carcinogenic potential, and preventative measures. Mutation Res.

[52] Dvorackova, 1. (1990). Aflatoxins and Human Health. Boca Raton, FL: CRC Press.

[53] Bennett, J. W. and Papa, K. E. (1988). The aflatoxigenic Aspergillus spp. Adv Plant Pathol. 6, 265–279.

[54] Bhatnagar, D., Ehrlich, K. C. & Cleveland, T. E. (1992). Oxidation-reduction reactions in biosynthesis of secondary metabolites. In Biosynthesis of Secondary Metabolites, chapter 10, pp. 255–286. Edited by Town: Publishers.

[55] Dutton, M. F. (1988). Enzymes and aflatoxin biosynthesis. Microbiol Rev. 52,274–295.

[56] Zaika, L. L. and Buchanan, R. L. (1987). Review of compounds affecting the biosynthesis of aflatoxins. J Food Prot 50, 691–708.

[57] Bhatnagar, D., Payne, G., Linz, 1. E. and Cleveland, T. E. (1995). Molecular Biology to Eliminate aflatoxins. INFORM.

[58] Park, D. L. and Liang, B. (1993). Perspectives on aflatoxin control for human food and animal feed. Trends Food Sci Technol4, 334–342.

[59] Park, D. L., Lee, L. S., Price, R. L. and Pohland, A. E. (1988). Review of the decontamination of aflatoxins by ammoniation: current status and regulation. J Assoc Of Anal Chem 71, 685–703.

[60] Ellis, W. O., Smith, 1. P. and Simpson, B. K. (1991). Aflatoxins in food; occurrence, biosynthesis, effects on organisms, detection, and methods for control. Crit Rev. Food Sci Nutr 30, 403–439.

[61] IARC (International Agency for Research on Cancer) (2012) Chemical agents and related occupations. In IARC Monographs on the Evaluation of Carcinogenic Risks to Humans; International Agency for Research on Cancer: Lyon (Fr), France,; Volume 100F, pp. 225–248.

[62] Bhatnagar, D., Cleveland, T. E. and Lillehoj, E. B. (1989). Enzymes in aflatoxin B1 biosynthesis: strategies for identifying pertinent genes. Mycopathologia 107, 75–83.

[63] Keller, N. P., Cleveland, T. E. and Bhatnagar, D. (1992b). A molecular approach towards understanding aflatoxin production. In Handbook.

[64] Linz, J. E. and Pestka, J. J. (1992). Mycotoxins: molecular mechanisms for control. In Aspergillus: Biology and Industrial Applications, pp. 217–231. Edited by J. Bennett and M. Klich. Stoneham, MA: Butterworth Publishing.

[65] Bennett, J. W. and Horowitz, P. C. (1979). Production of sclerotia by aflatoxigenic and nonaflatoxigenic strains of Aspergillus favus and A. parasiticus. Mycologia 71, 41 5–422.

[66] Skory, C. D., Chang, P.-K., Cary, J. and Linz, 1. E. (1992). Isolation and characterization of a gene from Aspergillus parasiticus associated with the conversion of versicolorin A to sterigmatocystin in aflatoxin

biosynthesis. Appl Environ Microbiol58, 3527–3537.

[67] Trail, F., Mahanti, N., Mehigh, R., Rarick, M., Liang, S.-H., Zhou, R. and Linz, 1. E. (1995). A physical and transcriptional map of the aflatoxin gene cluster and the functional disruption of a gene involved in the early part of the pathway. ApplEnviron Microbiol61, Albuquerque,New Mexico, August 1994.

[68] Price, R. L., J. H. Paulson, O. G. Lough, C. Gingg, and A. G. Kurtz. (1984). Aflatoxin Conversion by Dairy Cattle Consuming Naturally Contaminated Whole Cottonseed. Bulletin of the Department of Nutrition and Food Science, University of Arizona, Tucson. 16 pp.

[69] Stark, A. A., Y. Gal, and G. Shaulsky. (1990). Involvement of singlet oxygen in photoactivation of aflatoxins B1 and B2 to DNA-binding forms in vivo. Carcinogenesis 11:529–534.

[70] Ngindu, A., P. R. Kenya, D. M. Ocheng, T. N. Omonde, W. Ngare,D. Gatei, B. K. Johnson, J. A. Ngira, H. Nandwa, A. J. Jansen, J. N. Kaviti, and T. A. Siongok. (1982). Outbreak of acute hepatitis caused by aflatoxin poisoning in Kenya. Lancet 1:1346–1348.

[71] Hendrickse, R. G. (1985). The influence of aflatoxins on child health in the tropics with particular reference to kwashiorkor. Trans Royal Soc Trop Med Hyg 78:427–435.

[72] Nelson, D. B., R. Kimbrough, P. S. Landrigan, A. W. Hayes, G. C.Yang, and J. Benanides. (1980). Aflatoxin and Reye's syndrome: A case control study. Pediatrics 66:865–869.

[73] Yeh, G. S., M. C. Yu, C. C. Mo, S. Luo, M. J. Tong, and G. E. Hend-erson. (1989). Hepatitis B virus, aflatoxin, and hepatocellular carcinoma in southern Guangxi, China. Cancer Res 49:2506–2509.

[74] Scholl, P. and J. D. Groopman. (1995). Pp. 169–182. Epidemiology of Human Aflatoxin exposures and its Relationship to liver Cancer. In M. Eklund, J. L. Richard, and K. Mise (Eds.). Molecular Approaches to Food Safety: Issues Involving Toxic Microorganisms. Alaken, Inc., Fort Collins, Colorado.

[75] Busby, W. F. and G. N. Wogan. (1984). Aflatoxins. Pp. 945–1136. In C. E. Searle (Ed.). Chemical Carcinogens. American Chemical Society, Washington, D.C.

[76] Hoerr, F. J. and G. H. D'Andrea. (1983). Biological effects of aflatoxin in swine. Pp. 51–55. In U. L. Diener, R. L. Asquith, and J. W. Dickens (Eds.). Aflatoxin and Aspergillus flavus in Corn. Southern Cooperative Series Bulletin 279. Auburn University, Auburn, Alabama.

[77] Bodine, A. B., S. F. Fisher, and S. Gangjee. (1984). Effect of aflatoxin B1 and major metabolites on phytohemagglutinin-stimulated lymphoblastogenesis of bovine lymphocytes. J Dairy Sci 67:110–114.

[78] Cook, W. O., J. L. Richard, G. D. Osweiler, and D. W. Trampel. (1986). Clinical and pathologic changes in acute bovine aflatox-icosis: Rumen motility and tissue and fluid concentrations of aflatoxin B1 and M1. Am J Vet Res 47: 1817–1825.

[79] Veldman, A. J., A. C. Meijs, G. J. Borggreve, and J. J. Heeres-vander Tol. (1992). Carry-over of aflatoxins from cows' food to milk. Anim Prod 55:163–168.

[80] Osborne, D. J. and P. B. Hamilton. (1981). Decreased pancreatic digestive enzymes during aflatoxicosis. Poultry Sci 60:1818–1812.

[81] Hamilton, P. B. (1971). A natural and extremely severe occurrence of aflatoxicosis in laying hens. Poultry Sci 50:1880–1882.

[82] Huff, W. E., R. D. Wyatt, and P. B. Hamilton. (1975). Effects of dietary aflatoxin on certain egg yolk parameters. Poultry Sci 54:2014–2018.

[83] Miller, D. M., B. P. Stuart, W. A. Crowell, R. J. Cole, A. J. Goven, and J. Brown.(1978). Aflatoxicosis in swine: Its effect on immunity and relationship to salmonellosis. Am Assoc Vet Lab Diag 21:135–146.

[84] Pier, A. C., J. L. Richard, and J. R. Thurston. (1980b). Effects of aflatoxin on the mechanisms of immunity and native resistance. Pp. 301–309. In H.-J. Preusser (Ed.). Medical Mycology: Proceedings of the Mycological Symposia of the XII International Congress of Microbiology. Gustav Fischer Verlag, New York.

[85] Pier, A. C., M. E. McLaughlin, J. L. Richard, A. Baetz, and R. R.Dahlgren. (1985). In utero transfer of aflatoxin and selected ef Pestka, J. J. and G. S. Bondy. 1994a. Immunotoxic effects of mycotoxins. Pp. 339–358. In J. D. Miller and H. L. Trenholm (Eds.). Mycotoxins in Grain: Compounds Other than Aflatoxin. Eagan Press, St. Paul, Minnesota.

[86] Pestka, J. J. and G. S. Bondy. (1994a). Immunotoxic Effects of Mycotoxins. Pp. 339–358. In J. D. Miller and H. L. Trenholm (Eds.). Mycotoxins in Grain: Compounds Other than Aflatoxin. Eagan Press, St. Paul, Minnesota.

[87] Pestka, J. J. and G. S. Bondy. (1994b). Mycotoxin-induced Immune Modulation. Pp.163–182. In J. H. Dean, M. I. Luster, A. E. Munson, and I. Kimber (Eds.). Immunotoxicology and Immu-nopharmacology. Raven Press, New York.

[88] Ghosh, R. C., H. V. S. Chauhan, and G. J. Jha. (1991). Suppression of cell-mediated immunity by purified aflatoxin B1 in broiler chicks. Vet Immunol Immunopathol 28:165–172.

[89] Ghosh, R. C., H. V. S. Chauhan, and S. Roy. (1990). Immunosup-pression in broilers under experimental aflatoxicosis. Br Vet J 146:457–462.

[90] Kadian, S. K., D. R. Monga, and M. C. Goel. (1988). Effect of aflatoxin B1 on the delayed type hypersensitivity and phagocytic activity of reticuloendothelial system in chickens. Mycopathologia 104:33–36.

[91] Scott, T. R., S. M. Rowland, R. S. Rodgers, and A. B. Bodine. (1991). Genetic selection for aflatoxin B1 resistance influences chicken T-cell and thymocyte proliferation. Devel Comp Immunol 15:383–391.

[92] Raisuddin-Singh, K. P., S. I. A. Zaidi, A. K. Saxena, and P. K. Ray. (1990). Effects of aflatoxin on lymphoid cells of weanling rat. J Appl Toxicol 10: 245–250.

[93] Cusumano, V., G. B. Costa, and S. Seminara. (1990). Effect of aflatoxins on rat peritoneal macrophages. Appl Environ Microbiol 56:3482–3484.

[94] Neldon-Ortiz, D. L. and M. A. Qureshi. (1991). Direct and microsomal activated aflatoxin B1 exposure and its effects on turkey peritoneal macrophage functions in vitro. Toxicol Appl Pharmacol 109:432–442.

[95] Neldon-Ortiz, D. L. and M. A. Qureshi. (1992). The effects of direct and microsomal activated aflatoxin B1 on chicken peritoneal macrophages in vitro. Vet Immunol Immunopathol 31: 61–76.

[96] Singh, J., R. P. Tiwari, G. Singh, S. Singh, and D. V. Vadehra. (1987). Biochemical and immunological effects

of aflatoxin in rabbits. Toxicol Lett 35: 225–230.

[97] Thurston, J.R.,A.L.Baetz,N. R. Cheville, and J. L. Richard. (1980). Acute aflatoxicosis in guinea pigs: Sequential changes in serum proteins, complement, C4, and liver enzymes and histo-pathologic changes. Am J Vet Res 41:1272–1276.

[98] Pier, A. C. (1986). Immunomodulation in aflatoxicosis. Pp. 143–148. In J. L. Richard and J. L. Thurston (Eds.). Diagnosis of Mycotoxicoses. Martinus Nijhoff Publishers, Dordrecht, The Netherlands.

[99] Panangala, V. S., J. J. Giamgrone, U. L. Diener, N. D. Davis, F. J. Hoerr, *A. mitra*, R. D. Schultz, and G. R. Wilt. (1986). Effects of aflatoxin on the growth performance and immune responses of weanling swine. Am J Vet Res 47:2062–2067.

[100] Pier, A. C., E. L. Belden, J. A. Ellis, E. W. Nelson, and L. R. Maki. (1989). Effects of cyclopiazonic acid and aflatoxin singly and in combination on selected clinical, pathological and immunological responses of guinea pigs. Mycopathologia 105:135–142.

[101] Tung, H. T., W. E. Donaldson, and P. B. Hamilton. (1972). Altered lipid transport during aflatoxicosis. Toxicol Appl Pharmacol 22:97–104.

[102] Doerr, J. A., W. E. Huff, H. T. Tung, R. D. Wyatt, and P. B. Hamilton. (1974). A survey of T-2 toxin, ochratoxin, and aflatoxin for their effects on the coagulation of blood in young broiler chickens. Poultry Sci 53: 1728–1734.

[103] Wyatt, R. D., D. M. Briggs, and P. B. Hamilton. (1973). The effect of dietary aflatoxin on mature broiler breeder males. Poultry Sci 52:1119–1123.

[104] Lanza, G.M., K.W.Washburn, and R.D.Wyatt.(1980). Strain variation in hematological response of broilers to dietary aflatoxin. Poultry Sci 59:2686–2691.

[105] Dietert, R. R., S. E. Bloom, M. A. Qureshi, and U. C. Nanna. (1983). Hematological toxicology following embryonic exposure to aflatoxin B1. Proc Soc Exp Biol Med 173:481–485.

[106] Barnes, 5. E., Dola, T. P., Bennett, J. W. & Bhatnagar, D. (1994). Synthesis of sterigmatocystin on a chemically defined medium by species of Aspergillus and Chaetomium. Mycopathologia 125, 173–1 78.

[107] Townsend, C. A., McGuire, 5. M., Brobst, 5. W., Graybill, T. L., Pal,K. and Barry, C. E., 111. (1991). Examination of tetrahydro- and dihydrobisfuran formation in aflatoxin biosynthesis: from whole cells to purified enzymes. In Secondary-Metabofite Biognthesis and Metabolism, pp. 141–154. Edited by R. J. Petroski and S. P. McCormick. New York: Plenum Press.

[108] Yabe, K., Matsuyama, Y., Ando, Y., Nakajima, H. and Hamasaki, T. (1993). Stereochemistry during aflatoxin biosynthesis: conversion of norsolorinic acid to averufin. Appf Environ Microbiof 59,

[109] Bhatnagar, D., Ullah, A. H. J. andCleveland, T. E. (1988). Purification and characterization of a methyltransferase from Aspergillus parasiticus SRRC 163 involved in the aflatoxin biosynthetic pathway. Prep Biochem 18, 321–349.

[110] Keller, N. P., Dischinger, H. C., Jr., Bhatnagar, D., Cleveland, T. E. and Ullah, A. H. J. (1992c). Purification of a 40-kilodalton methyl- transferase active in the aflatoxin biosynthetic pathway. Appl Environ Microbiol59, 479484.

[111] Bhatnagar, D. and Cleveland, T. E. (1990). Purification and characterization of a reductase from

Aspergillus parasiticus SRRC 2043 involved in aflatoxin biosynthesis. FASEB J 4, 2727.

[112] Chuturgoon, A. A. and Dutton, M. F. (1991). The affinity purification and characterization of a dehydrogenase from Aspergillus parasiticus involved in aflatoxin B, biosynthesis. Prep Biochem 21, 125–140.

[113] Lin, B.-K. and Anderson, J. A. (1992). Purification and properties of versiconal cyclase from Aspergillus parasiticus. Arch Biocbem Biophys??????

[114] Matsushima, KA., Ando, Y., Hamasaki, T. and Yabe, K. (1994). Purification and characterization of two versiconal hemiacetal acetate reductases involved in aflatoxin biosynthesis. Appl Environ Microbiol 60, 2561–2567.

[115] Horng, J. S., Chang, P.-K., Pestka, J. J. and Linz, J. E. (1990). Development of a homologous transformation system for Aspergillus parasiticus with the gene encoding nitrate reductase. Mol and Gen Genet 224, 294–296.

[116] Skory, C. D., Horng, J. S., Pestka, 1. J. and Linz, J. E. (1990). A transformation system for Aspergillus parasiticus based on the homologous gene involved in pyrimidine biosynthesis (P_yrG).Appl Environ Microbiol56, 331 5–3320.

[117] Woloshuk, C., Seip, E., Payne, G. and Adkins, C. (1989). Gene transformation system for the aflatoxin-producing fungus Aspergillus flavus. Appl Environ Microbiof 55, 86–90.

[118] Chang, P.-K., Skory, C. D. and Linz, J. E. (1992). Cloning of a gene associated with aflatoxin B1 biosynthesis in Aspergillus parasiticus. Curr Genet 21, 231–233.

[119] Lee, L. S., Bennett, J. W., Goldblatt, L. A. and Lundin, R. E. (1970). Norsolorinic acid from a mutant strain of Aspergillus parasiticus. J A m Oil Cbem Soc 48, 93–94.

[120] Keller, N. P., Kantz, N. 1.81 Adams, T. H. (1994). Aspergillus nidulans verA is required for production of the mycotoxin sterigmatocystin. Appl Environ Microbiol 60, 1444–1450.

[121] Trail, F., Chang, P.-K., Cary, 1. and Linz, J. E. (1994). Structural and functional analysis of the nor- 1 gene involved in the biosynthesis of aflatoxins by Aspergillus parasiticus. Appl Environ Microbiof 60,

[122] Liang, S.-H. and Linz, J. E. (1994). Structural and functional characterization of the ver- 1 genes and proteins from Aspergillus parasiticus associated with the conversion of versicolorin A to sterigmatocystin in aflatoxin biosynthesis. Proceedings of Current Issnes in Food Safety. National Food Safety Toxicology Center, Michigan State University, October 1994.

[123] Zhou, R. and Linz, J. E. (1994). Expression of a norsolorinic acid reductase from Aspergilfus parasiticus in *Escherichia coli* strain DH5a and development of an enzyme activity assay. Proceedings of Current Issues in Food Safety. National Food Safety and Toxicology Center, Michigan State University, October 1994.

[124] Mahanti, N., Bhatnagar, D. and Linz, 1. E. (1994). Identification and disruption of a gene involved in the aflatoxin biosynthetic pathway of Aspergillus parasiticus. Proceedings of the American Plytopathology Society National Meeting, Albuquerque, New Mexico, August 1994.

[125] Kottig, H., Rottner, G., Beck, K., Schweizer, M. and Schweizer, E. (1991). The pentafunctional FASl genes of Saccbaromyces cerevisiae and Yarrowia lipohtica are co-linear and considerably

longer than previously estimated. Mol and Gen Genet 226, 310–314.

[126] Yu, J., Cary, J. W., Bhatnagar, D., Cleveland, T. E., Keller, N. P. and Chu, F. S. (1993). Cloning and characterization of a cDNA from Aspergillus parasiticus encoding an 0-methyltransferase involved in aflatoxin biosynthesis. Appl Environ Microbiof 59, 3564–3571.

[127] Feng, G. H., Chu, F. S. and Leonard, T. J. (1992). Molecular cloning of genes related to aflatoxin biosynthesis by differential screening. Appl Environ Microbiol58, 455–460.

[128] Luchese, R. H. and Harrigan, W. F. (1993). Biosynthesis of aflatoxin - the role of nutritional factors. J Appl Bacteriol74, 5–14.

[129] Buchanan, R. L., Jones, 5. B., Gerasimowicz, W. V., Zaika, L. L., Stahl, H. G. and Ocker, L. A. (1987). Regulation of aflatoxin biosynthesis: assessment of the role of cellular energy status as a regulator of the induction of aflatoxin production. Appl Environ Microbiol53, 1224–1231.

[130] Anderson, J. A. and Green, L. D. (1994). Timing of appearance of versiconal hemiacetal acetate esterase and versiconal cyclase activity in cultures of Aspergillus parasiticus. Mycopathologia 126, 169–1 72.

[131] Chuturgoon, A. A., Dutton, M. F. and Berry, R. K. (1990). The preparation of an enzyme associated with aflatoxin biosynthesis by affinity chromatography. Biochem Biopbys Res Commun 166, 38–42.

[132] Cleveland, T. E. and Bhatnagar, D. (1990). Evidence for de novo synthesis of an aflatoxin pathway methyltransferase near the cessation of active growth and the onset of aflatoxin biosynthesis in Aspergillus parasiticus mycelia. Can J Microbiol36, 1–5.

[133] Skory, C. D., Chang, P.-K. and Linz, 1. E. (1993). Regulated expression of the nor-1 and ver-1 genes associated with aflatoxin biosynthesis. Appl Environ Microbiol59, 1642–1 646.

[134] Payne, G. A., Nystrom, G. J., Bhatnagar, D., Cleveland, T. E. and Woloshuk, C. P. (1993). Cloning of the afl-2 gene involved in aflatoxin biosynthesis from Aspergillus flavus. Appl Environ Microbiol Penington Center Nutrition Series, vol. I. Baton Rouge: Louisiana State University.

[135] Woloshuk, C. P., Foutz, K. R., Brewer, 1. F., Bhatnagar, D., Cleveland, T. E. and Payne, G. A. (1994). Molecular characterization of ajR, a regulatory locus for aflatoxin biosynthesis. Appl Environ Microbiof 60, 2408–2414.

[136] Papa, K. E. (1984). Genetics of Aspergillus flavus: linkage of aflatoxin mutants. Can J Microbiol 30, 68–73.

[137] Bhatnagar, D., Yu, J., Chang, P.-K., Cleveland, T. E., Cary, 1. W., Linz, J. E. and Payne, G. A. (1994). Molecular regulation of aflatoxin biosynthesis: comparative mapping of aflatoxin pathway gene clusters in the aflatoxigenic fungi Aspergillus flavus and A. parasiticus. International Congress of Biochemistry and Mofecular Biology, New Delhi, India.

[138] Mayorga, M. E. & Timberlake, W. E. (1992). The developmentally regulated Aspergillus nidulans w A gene encodes a polypeptide homologous to polyketide and fatty acid synthases. Mol& Gen Genet, 235, 205–212.

[139] Hopwood, D. A. and Khosla, C. (1992). Genes for polyketide secondary metabolic pathways in microorganisms and plants. In SecondaT Metabolites: their Function and Evolution, Ciba Foundation Symposium vol. 171, pp. 88–112. Edited by D. J. Chadwick and.

[140] Martin, 1. F. and Liras, P. (1989). Organization and expression of genes

involved in the biosynthesis of antibiotics and other secondary metabolites. Annu Rev. Microbiol43, 173–206.

[141] Aharonowitz, Y. and Cohen, G. (1992). Penicillin and cephalosporin biosynthetic genes:structure, organization, regulation, and evolution. Annu Rev. Microbiol46, 461–495.

[142] Montenegro, E., Fierro, F., Fernandez, F. J., Gutierrez, 5. & Martin, J. F. (1992). Resolution of chromosomes I11 and VI by pulsed-field gel electrophoresis shows that the penicillin biosynthetic pathway genes pcbAB, pcbC, and penDE are clustered on chromosome VI (3.0 megabases). J Bacterioll74, 7063–7067.

[143] Hohn, T. M., McCormick, 5. P. and Desjardins, A. E. (1993). Evidence for a gene cluster involving trichothecene-pathway biosynthetic genes in *Fusarium sporotrichioides*. Curr Genet 24, 291–295.

[144] Kimura, N. and Tsuge, T. (1993). Gene cluster involved in melanin biosynthesis of the filamentous fungus *Alternaria alternata*. J Bacterioll75, 4427–4435.

[145] Cavalli, G. and Thoma, F. (1993). Chromatin transitions during activation and repression of galactose-regulated genes in yeast. EMBO J 12,4603–4613.

[146] Gross, D.S., Adams, C. C., Lee, S. and Stentz, B. (1993). A critical role for heat shock transcription factor in establishing a nucleosome free region over the TATA-initiation site of the yeast HSP82 heat shock gene. EMBO J 12, 3931–3945.

[147] Wolffe, A. P. (1994). Nucleosome positioning and modification: chromatin structures that potentiate transcription. Trends Biof Sci 19, 240–244.

[148] Keller, N.P., Cleveland, T.E. and Bhatnagar, D. (1992a). Variable electrophoretic karyo-types in Aspergillus flavus and Aspergillus parasiticus.Curr Genet 21, 371–375.

[149] Leaich, L. L. and Papa, K. E. (1974). Aflatoxins in mutants of Aspergillus flavus. Mycopatbol Mycol Appl52, 223–229.

[150] Woloshuk, C. P. and Yousibova, G. L. (1994). aj-1 in Aspergillus flavus effects the expression of aflatoxin genes. Proceedings of the American Plytopathology Society National Meeting, Albuquerque, New Mexico, August 1994.

[151] Trail, F., Wu, T.4. and Linz, J.E. (1994).Identification of regulatory elements in two genes involved in aflatoxin biosynthesis.Proceedings of the American Plytopa-thofogy Socieo National Meeting, Albuquerque,New Mexico, August 1994.

[152] Wu, T.4. and Linz, J. E. (1994). Transcriptional analysis of genes involved in aflatoxin production. Proceedings of Current Issues in Food Safety. National Food Safety Toxicology Center, Michigan State University, October 1994.

[153] Cotty, P. J. & Bhatnagar, D. (1994). Variability among toxigenic Aspergillusj favus strains in ability to prevent aflatoxin contamination and production of aflatoxin biosynthetic pathway enzymes. Appl Environ Microbiol60, 2248–2251.

[154] Rarick, M.,Thomas, R., Skory, C. D. and Linz, J. E. (1994). Identification and analysis of the aflatoxin biosynthetic genes nor-1 and ver- 1 in the commercial species Aspergillus sojae and A. otypae as well as toxigenic and nontoxigenic strains of A. flavus. Proceedings of Current Issues in Food Safety. National Food Safety and Toxicology Center, Michigan State University, October 1994.

[155] Brown, D. W., Hauser, F. M., Tommasi, R., Corlett, 5. and Salvo, J. J. (1993).Structural elucidation of a putative conidial pigment intermediate in Aspergillus parasiticus. Tetrahedron Lett 34, 41 9–422.

[156] Brown, D. W. and Salvo, J. J. (1994). Isolation and characterization of sexual spore pigments from. Aspergillus nidulans. Appl Environ Microbiol 60, 979–983.

[157] Vidal-Cros, A., Viviani, F., Labesse, G., Boccara, M. and Gaudry, M. (1994). Polyhydroxynapthalene reductase involved in melanin biosynthesis in Magnaporthe grisea. Eur J Biochem 219, 985–992.

Chapter 2

# Aflatoxins: Food Safety, Human Health Hazards and Their Prevention

*Enespa and Prem Chandra*


## Abstract

Aflatoxins (AFTs) are group of secondary metabolites produced by filamentous fungi such as *Aspergillus flavus, A. parasiticus, A. nomius*, and *Emericella nidulans*. AFTs contaminate foods, feeds, other raw ingredients used to produce them and that pose a significant threat to human health. These toxins designated as aflatoxin B1 (AFB1), aflatoxin B2 (AFB2), aflatoxin G1 (AFG1), and aflatoxin G2 (AFG2), aflatoxin M1 (AFM1) and aflatoxin M2 (AFM2) are hydroxylated metabolites form of AFB1 and AFB2 are known as difuranocoumarin compounds. Naturally, these AFs have carcinogenic, teratogenic and mutagenic effects and caused several metabolic disorders such as aflatoxicosis in domestic animals and humans worldwide. For the increasing in cancer incidences these risk factors are liable. AFB1 is 1000 times more potent hepatocarcinogen found in food then benzo (α) pyrene carcinogen. This chapter offers contamination sources, effects and their controlling approaches to confirm the food safety.


**Keywords:** Aflatoxin, health, risk assessment, aflatoxicosis, teratogen, carcinogen, mutation, hepatocellular carcinoma

## 1. Introduction

The fungi *Aspergillus flavus, Aspergillus parasiticus*, *Aspergillus nomius* and *Aspergillus tamari* produced aflatoxins are naturally secondary metabolites bisfuranocoumarin compounds [1, 2]. In agriculture *A. flavus* is a mutual contaminant and *A. pseudotamari A. bombycis*, *A. ochraceus*, and *A. nomius* are normally aflatoxin-producing species. *A. minisclerotigenes* and *A. arachidicola* are two another newly defined aflatoxigenic species [3]. Aflatoxins - B1, B2, G1 and G2 are four common contaminants of food products. Aflatoxins biosynthetically arise through polyhydroxy anthraquinone intermediates are acetate-derived decaketides. *A. flavus* and *A. parasiticus* species are found universally in the soil and air and grow at temperatures between 22 and 35°C [4, 5]. Aflatoxins classified as teratogenic, genotoxic, carcinogenic and invisible poisons by the World Health Organization (WHO). The multiple staple foods, cash crops such as maize, tree nuts, cassava, millet, peanuts, wheat and a range of spices contaminated by aflatoxins. In the milk, eggs, and meat from animals fed contaminated feed. Aflatoxins have been also detected in eggs, milk, and meet using contaminated feed [6, 7]. The drought and pests attacks endangered to stress factors of crops when preharvest occurrence of aflatoxin increases. With poor drying, storage and handling contamination spikes after post harvesting. Aflatoxins symbolize an excessive health and socio-economic issues for both industrialized and underdeveloped countries [8, 9]. At any stage of food production contamination can occur from pre-harvest to storage. It can be carcinogenic, hepatotoxic, teratogenic, and mutagenic at very small concentrations to human health by ingestion, inhaled, or absorbed through the skin [10, 11]. In several countries aflatoxins causes aflatoxicosis. In 1960, the aflatoxin causes Turkey X disease which is known as hepatic necrosis. High levels of aflatoxin and chronic hepatitis B virus (HBV) infection both exposed individually which increased liver cancer risk greatly in several parts of the world in Asia and sub-Saharan Africa [12, 13]. Aflatoxins and other toxins are analyzed in agricultural products by the Food and Agricultural Organization (FAO) and WHO. These toxins cannot be destroyed after contaminations of foods by the usual cooking processes. Furthermore, these toxins partially or completely eliminated from food using by physical, chemical and biological methods can be applied and assurance the food safety and health concerns of users [14, 15]. Hazard analysis of critical control points (HACCP) and good manufacturing practices are the recent advances have been developed keep final food products safe and healthy. An overview of aflatoxigenic fungi, their health hazards to humans and livestock, the biosynthesis of aflatoxins and their chemistry, along with their variety in existence are discussed in this chapter.

## 2. Source of aflatoxins

A number of airborne conidia and propagules that infect plants like cotton created by *A. flavus* [16]. During harvest in the agriculture form, in storage conditions, and during processing grains can be infected by *A. flavus*, *A. parasiticus* and are commonly isolated from corn, cottonseed, peanuts, and tree nuts (**Figure 1**).

*Aspergillus flavus* can grow at temperatures ranging between 12 and 48°C and consisted of mycelium, conidia, or sclerotia [17]. AFB1, AFB2 produces by *A. flavus* but AFG1, and AFG2, AFB1, and AFB2 are produces by *A. parasiticus* and *A. nomius* fungal isolates [18]. The hydroxylated metabolites which is known as AFM1 and AFM2 produced by AFB1 and AFB2 (**Figure 2**). AFB2 and AFG2 are manufactured

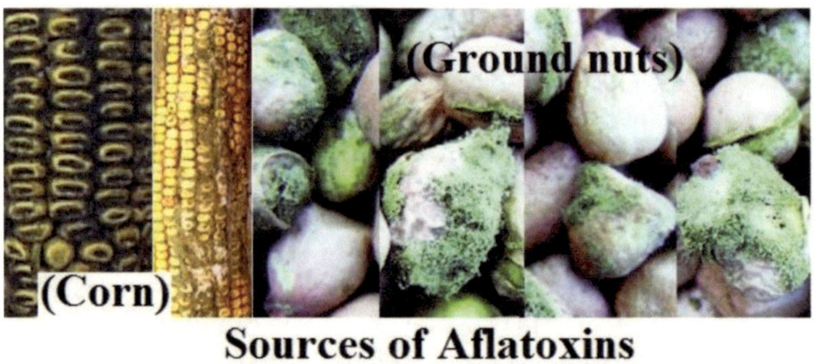


**Figure 1.**
*Source of aflatoxins in depicted in ground nuts and corn.*

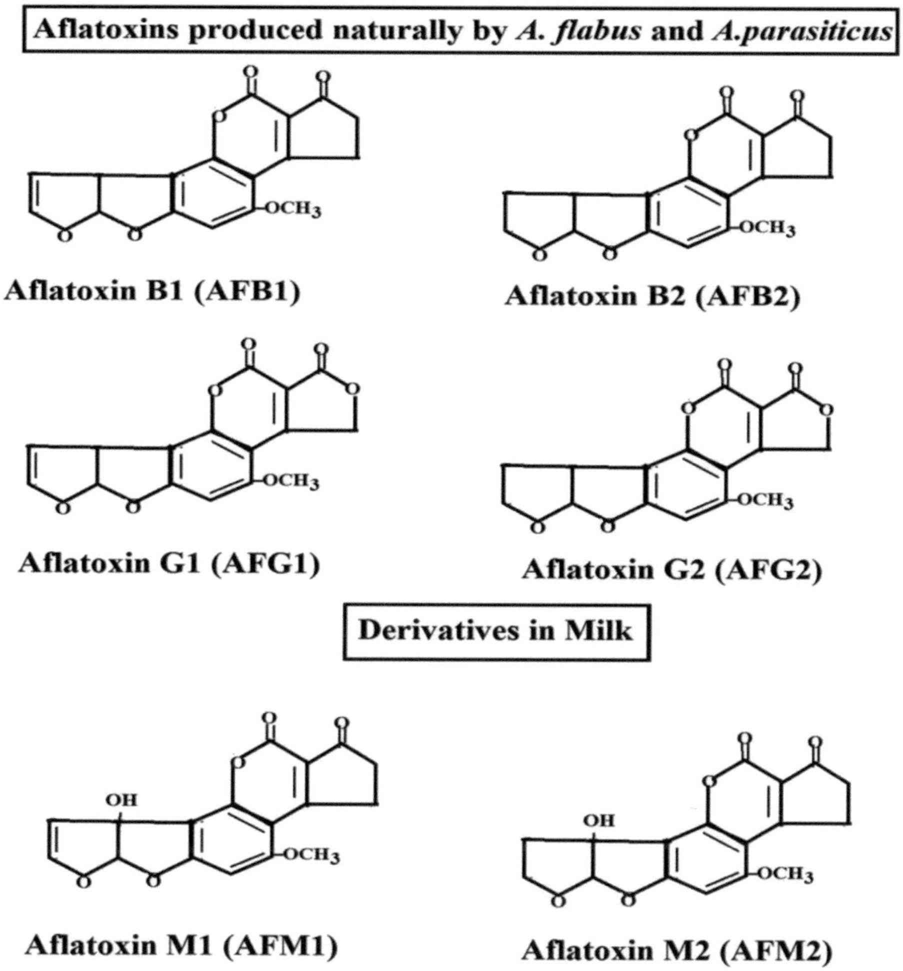


**Figure 2.**
*Aflatoxin produced by* A. flabus *and* A. parasiticus *showing chemical structure.*

at one-tenth to one-third of the amount of AFB1 and AFG1, correspondingly. And in largest quantities of AFB1 is produced in several strains [19, 20].

After classification by the International Agency for Research on Cancer (IARC) in 1987 (Category 1A) the aflatoxin B1 is as carcinogen, and AFM1 is a potentially carcinogenic substance with a toxicity range of AFB1 > AFG1 > AFB2 > AFG2 according to Category 2B. Aflatoxin detected in food in majority that ultimately harms to human and animal health among the mycotoxins affecting food and feed [21, 22]. Under the culture conditions most of the species produced major mycotoxin known as aflatoxin B1. AFB1 and AFB2 are named because of their strong blue fluorescence under UV light, whereas AFG1 and AFG2 fluoresces greenish yellow [23]. The B-toxins are categorized by the fusion of a cyclopentenone ring to the lactone ring of the coumarin structure, while G-toxins contained and additional fused lactone ring. In human other metabolites of AFB1 include Aflatoxin Q1 (AFQ1), aflatoxicol (AFL), AFM1, AFB2 and AFB1–2, 2-dihydrodiol. Both un-metabolized (B1, B2, G1, G2) as well as metabolized forms (aflatoxicol, M1 and M2) of aflatoxins get excreted in urine, stool and milk [24, 25].

## 3. Gene for aflatoxin production

Several genes and their enzymes are involved for the production of sterigmatocystin (ST) dihydrosterigmatocystin (DHST) (**Figure 3**) known as aflatoxins precursors [26, 27]. During the biosynthesis of aflatoxin gene nor-1 was first cloned in *A. parasiticus* named after the product formed by the gene. According to substrate product formed these genes entitled as Nor-1 (norsolorinic acid [NOR]), norA, norB, avnA (averanti [AVN]), avfA (averufin [AVF]), ver-1 (versicolorin A [VERA]), verA and verB while those based on enzyme functions fas-2 (FAS alpha subunit), fas-1 (FAS beta subunit), pksA (PKS), adhA (alcohol dehydrogenase), estA (esterase), vbs (VERB synthase), dmtA (mt-I; O-methyltransferase I), omtA (O-methyltransferase A), ordA (oxidoreductase A), cypA (cytochrome P450 monooxygenase), cypX (cytochrome P450 monooxygenase), and moxY (monooxygenase) [28, 29]. In *A. flavus* [30] primarily the aflatoxin regulatory gene was named afl-2 and in *A. parasiticus* named apa-2 [31]. But in *A. flavus, A. parasiticus*, and *A. nidulans* it is symbolized as aflR due to its part as a transcriptional activator. AflA (fas-2), aflB (fas-1), and aflC (pksA) accountable for conversion of acetate to NOR reported in earlier observations [32, 33]. Furthermore, in *A. parasiticus* for NOR biosynthesis as well as aflatoxin production the uvm8 gene was reported to be essential. From *Saccharomyces cerevisiae* the amino acid of sequence gene is related to the beta subunit of FASs (FAS1) [34]. During aflatoxin synthesis FAS forms the polyketide backbone and

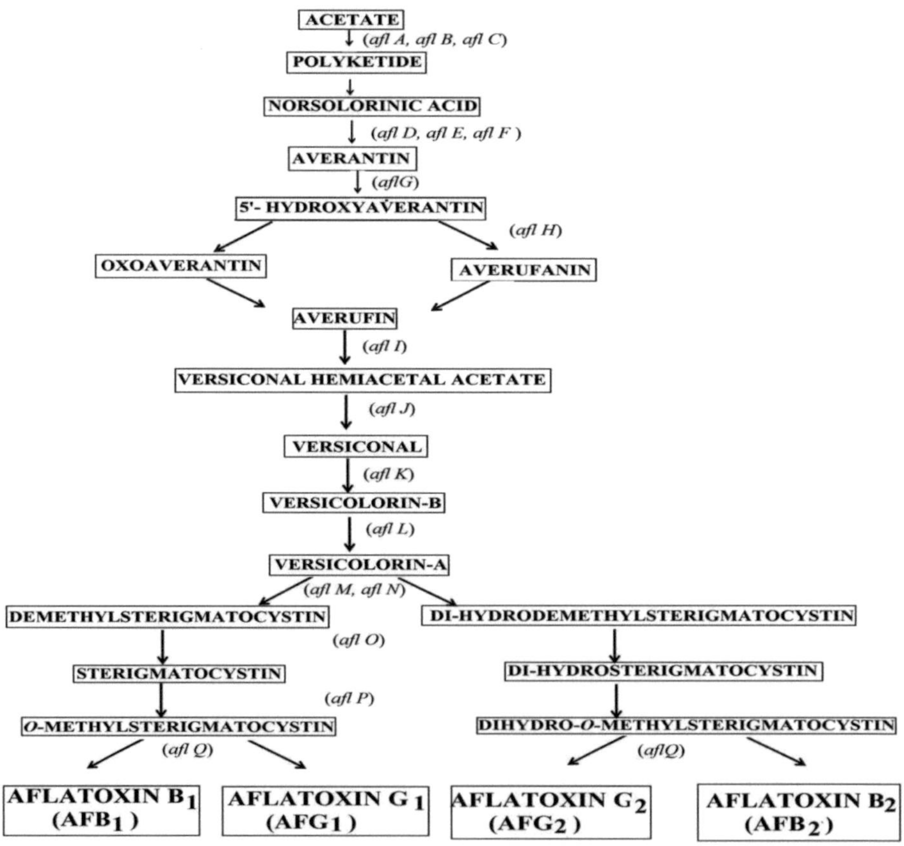


**Figure 3.**
*Pathway of AFB1, AFB2, AFG1, and AFG2 production.*

uvm8 gene known as fas-1 [35]. In *A. nidulans* the fatty acid syntheses (FASs) is responsible for sterigmatocystin (ST) biosynthesis and recognized as stcJ and stcK gene which encoded as FAS-2 and FAS-1 subunits [36].

## 4. Aflatoxin biosynthesis and regulation

The aflatoxin biosynthesis is very sophisticated [37], *A. flavus* and *A. parasiticus*, are extremely homologous and the genes of AF biosynthesis generally known as AF producers. The order of 25 genes within the aflatoxin gene clusters in two organisms has been displayed to be same [38]. Approximately 23 enzymatic reactions steps are involved in the AF biosynthetic pathway and recent investigations have revealed that about 30 clustered genes in AF biosynthesis mechanism. In *A. flavus* the pathway for AF biosynthesis are encoded by the 75 kb gene cluster for the gene encoding [39]. Within the gene cluster 29 AF biosynthetic genes have been identified [40] and exposed their functions. At least 21 enzymatic reactions consisted in the entire AF biosynthetic pathway. In the genome of *A. flavus* and *A. parasiticus* the AF pathway genes clustered in one locus expressed simultaneously [41]. The AF structural genes are the complex process in the expression and controlled by the acting regulatory genes are aflR located of the AF gene cluster in the middle. Adjacent to aflR gene aflS was found to be relating with aflR and sharing in the transcription regulation [42]. Another gene involved in regulation of the aflatoxin gene expression non-coded by the aflatoxin gene cluster. LaeA and VeA positively regulate aflatoxin production known as global regulators. In *A. flavus* and *A. parasiticus* strains deletion of VeA caused disruption in aflatoxin manufacturing [43, 44]. In *A. flavus* hundreds of genes are regulated by VeA such as secondary metabolite and developmental gene clusters also influenced by presence or absence of light [45, 46]. To form protein complex designated velvet, putative methyltransferase LaeA and the velvet protein VeA to interact with each other have been shown. For the synthesis of AF, cyclopiazonic acid and aflatrem require to regulate the expression of several crucial genes interacts with velvet domain containing proteins and global regulator VeA [47, 48]. In DNA methyltransferase the dmtA mutants deficient revealed diminished asexual reproduction and aflatoxin biosynthesis. The dmtA mutants scarce in DNA methyltransferase exhibited reduced asexual reproduction. In contrast with wild-type strain *A. flavus* and aflatoxin biosynthesis signifying the dmtA hit valuable in the aflatoxin cluster of transcriptional level of genes [49, 50]. Furthermore, in the seed infection dmtA deletion induced such changes, resulted more conidia formation in crop seeds comparison to wild type strain. By the transcription factor NsdC the asexual growth and AF manufacture were regulated. In *A. flavus*, transcription factor is a key controller in aflatoxin metabolism and conidia formation both, transcriptional regulator nsdC have elevated its role [51, 52].

## 5. Aflatoxins and their structural diversity

The polyketide pathway synthesized difuranocournarins/difurocoumarins and known as aflatoxins structurally and consist of a coumarin nucleus (**Figure 4A** and **B,** black in middle) to attached a difuran moiety in one side (**Figure 4A**, left in green) and a pentene ring (**Figure 4A**, in red on right side) or a hexane lactone ring in the other side (**Figure 4B**, red on the right side) [53]. They fall in to two main groups on this basis aflatoxins: (i) difurocoumarocyclopentenones contained usually aflatoxin B series and their byproducts (**Figure 4A**), and (ii) difurocoumarolactones with aflatoxin G series as the main agents, counting AFG1, AFG2, AFGM1, AFGM2, and AFG2a

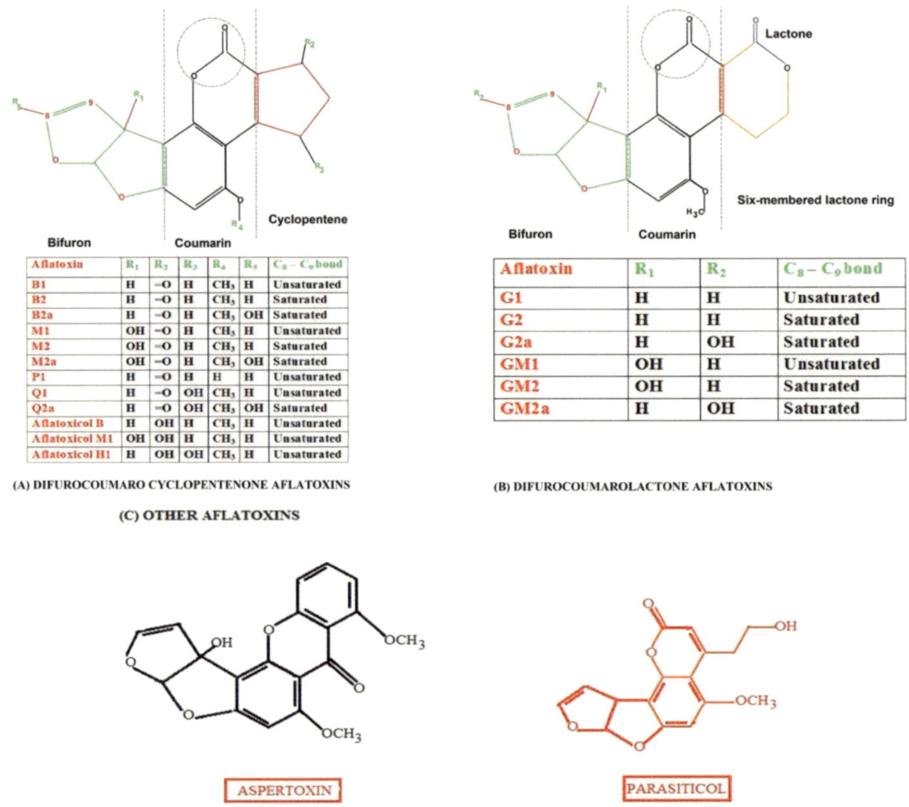


| Aflatoxin | $R_1$ | $R_2$ | $R_3$ | $R_4$ | $R_5$ | $C_8 - C_9$ bond |
|---|---|---|---|---|---|---|
| B1 | H | =O | H | $CH_3$ | H | Unsaturated |
| B2 | H | =O | H | $CH_3$ | H | Saturated |
| B2a | H | =O | H | $CH_3$ | OH | Saturated |
| M1 | OH | =O | H | $CH_3$ | H | Unsaturated |
| M2 | OH | =O | H | $CH_3$ | H | Saturated |
| M2a | OH | =O | H | $CH_3$ | OH | Saturated |
| P1 | H | =O | H | H | H | Unsaturated |
| Q1 | H | =O | OH | $CH_3$ | H | Unsaturated |
| Q2a | H | =O | OH | $CH_3$ | OH | Saturated |
| Aflatoxicol B | H | OH | H | $CH_3$ | H | Unsaturated |
| Aflatoxicol M1 | OH | OH | H | $CH_3$ | H | Unsaturated |
| Aflatoxicol H1 | H | OH | OH | $CH_3$ | H | Unsaturated |

| Aflatoxin | $R_1$ | $R_2$ | $C_8 - C_9$ bond |
|---|---|---|---|
| G1 | H | H | Unsaturated |
| G2 | H | H | Saturated |
| G2a | H | OH | Saturated |
| GM1 | OH | H | Unsaturated |
| GM2 | OH | H | Saturated |
| GM2a | H | OH | Saturated |

**Figure 4.**
*Aflatoxins chemical structures (A) Difurocoumarocyclopentenone (B) Difurocoumarolactone (C) Aspertoxin, a difuranoxanthane, and parasiticol, lacking the lactone ring of its parent aflatoxin G1, are occasionally considered as standalone mycotoxins.*

(**Figure 4B**). Parasiticol usually known as aflatoxin $B_3$ considered as a member of the latter group despite the lack of the characteristic six-membered lactone ring (**Figure 4C**, right).

## 6. Conditions for manufacturing of aflatoxin B1

Aflatoxins are usually associated with drought stress often occurs in various crop in the agriculture field before harvest. During the rainy seasons the poor storage conditions can increase the aflatoxins concentration. And these conditions developed chiefly in humid and hot regions where humidity and high temperature are optimal for growth of molds and for production toxin [54]. Several factors provide an ideal environment which promotes the growth of fungi. The principal climatic circumstances such as erratic rainfall, drought, more temperature between 20 and 35°C and more humidity (40–89%), provides a suitable environment for the molds growth and aflatoxins production. In proper dried and stored foods the molds cannot grow properly [55].

## 7. Permitted levels of aflatoxin

Food and Drug Administration (FDA) permitted an entire quantity of 0.5 g/kg or 50 ng/l in milk and 20 ng/g in livestock feed in US. The permitted levels of aflatoxin M1 in milk, milk products and baby food are 0.005 mg/kg in European countries. Various regulations for permitted levels of aflatoxin in livestock feed sets by other countries [56, 57]. For example the permitted levels of aflatoxin from 0.05 to 0.5 μg/kg setup by European Union (EU). The environmental factors like weather conditions are effective the determining acceptable levels of aflatoxin. In tropical countries the permitted levels of this toxin are more compared to cold countries [58, 59].

## 8. Biochemical mechanisms of aflatoxin carcinogenesis

### 8.1 Biotransformation of aflatoxins

Aflatoxins biotransformation is interconnected closely with their toxic and carcinogenic effects. Therefore, in species sensitivities to aflatoxin B1 (AFB1) - induced carcinogenesis the biotransformation pathways of aflatoxin are hazardous [60]. To the reactive AFB1–8, 9-epoxide requires microsomal oxidation of AFB1 to utilize its hepatocarcinogenic effects. AFBO serves as a critical pathway for AFB1 detoxification may be conjugated enzymatically with GSH (**Figure 5**). To form the primary AFB1-DNA adduct, 8, 9-dihydro-8- (N7-guanyl)-9-hydroxyaflatoxin B1 (AFB1-N7-Gua) when the epoxide reacts with DNA. And it can break down into the apurinic (AP) site or the AFB1-formamidopyrimidine (FAPY) adduct are the two secondary lesions. AFB1-N7-Gua adducts causes G to T mutations has been observed in *Escherichia coli* [61]. In blocked replication AFB1-FABY also resulted. In single-stranded DNA blocks replication the dominant species whereas the AFB1-FABY form present normally in double-stranded DNA is mutagenic [62].

### 8.2 Aflatoxins and their health consequences

The aflatoxin is an international food safety concern documented by WHO. Being the population with rural survival in developing countries aflatoxin exposure caused natural and environmental hazards and is most at risk and due to global food safety concern. The liver organ targeted specifically using aflatoxin [63]. Aflatoxins comprise fever, malaise, abdominal pain; vomiting, hepatitis and anorexia are early symptoms of hepatotoxicity of liver. Acute poisoning is rare and exceptional but the immunosuppressive and carcinogenic effects caused due to chronic toxicity by aflatoxins [64].

### 8.3 Aflatoxins related diseases

After consumption of mold damaged corn exposed to 2–6 mg of aflatoxin daily for approximately one month and caused aflatoxicosis characterized portal hypertension, jaundice, ascites and other signs of hepatic failure has been determined in humans. Liver cancer, kwashiorkor, Reye's syndrome including hepatotoxicity has been connected with nutritional contamination with aflatoxins caused adverse human health effects [65, 66].

### 8.4 Aflatoxicosis

Aflatoxins caused human intoxication via contact, ingestion and inhalation which affects the internal organs of the body such as salivary glands, colon, liver, kidney, stomach and lungs and skin. The gastrointestinal tract rapidly absorbs aflatoxin B1 after ingestion and metabolized in the liver [67]. Aflatoxins irreversibly

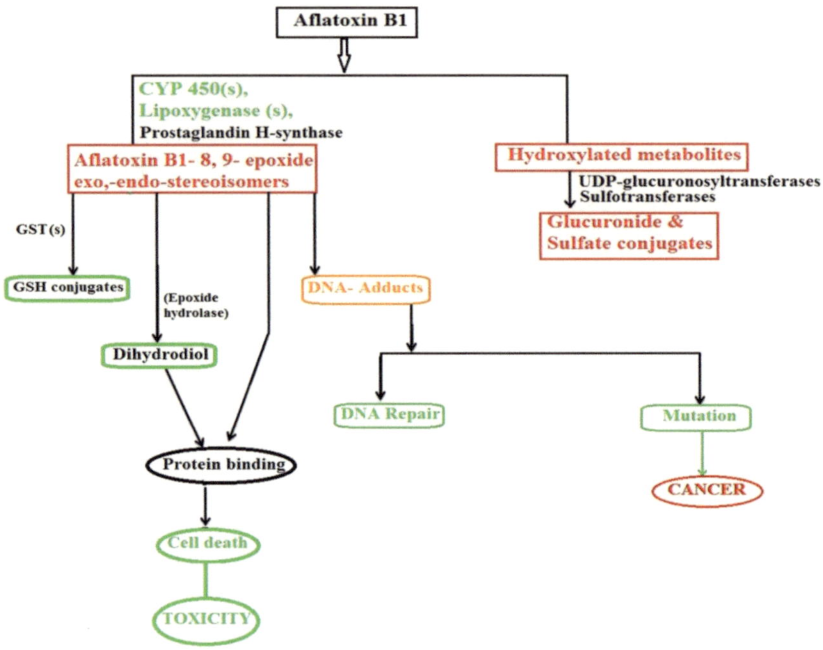


**Figure 5.**
*Overview of bio-transformational pathways for aflatoxin B1.*

bind to proteins and DNA bases after ingestion 1–3% and form aflatoxin B1-lysine in albumin. Protein and DNA bases disruption in hepatocytes causes liver toxicity. In a long period of time very small doses of aflatoxins ingestion caused chronic exposure. And acute aflatoxicosis determined after higher doses of aflatoxins. B1 > G1 > B2 > G2 is the order of potency for acute and chronic toxicity. AFB1 is not toxic itself, but it produces metabolites are more toxic, and its successive metabolism governs acute and chronic both toxicity [68, 69].

## 9. Gastrointestinal cancer and other cancers

In association with other mycotoxins AFB1 effects on Caco-2 cells were evaluated alone. Owing a cytotoxic effect at the concentration of 19.28 M, AFB1 resulted the third more cytotoxic among tested mycotoxin. To verify its effect on genotoxicity and DNA damage HCT116 colorectal cancer cells were treated with AFB1 (3–5 M) in another study [70].

### 9.1 Liver cancer

The improved risk of liver cancer is interrelated to AFB1 exposure revealed in earlier report. AFB1 is resulted to be an important hepatocarcinogenic. AFB1 induces the formation of DNA adducts that contribute to liver cancer formation indicated in 2002 to belong to Group 1 of the carcinogens [21]. With 4.6–28.2% of hepatocellular carcinoma (HCC) cases globally attributed to AFB1 exposure, Likewise, in AFB1-exposed people Hepatitis B virus (HBV) can increase the risk of HCC by 30-fold. Acute hepatitis caused by high exposure concentrations and as a result the chronic exposure causes the increase of liver cancer [71].

## 10. Possible mechanisms for the interaction between aflatoxin B1 and hepatitis B virus

To the carcinogenic effects of AFB1 the Hepatitis B virus infection may directly or indirectly sensitize hepatocytes. To bind to DNA causing changes AFB1–8, 9- epoxide has been displayed that increase the threat of assimilation of viral DNA and hence malignant transformation [72]. With heavy exposure to AFB1 the 249ser mutation is made-up to be a primary and early genetic event in hepatocarcinogenesis this mutation is present in 36.3 to 66% of patients. In sequences of the virus the HBV x gene is frequently included that are incorporated into the cellular DNA [73]. For removing AFB1-DNA adducts nuclear excision repair is accountable normally and is introverted by HBV x protein, approving the determination of present mutations or impaired DNA. To uncontrolled cell proliferation it may also contribute [74].

The p21waf1/cip1 transcription is initiated by HBVx protein in a dose-dependent method in the presence of functional p53 which induces cell cycle arrest, though the transcription is inhibited by HBV x protein when p53 is absent or present at a low level [75]. In transgenic mice in the total frequency of DNA mutations in transgenic mice the expression of HBVx protein also correlates and a 2-fold growth in the incidence of the 249 ser mutation exposed to AFB1. For an interaction between AFB1 and HBV another possible mechanism is that improved hepatocyte necrosis and propagation resultant from HBV infection increase the possibility of AFB1 mutations, comprising 249ser, and the successive clonal development of cells covers these mutations [76]. Generation of oxygen and nitrogen reactive species is the results of chronic inflammatory hepatic disease from HBV infection. Latter both are mutagenic, increased oxidative stress shown to induce 249ser mutations. In hepatocarcinogenesis altered methylation of genes may play an important role. Between ras association domain gene 1A (RASSF1A) methylation status and the level of AFB1-DNA adducts in HCC tissues a statistically significant association exists [62].

### 10.1 Potential mechanisms

Through liver toxicity the aflatoxin exposure may interrupt the pathway of insulin-like growth factors (IGF). Lower IGF1 levels described about 16% effect of aflatoxin on child height displayed in a path analysis. In another prospective device include the immunosuppressive effect of aflatoxin exposure for the aflatoxin child growth weakening that may upturn the susceptibility of infection, subsequently ruining the nutrition grade through appetite reduction and decrease the nutrient absorption [77]. Moreover, it is proposed that exposure to aflatoxin may stimulate the intestinal damage due to inhibition of protein synthesis. Consequently, the absorption of essential nutrients reduced and later impaired the growth. If the affiliation among impaired child growth and aflatoxin exposure is in fact causal it is challenging to establish on bases of above given evidence [78, 79].

### 10.2 Impaired child growth

During pregnancy dietary intake plays a necessary role in the child's future health status. Malnutrition and child growth impairment are major public health burdens in sub-Saharan Africa. At different time points the impact of aflatoxin on growth impairment has been investigated [80].

### 10.3 In utero exposure

Aflatoxin exposure can occur in utero through a trans-placental pathway have demonstrated in several observations. Lower birth weights and stunted child growth have been associated with higher exposure levels of aflatoxins in utero. The consequences of in utero exposure to aflatoxin analyzed on the white blood cell DNA global methylation level in children aged 2–8 months [81].

### 10.4 Exposure via breast milk

Breast milk is the potential source of aflatoxin exposure for very young infants. The hydroxylated metabolite AFM1 is analyzed in breast milk following ingestion of foods contaminated with AFB1 after 12 to 24 hours. In the breast milk samples of lactating Iranian women the AFM1 concentrations analyzed were negatively associated with their infants' HAZ scores (correlation coefficient $\beta = -0.31$, $P = 0.01$) during the breast feeding their children exclusively [82, 83]. Along with anthropometric data the breast milk samples were collected at the first, third and fifth month following birth. And the AFM1 was analyzed in breast milk samples of 143 lactating mothers, and growth impairment in their infants fewer than 6 months of age in Northern Tanzania. AFM1 concentrations ranging from 0.01 to 0.55 ng/mL detected in all the collected samples. The potential for exposure of AFM1 from breast milk contributing to child growth impairment observed in this analysis [9, 84].

### 10.5 Immune suppression

In several animal species it is investigated that the immunosuppressive effects of aflatoxin reduced antibody production and cell-mediated immunity and increased the susceptibility to contagious diseases. The sIgA protects against infectious diseases and uptake of harmful micro-organisms is an important component of the mucosal barrier [85, 86]. The IgA (sIgA) antibody reduced in children with detectable AF-alb concentrations in their blood ($n = 432$) associated to those with non-detectable levels ($n = 32$) accompanied in a study in Gambia. Aflatoxin exposure reduced level of sIgA and could be a prospective mechanism for the impaired child growth that was also detected in this cohort [87, 88]. The AF-alb adduct biomarker measured high levels of aflatoxin exposure in a study of Ghanaian adults associated to those exposed to low levels of aflatoxin, had expressively lower percentages of CD3 + CD69 and CD19 + CD69 cells, and lesser percentages of CD8+ type T lymph cells that restricted perforin or both perforin and granzyme A [89]. Moreover, after modification for age and other immune parameters the negative relations were detected between CD3 + CD69 and CD19 + CD69 cells and AF-alb concentrations. Reductions in these immunological parameters could consequently lead to impaired cell-mediated immunity increasing susceptibility to infectious diseases [90–92].

## 11. Prevention and monitoring of aflatoxins in the food supply

During the harvest, production, storage, transport, and processing, make it problematic to eliminate prospective contamination sources of aflatoxin producing fungi in food crops. In the food supply chain the prevention of aflatoxin production is very challenging [93, 94]. Several techniques can be used to decrease risk contamination during agricultural farming and storing. For toxin-constructing molds on seeds or in storage bowls, expending genetically resistant varieties of harvests, good practices for agronomic developments such as suitable time of irrigation and harvest, bio controls, and chemical controls [95]. For toxin-producing molds on seeds or in storing containers, using hereditarily resistant selections of crops, good agronomic performs such as suitable scheduling of irrigation and harvest, biological controls (atoxigenic strains of *A. flavus* uses), and chemical controls (fungicides application) common preharvest approaches holds analysis [96, 97]. To mold spores can reduce the risk, controlling moisture content and minimizing exposure during harvest. During storage to regulate moisture content and temperature industrial farming operations often use sophisticated equipment to mechanically dry crops [98]. For preventing aflatoxin formation farmers must consider alterations in climate, weather, crop varieties and types, and postharvest arrangement in adapting plans. Most industrialized countries to limit human exposure consistently screened for the level of aflatoxins in cultivated crops and food products [13]. The Food and Drug Administration and the U.S. Department of Agriculture monitor food provisions to assurance compliance with stringent directing restrictions first put into place in 1971, in the United States. Under tough procedures before being acceptable into food supply foods adulterated with aflatoxins above the allowable parameters must be renovated [99, 100]. Consequently, In the United States, no epidemics of acute aflatoxicosis have been documented.

## 12. Promising technologies for aflatoxin control

In crop production good management practices, handling, drying and storage is necessary but not sufficient for control. Because molds growth affected by several environmental factors that yields aflatoxins control is thus complex [13, 101]. For diverse production environments for integrating resistance along with required agronomic features. Both host resistance and enhanced management will require long-term efforts in research and extension for some progress is being made. To reduce the levels of aflatoxins rising during the harvesting and storage biocontrol offers a preventative measure [102, 103]. This expertise is used in United States commonly and also adopted for tropical maize and groundnuts. This newest skill technique has potential to reduce aflatoxins extensively at their initial source: in farmers' fields indicates by the field trials. Such apparatuses would expedite both public observing for aflatoxins as well as the improvement of marketable for amended-excellence grain. These new determination and diagnostic tools development are inexpensive, more dependable, and easily used in agriculture [104, 105].

## 13. Economic impact of aflatoxins

Aflatoxins producing fungal species such as *Aspergillus* sp. that grows and produces aflatoxins as byproducts in universal climates but commonly grown in humid and warm climatic conditions [106]. But most foodstuffs especially peanut and maize harvested in tropical countries are contaminated easily with aflatoxins. Human and animal feeds pose serious health and economic risks globally due to aflatoxin contamination. The economic impact is difficult to measure of aflatoxin contamination [107]. Developing countries of tropical and sub-tropical regions negative impact on health, economy, and social life are greater. The countries such as Gambia, Uganda, Kenya, and Tanzania, China, Thailand, Vietnam, India and

Indonesia have been classically connected with more occurrences of aflatoxins in agricultural products and foodstuffs. In U.S. $225 million/yr. impact have been estimated in maize due to aflatoxins, and in peanuts $25.8 million losses were assessed during 1993 to 1996 per year [78, 108].

## 14. Conclusions

In both humans and animals chronic consumption of aflatoxin-contaminated foods is a common problem. Aflatoxin exposure is the result of staple cereal crops contamination and is an important food safety issue in various countries. Acute toxicity can be lethal due to very high exposure. At any stage such as in utero, and increases during weaning naturally the chronic exposure can occur. HBV infection co-exists aflatoxin is an established risk factor, which causes the health impacts like child growth impairment and immune suppression and liver cancer. Due to aflatoxin exposure the immunosuppressive effects could increase susceptibility to contagious diseases, like diarrhea, and leading to impaired child growth due to reducing nutrient absorption. In China, Liver cancer risk has been reduced suggestively over current periods as a result of HBV vaccination and nutritional changes that reduced aflatoxin exposure. In under developing countries of south East Asia and sub-Saharan Africa where there is poor food harvesting, processing and storing thus permitting the growth of mold on them several body organs can affect due to aflatoxins.


## Author details

Enespa[1] and Prem Chandra[2*]

1 Department Plant Pathology, School of Agriculture, Sri Mahesh Prasad Degree College, University of Lucknow, Lucknow, UP, India

2 Food Microbiology and Toxicology Laboratory, Department of Environmental Microbiology, School for Earth and Environmental Sciences, B. B. Ambedkar (A Central) University, Lucknow, UP, India

*Address all correspondence to: p.chandrabbau@gmail.com

## References

[1] Uka, V., Cary, J. W., Lebar, M. D., Puel, O., De Saeger, S. & Diana Di Mavungu, J. (2020). Chemical repertoire and biosynthetic machinery of the *Aspergillus flavus* secondary metabolome: A review. *Comprehensive Reviews in Food Science and Food Safety*, 19(6), 2797-2842.

[2] Thanaboripat, D. (2002). Importance of aflatoxins. *CURRENT APPLIED SCIENCE AND TECHNOLOGY*, *2*(1), 38-45.

[3] Varga, J., Frisvad, J. C. & Samson, R. A. (2011). Two new aflatoxin producing species and an overview of *Aspergillus* section Flavi. *Studies in Mycology*, 69, 57-80.

[4] Abbas, H. K., Wilkinson, J. R., Zablotowicz, R. M., Accinelli, C., Abel, C. A., Bruns, H. A. & Weaver, M. A. (2009). Ecology of *Aspergillus flavus*, regulation of aflatoxin production, and management strategies to reduce aflatoxin contamination of corn. *Toxin reviews*, *28*(2-3), 142-153.

[5] Reiter, E., Zentek, J. & Razzazi, E. (2009). Review on sample preparation strategies and methods used for the analysis of aflatoxins in food and feed. *Molecular nutrition & food research*, *53*(4), 508-524.

[6] Kumar, P., Mahato, D. K., Kamle, M., Mohanta, T. K. & Kang, S. G. (2017). Aflatoxins: a global concern for food safety, human health and their management. *Frontiers in microbiology*, *7*, 2170.

[7] Granados-Chinchilla, F., Redondo-Solano, M. & Jaikel-Víquez, D. (2018). Mycotoxin contamination of beverages obtained from tropical crops. *Beverages*, 4(4), 83.

[8] Wild, C. P. (2007). Aflatoxin exposure in developing countries: the critical interface of agriculture and health. *Food and Nutrition Bulletin*, *28*, S372-S380.

[9] Williams, J. H., Phillips, T. D., Jolly, P. E., Stiles, J. K., Jolly, C. M. & Aggarwal, D. (2004). Human aflatoxicosis in developing countries: a review of toxicology, exposure, potential health consequences, and interventions. *The American journal of clinical nutrition*, *80*(5), 1106-1122.

[10] Omotayo, O. P., Omotayo, A. O., Mwanza, M. & Babalola, O. O. (2019). Prevalence of mycotoxins and their consequences on human health. *Toxicological research*, 35(1), 1-7.

[11] Peles, F., Sipos, P., Győri, Z., Pfliegler, W. P., Giacometti, F., Serraino, A. & Pócsi, I. (2019). Adverse effects, transformation and channeling of aflatoxins into food raw materials in livestock. *Frontiers in microbiology*, *10*, 2861.

[12] Kensler, T. W., Roebuck, B. D., Wogan, G. N. & Groopman, J. D. (2011). Aflatoxin: a 50-year odyssey of mechanistic and translational toxicology. *Toxicological sciences*, 120, S28-S48.

[13] Benkerroum, N. (2020a). Aflatoxins: Producing-molds, structure, health issues and incidence in Southeast Asian and Sub-Saharan African countries. *International journal of environmental research and public health*, *17*(4), 1215.

[14] Cinar, A. & Onbaşı, E. (2019). Mycotoxins: The hidden danger in foods. In Mycotoxins and food safety. *Intech Open*. (pp. 114). DOI: http://dx.doi.org/10.5772/intechopen.89001

[15] Surai, P., Mezes, M., Fotina, T. I. & Denev, S. D. (2010). Mycotoxins in human diet: a hidden danger. In *Modern*

*Dietary Fat Intakes in Disease Promotion* (pp. 275-303). Humana Press, Totowa, NJ.

[16] Horn, B. W. (2003). Ecology and population biology of aflatoxigenic fungi in soil. *Journal of Toxicology: Toxin Reviews*, *22*(2-3), 351-379.

[17] Frawley, D., Greco, C., Oakley, B., Alhussain, M. M., Fleming, A. B., Keller, N. P. & Bayram, Ö. (2020). The tetrameric pheromone module SteC-MkkB-MpkB-SteD regulates asexual sporulation, sclerotia formation and aflatoxin production in Aspergillus flavus. *Cellular microbiology*, *22*(6), e13192.

[18] Matumba, L., Sulyok, M., Njoroge, S. M., Ediage, E. N., Van Poucke, C., De Saeger, S. & Krska, R. (2015). Uncommon occurrence ratios of aflatoxin B 1, B 2, G 1, and G 2 in maize and groundnuts from Malawi. *Mycotoxin research*, *31*(1), 57-62.

[19] Santacroce, M. P., Conversano, M. C., Casalino, E., Lai, O., Zizzadoro, C., Centoducati, G. & Crescenzo, G. (2008). Aflatoxins in aquatic species: metabolism, toxicity and perspectives. *Reviews in Fish Biology and Fisheries*, 18(1), 99-130.

[20] Bedoya-Serna, C. M., Michelin, E. C., Massocco, M. M., Carrion, L. C., Godoy, S. H., Lima, C. G. & Fernandes, A. M. (2018). Effects of dietary aflatoxin B1 on accumulation and performance in matrinxã fish (*Brycon cephalus*). *PloS one*, *13*(8), e0201812.

[21] Marchese, S., Polo, A., Ariano, A., Velotto, S., Costantini, S. & Severino, L. (2018). Aflatoxin B1 and M1: Biological properties and their involvement in cancer development. *Toxins*, 10(6), 214.

[22] Bbosa, G. S., Kitya, D., Lubega, A., Ogwal-Okeng, J., Anokbonggo, W. W. & Kyegombe, D. B. (2013). Review of the biological and health effects of aflatoxins on body organs and body systems. *Aflatoxins-recent advances and future prospects*, *12*, 239-265.

[23] Nazhand, A., Durazzo, A., Lucarini, M., Souto, E. B. & Santini, A. (2020). Characteristics, occurrence, detection and detoxification of aflatoxins in foods and feeds. *Foods*, *9*(5), 644.

[24] Goeger, D. E., Anderson, K. E. & Hsie, A. W. (1998). Coumarin chemo protection against aflatoxin B1-induced gene mutation in a mammalian cell system: A species difference in mutagen activation and protection with chick embryo and rat liver S9. *Environmental and molecular mutagenesis*, 32(1), 64-74.

[25] Guan, S., Ji, C., Zhou, T., Li, J., Ma, Q. & Niu, T. (2008). Aflatoxin B1 degradation by Stenotrophomonas maltophilia and other microbes selected using coumarin medium. *International journal of molecular sciences*, *9*(8), 1489-1503.

[26] Yu, J., Chang, P. K., Ehrlich, K. C., Cary, J. W., Bhatnagar, D., Cleveland, T. E. & Bennett, J. W. (2004). Clustered pathway genes in aflatoxin biosynthesis. *Applied and environmental microbiology*, *70*(3), 1253-1262.

[27] Yu, J. (2012). Current understanding on aflatoxin biosynthesis and future perspective in reducing aflatoxin contamination. *Toxins*, *4*(11), 1024-1057.

[28] Abdel-Hadi, A., Carter, D. & Magan, N. (2010). Temporal monitoring of the nor-1 (aflD) gene of *Aspergillus flavus* in relation to aflatoxin B1 production during storage of peanuts under different water activity levels. *Journal of Applied Microbiology*, 109(6), 1914-1922.

[29] Do, J. H. & Choi, D. K. (2007). Aflatoxins: detection, toxicity, and biosynthesis. *Biotechnology and Bioprocess Engineering*, *12*(6), 585-593.

[30] Payne G. A., Nystrom G. J., Bhatnagar D., Cleveland T. E., Woloshuk C. P. (1993). Cloning of the afl-2 gene involved in aflatoxin biosynthesis from *Aspergillus flavus*. *Appl. Environ. Microbiol*. 59 156-162.

[31] Yu, J., Whitelaw, C. A., Nierman, W. C., Bhatnagar, D. & Cleveland, T. E. (2004). *Aspergillus flavus* expressed sequence tags for identification of genes with putative roles in aflatoxin contamination of crops. *FEMS Microbiology Letters*, 237(2), 333-340.

[32] Hoffmeister, D. & Keller, N. P. (2007). Natural products of filamentous fungi: enzymes, genes, and their regulation. *Natural product reports*, *24*(2), 393-416.

[33] Yu, J. & Ehrlich, K. C. (2011). Aflatoxin biosynthetic pathway and pathway genes (pp. 41-66). *INTECH* Open Access Publisher.

[34] Minto, R. E. & Townsend, C. A. (1997). Enzymology and molecular biology of aflatoxin biosynthesis. *Chemical reviews*, *97*(7), 2537-2556.

[35] Mahanti, N., Bhatnagar, D., Cary, J. W., Joubran, J. & Linz, J. E. (1996). Structure and function of fas-1A, a gene encoding a putative fatty acid synthetase directly involved in aflatoxin biosynthesis in *Aspergillus parasiticus*. *Applied and environmental microbiology*, 62(1), 191-195.

[36] Brown, D. W., Adams, T. H. & Keller, N. P. (1996). *Aspergillus* has distinct fatty acid synthases for primary and secondary metabolism. *Proceedings of the National Academy of Sciences*, 93(25), 14873-14877.

[37] Yang, K., Zhuang, Z., Zhang, F., Song, F., Zhong, H., Ran, F. & Wang, S. (2015). Inhibition of aflatoxin metabolism and growth of *Aspergillus flavus* in liquid culture by a DNA methylation inhibitor. *Food Additives & Contaminants*: Part A, 32(4), 554-563.

[38] Caceres, I., Khoury, A. A., Khoury, R. E., Lorber, S., Oswald, I. P., Khoury, A. E. & Bailly, J. D. (2020). Aflatoxin biosynthesis and genetic regulation: a review. *Toxins,* 12(3), 150.

[39] Šimončicová, J., Kaliňáková, B. & Kryštofová, S. (2017). Aflatoxins: biosynthesis, prevention and eradication. *Acta Chimica Slovaca*, 10(2), 123-131.

[40] Yabe, K. & Nakajima, H. (2004). Enzyme reactions and genes in aflatoxin biosynthesis. *Applied microbiology and biotechnology,* 64(6), 745-755.

[41] Georgianna, D. R. & Payne, G. A. (2009). Genetic regulation of aflatoxin biosynthesis: from gene to genome. *Fungal Genetics and Biology*, 46(2), 113-125.

[42] Sohrabi, N. & Taghizadeh, M. (2018). Molecular identification of aflatoxigenic Aspergillus species in feedstuff samples. *Current medical mycology*, 4(2), 1.

[43] Adhikari, B. N., Bandyopadhyay, R. & Cotty, P. J. (2016). Degeneration of aflatoxin gene clusters in *Aspergillus flavus* from Africa and North America. Amb Express, 6(1), 1-16.

[44] Cary, J. W., Han, Z., Yin, Y., Lohmar, J. M., Shantappa, S., Harris-Coward, P. Y. & Calvo, A. M. (2015). Transcriptome analysis of *Aspergillus flavus* reveals veA-dependent regulation of secondary metabolite gene clusters, including the novel aflavarin cluster. Eukaryotic cell, 14(10), 983-997.

[45] Dhingra, S., Lind, A. L., Lin, H. C., Tang, Y., Rokas, A. & Calvo, A. M. (2013). The fumagillin gene cluster, an example of hundreds of genes under veA control in *Aspergillus fumigatus*. *PLoS One*, 8(10), e77147.

[46] Martín, J. F. (2017). Key role of LaeA and velvet complex proteins on

expression of β-lactam and PR-toxin genes in *Penicillium chrysogenum*: cross-talk regulation of secondary metabolite pathways. *Journal of Industrial Microbiology and Biotechnology*, 44(4-5), 525-535.

[47] Yin, W. & Keller, N. P. (2011). Transcriptional regulatory elements in fungal secondary metabolism. Journal of Microbiology, 49(3), 329-339.

[48] Yang, K., Liang, L., Ran, F., Liu, Y., Li, Z., Lan, H. & Wang, S. (2016). The DmtA methyltransferase contributes to *Aspergillus flavus* conidiation, sclerotial production, aflatoxin biosynthesis and virulence. *Scientific reports*, 6(1), 1-13.

[49] Yuan, J., Li, D., Qin, L., Shen, J., Guo, X., Tumukunde, E. & Wang, S. (2019). HexA is required for growth, aflatoxin biosynthesis and virulence in *Aspergillus flavus*. *BMC Molecular biology*, 20(1), 1-13.

[50] Ludovici, M., Ialongo, C., Reverberi, M., Beccaccioli, M., Scarpari, M. & Scala, V. (2014). Quantitative profiling of oxylipins through comprehensive LC-MS/MS analysis of *Fusarium verticillioides* and maize kernels. *Food Additives & Contaminants*: Part A, 31(12), 2026-2033.

[51] Lan, H., Wu, L., Fan, K., Sun, R., Yang, G., Zhang, F. & Wang, S. (2019). Set3 is required for asexual development, aflatoxin biosynthesis, and fungal virulence in *Aspergillus flavus*. *Frontiers in Microbiology*, 10, 530.

[52] Pietiäinen, M., Kontturi, J., Paasela, T., Deng, X., Ainasoja, M., Nyberg, P. & Teeri, T. H. (2016). Two polyketide synthases are necessary for 4-hydroxy-5-methylcoumarin biosynthesis in *Gerbera hybrida*. *The Plant Journal*, 87(6), 548-558.

[53] Cotty, P. J. & Jaime-Garcia, R. (2007). Influences of climate on aflatoxin producing fungi and aflatoxin contamination. *International Journal of food microbiology*, 119(1-2), 109-115.

[54] Waliyar, F., Osiru, M., Ntare, B. R., Kumar, K., Sudini, H., Traore, A. & Diarra, B. (2015). Post-harvest management of aflatoxin contamination in groundnut. *World Mycotoxin Journal*, 8(2), 245-252.

[55] Battacone, G., Nudda, A., Palomba, M., Mazzette, A. & Pulina, G. (2009). The transfer of aflatoxin M1 in milk of ewes fed diet naturally contaminated by aflatoxins and effect of inclusion of dried yeast culture in the diet. Journal of Dairy Science, 92(10), 4997-5004.

[56] Omar, S. S. (2016). Aflatoxin M1 levels in raw milk, pasteurized milk and infant formula. *Italian Journal of food safety*, 5(3).

[57] Puga-Torres, B., Salazar, D., Cachiguango, M., Cisneros, G. & Gómez-Bravo, C. (2020). Determination of aflatoxin M1 in raw milk from different provinces of Ecuador. *Toxins,* 12(8), 498.

[58] Anukul, N., Vangnai, K. & Mahakarnchanakul, W. (2013). Significance of regulation limits in mycotoxin contamination in Asia and risk management programs at the national level. *Journal of food and drug analysis*, 21(3), 227-241.

[59] Wild, C. P. & Turner, P. C. (2002). The toxicology of aflatoxins as a basis for public health decisions. *Mutagenesis,* 17(6), 471-481.

[60] Tang, M. S., Wang, H. T., Hu, Y., Chen, W. S., Akao, M., Feng, Z. & Hu, W. (2011). Acrolein induced DNA damage, mutagenicity and effect on DNA repair. *Molecular nutrition & food Research*, 55(9), 1291-1300.

[61] Kew, M. C. (2003). Synergistic interaction between aflatoxin B1 and

hepatitis B virus in hepatocarcinogenesis. *Liver international*, 23 (6), 405-409.

[62] Grace, D., Mahuku, G., Hoffmann, V., Atherstone, C., Upadhyaya, H. D. & Bandyopadhyay, R. (2015). International agricultural research to reduce food risks: case studies on aflatoxins. *Food Security*, 7(3), 569-582.

[63] Mekuria, A. N., Routledge, M. N., Gong, Y. Y. & Sisay, M. (2020). Aflatoxins as a risk factor for liver cirrhosis: a systematic review and meta-analysis. *BMC Pharmacology and Toxicology*, 21, 1-8.

[64] Farombi, O. E. (2006). Aflatoxin contamination of foods in developing countries: Implications for hepatocellular carcinoma and chemo preventive strategies. *African Journal of Biotechnology*, 5(1), 1-14.

[65] Magnussen, A. & Parsi, M. A. (2013). Aflatoxins, hepatocellular carcinoma and public health. *World Journal of Gastroenterology*: WJG, 19(10), 1508.

[66] Lizárraga-Paulín, E. G., Moreno-Martínez, E. & Miranda-Castro, S. P. (2011). Aflatoxins and their impact on human and animal health: an emerging problem. *Aflatoxins-Biochemistry and Molecular Biology*, 13, 255-282.

[67] Kowalska, A., Walkiewicz, K., Kozieł, P. & Muc-Wierzgoń, M. (2017). Aflatoxins: characteristics and impact on human health. *Postepy higieny i medycyny doswiadczalnej* (Online), 71, 315-327.

[68] Wild, C. P., Garner, R. C., Montesano, R. & Tursi, F. (1986). Aflatoxin B 1 binding to plasma albumin and liver DNA upon chronic administration to rats. *Carcinogenesis*, 7(6), 853-858.

[69] Zhang, J., Zheng, N., Liu, J., Li, F. D., Li, S. L. & Wang, J. Q. (2015). Aflatoxin B1 and aflatoxin M1 induced cytotoxicity and DNA damage in differentiated and undifferentiated Caco-2 cells. *Food and Chemical Toxicology*, 83, 54-60.

[70] Ozakyol, A. (2017). Global epidemiology of hepatocellular carcinoma (HCC epidemiology). *Journal of Gastrointestinal Cancer*, 48(3), 238-240.

[71] Ming, L., Thorgeirsson, S. S., Gail, M. H., Lu, P., Harris, C. C., Wang, N. & Sun, Z. (2002). Dominant role of hepatitis B virus and cofactor role of aflatoxin in hepatocarcinogenesis in Qidong, China. *Hepatology*, *36*(5), 1214-1220.

[72] Zekri, A. R., Bahnassy, A. A., Madbouly, M. S., Asaad, N. Y., El-Shehaby, A. M. & Alam El Din, H. M. (2006). p53 mutation in HCV-genotype-4 associated hepatocellular carcinoma in Egyptian patients. *J Egypt Natl Canc Inst*, 18(1), 17-29.

[73] Feng, W. H., Xue, K. S., Tang, L., Williams, P. L. & Wang, J. S. (2017). Aflatoxin B1-induced developmental and DNA damage in *Caenorhabditis elegans*. *Toxins*, *9*(1), 9.

[74] Park, U. S., Park, S. K., Lee, Y. I., Park, J. G. & Lee, Y. I. (2000). Hepatitis B virus-X protein up regulates the expression of p21 wafl/cipl and prolongs G1→ S transition via a p53-independent pathway in human hepatoma cells. *Oncogene,* 19(30), 3384-3394.

[75] Madden, C. R., Finegold, M. J. & Slagle, B. L. (2002). Altered DNA mutation spectrum in aflatoxin b1-treated transgenic mice that express the hepatitis B virus x protein. *Journal of Virology,* 76(22), 11770-11774.

[76] Castelino, J. M., Routledge, M. N., Wilson, S., Dunne, D. W., Mwatha, J. K., Gachuhi, K. & Gong, Y. Y. (2015). Aflatoxin exposure is inversely

associated with IGF1 and IGFBP3 levels in vitro and in Kenyan schoolchildren. *Molecular nutrition & food research*, 59(3), 574-581.

[77] Smith, L. E., Stoltzfus, R. J. & Prendergast, A. (2012). Food chain mycotoxin exposures, gut health, and impaired growth: a conceptual framework. *Advances in Nutrition*, *3*(4), 526-531.

[78] Benkerroum, N. (2020b). Chronic and acute toxicities of aflatoxins: Mechanisms of action. *International J Environmental Research and Public Health*, 17(2), 423.

[79] Adaku Chilaka, C. & Mally, A. (2020). Mycotoxin Occurrence, Exposure and Health Implications in Infants and Young Children in Sub-Saharan Africa: *A Review. Foods*, 9(11), 1585.

[80] Smith, L. E., Prendergast, A. J., Turner, P. C., Humphrey, J. H. & Stoltzfus, R. J. (2017). Aflatoxin exposure during pregnancy, maternal anemia, and adverse birth outcomes. *The American journal of tropical medicine and hygiene*, *96*(4), 770-776.

[81] Shuaib, F. M., Jolly, P. E., Ehiri, J. E., Yatich, N., Jiang, Y., Funkhouser, E. & Williams, J. H. (2010). Association between birth outcomes and aflatoxin B1 biomarker blood levels in pregnant women in Kumasi, Ghana. *Tropical Medicine & International Health*, 15(2), 160-167.

[82] Eze, U. A., Routledge, M. N., Okonofua, F. E., Huntriss, J. & Gong, Y. Y. (2018). Mycotoxin exposure and adverse reproductive health outcomes in Africa: A review. *World Mycotoxin Journal,* 11(3), 321-339.

[83] Maleki, F., Abdi, S., Davodian, E., Haghani, K. & Bakhtiyari, S. (2015). Exposure of infants to aflatoxin M1 from mother's breast milk in Ilam, Western Iran. *Osong public health and research perspectives*, 6(5), 283-287.

[84] Bouhet, S. & Oswald, I. P. (2005). The effects of mycotoxins, fungal food contaminants, on the intestinal epithelial cell-derived innate immune response. *Veterinary immunology and Immunopathology*, 108(1-2), 199-209.

[85] Park, S. H., Kim, D., Kim, J. & Moon, Y. (2015). Effects of mycotoxins on mucosal microbial infection and related pathogenesis. *Toxins*, *7*(11), 4484-4502.

[86] Corthésy, B. (2013). Multi-faceted functions of secretory IgA at mucosal surfaces. *Frontiers in Immunology*, 4, 185.

[87] James-Ellison, M. Y., Roberts, R., Verrier-Jones, K., Williams, J. D. & Topley, N. (1997). Mucosal immunity in the urinary tract: changes in sIgA, FSC and total IgA with age and in urinary tract infection. *Clinical Nephrology*, 48(2), 69-78.

[88] Cysewski, S. J., Wood, R. L., Pier, A. C. & Baetz, A. L. (1978). Effects of aflatoxin on the development of acquired immunity to swine erysipelas. *American Journal of Veterinary Research*, 39(3), 445-448.

[89] Jiang, Y. I., Jolly, P. E., Ellis, W. O., Wang, J. S., Phillips, T. D. & Williams, J. H. (2005). Aflatoxin B1 albumin adduct levels and cellular immune status in Ghanaians. *International Immunology*, 17(6), 807-814.

[90] Chen, G., Gong, Y. Y., Kimanya, M. E., Shirima, C. P. & Routledge, M. N. (2018). Comparison of urinary aflatoxin M1 and aflatoxin albumin adducts as biomarkers for assessing aflatoxin exposure in Tanzanian children. *Biomarkers*, *23*(2), 131-136.

[91] Arce-López, B., Lizarraga, E., Vettorazzi, A. & González-Peñas, E. (2020). Human biomonitoring of

mycotoxins in blood, plasma and serum in recent years: a review. *Toxins*, *12*(3), 147.

[92] Udomkun, P., Wiredu, A. N., Nagle, M., Müller, J., Vanlauwe, B. & Bandyopadhyay, R. (2017). Innovative technologies to manage aflatoxins in foods and feeds and the profitability of application–A review. *Food control*, 76, 127-138.

[93] Lavkor, I. & Var, I. (2017). The control of aflatoxin contamination at harvest, drying, pre-storage and storage periods in peanut: The new approach. Aflatoxin-control, analysis, detection and health risks, 45-64.

[94] El-Ramady, H. R., Domokos-Szabolcsy, É., Abdalla, N. A., Taha, H.S. & Fári, M. (2015). Postharvest management of fruits and vegetables storage. In Sustainable agriculture reviews (pp. 65-152). Springer, Cham.

[95] Achar, P. N., Quyen, P., Adukwu, E. C., Sharma, A., Msimanga, H. Z., Nagaraja, H. & Sreenivasa, M. Y. (2020). Investigation of the Antifungal and Anti-Aflatoxigenic Potential of Plant-Based Essential Oils against *Aspergillus flavus* in Peanuts. *Journal of Fungi*, 6(4), 383.

[96] Agriopoulou, S., Stamatelopoulou, E. & Varzakas, T. (2020). Advances in occurrence, importance, and mycotoxin control strategies: Prevention and detoxification in foods. *Foods*, 9(2), 137.

[97] Díaz-Valderrama, J. R., Njoroge, A. W., Macedo-Valdivia, D., Orihuela-Ordóñez, N., Smith, B. W., Casa-Coila, V. & Baributsa, D. (2020). Postharvest practices, challenges and opportunities for grain producers in Arequipa, Peru. *Plos One*, 15(11), e0240857.

[98] Lopes, L. O., Silva, R., Guimarães, J. T., Coutinho, N. M., Castro, B. G., Pimentel, T. C. & Cruz, A. G. (2020). Food defense: Perceptions and attitudes of Brazilian dairy companies. *Journal of Dairy Science*, 103(9), 8675-8682.

[99] Watner, C. (2020). Who Should Decide What Goes into a Can of Tomatoes? Food Laws from a Voluntaryist Perspective. *Journal of Libertarian Studies*, 24(1), 188-205.

[100] Migwi, B., Mutegi, C., Mburu, J., Wagacha, J., Cotty, P., Bandyopadhyay, R. & Manyong, V. M. (2020). Assessment of willingness-to-pay for Aflasafe KE01, a native biological control product for aflatoxin management in Kenya. *Food Additives & Contaminants*: Part A, 37(11), 1951-1962.

[101] Min, L., Li, D., Tong, X., Sun, H., Chen, W., Wang, G. & Wang, J. (2020). The challenges of global occurrence of aflatoxin M1 contamination and the reduction of aflatoxin M1 in milk over the past decade. *Food Control*, 107352.

[102] Qin, P. W., Xu, J., Jiang, Y., Hu, L., van der Lee, T., Waalwijk, C. & Xu, X. D. (2020). Survey for toxigenic Fusarium species on maize kernels in China. *World Mycotoxin Journal*, *13*(2), 213-224.

[103] Palumbo, R., Gonçalves, A., Gkrillas, A., Logrieco, A., Dorne, J. L., Chiara, D. A. & Battilani, P. (2020). Mycotoxins in maize: mitigation actions, with a chain management approach. *Phytopathologia Mediterranea*, 59 (1), 5-28.

[104] Agbetiameh, D., Ortega-Beltran, A., Awuah, R. T., Atehnkeng, J., Elzein, A., Cotty, P. J. & Bandyopadhyay, R. (2020). Field efficacy of two atoxigenic biocontrol products for mitigation of aflatoxin contamination in maize and groundnut in Ghana. *Biological Control*, 150, 104351.

[105] Ncube, J. & Maphosa, M. (2020). Current state of knowledge on groundnut aflatoxins and their management from a plant breeding

perspective: Lessons for Africa. *Scientific African*, *7*, e00264.

[106] Zhang, K. & Banerjee, K. (2020). A Review: Sample Preparation and Chromatographic Technologies for Detection of Aflatoxins in Foods. *Toxins*, *12*(9), 539.

[107] Rashed, W. M., Kandeil, M. A. M., Mahmoud, M. O. & Ezzat, S. (2020). Hepatocellular Carcinoma (HCC) in Egypt: A comprehensive overview. *Journal of the Egyptian National Cancer Institute*, *32*(1), 1-11.

[108] Ayo, E. M., Matemu, A., Laswai, G. H. & Kimanya, M. E. (2018). Socioeconomic characteristics influencing level of awareness of aflatoxin contamination of feeds among livestock farmers in Meru district of Tanzania. *Scientifica*, *2018*. Article ID 3485967

Chapter 3

# The Role of Socio-Economic Factors and Indigenous Knowledge Practices on the Mycotoxigenic Fungi Contamination of Food

*Esiegbuya Daniel Ofeoritse and Ojieabu Amarachi*

## Abstract

Indigenous methods of food processing in Nigeria are influenced by a wide range of socioeconomic factors and indigenous knowledge practices which support mycotoxingenic fungal contamination of processed food. Some of the socioeconomic factors include level of education, methods of skill acquisition, methods of food vending in market places, methods of food handling and storage, hygienic practices and poor water supply. The uses of indigenous knowledge in food processing are important because its application serve as a source of livelihood improvements, sustainability of indigenous food and eradication of food shortage. The limitation of the application of indigenous knowledge in food processing encourages mycotoxins contamination of foods. This is as a result of the poor hygienic conditions of the processing utensils, processing environments and methods of packaging the processed food. Due to the absence of policies in monitoring the quality of indigenously processed foods in market places and the risk associated with indigenous methods of food processing, there is the need for government agencies to address these issues through policy assessment in the areas of operations, inspection and enforcement and training so as to effectively harness the benefits of indigenous knowledge in food processing for national development.

**Keywords:** socio-economic, indigenous knowledge, policies, interventions, mycotoxigenic fungi

## 1. Introduction

Fungi are ubiquitous in nature and produce a wide range of toxins on food substances. The toxins produced by fungi have been documented to be harmful to both man and animals [1, 2]. The pre and postharvest conditions reported to enhance mycotoxins production on food by fungi according to Atanda et al. [1] include climatic conditions, nutrient availability for the fungi, soil types and conditions, time of harvesting, pest infestation, drying condition and duration, storage factors, sanitation, traditional processing methods, substrate types and lack of awareness by a majorly farmers, food handlers and processors.

Exposure to mycotoxins may cause diseases such as primary hepatocellular carcinoma, anemia, immunodeficiency, liver cirrhosis, infertility, stunting and being underweight and nephropathy [2]. The adverse effect of cases of individuals with symptoms similar to these diseases is not well documented especially in developing countries when compared to the incidence and prevalence of mycotoxins in staple foods such as maize, groundnut, rice, peanut etc. In the work of Darwish et al. [2], the author's highlighted the distribution of mycotoxins across different staple foods, feeds and drinks in Africa and the amount and type of mycotoxin present in them. Accordingly, to the authors the percentage distribution of the different types of mycotoxins are aflatoxin 43.75%, ochratoxins 12.5%, fuminosin 21.87%, zearalenone 9.375%, deoxynivalenol 6.25% and beauvericin 12.5%.

However, there are scarcely documented medical reports linking mycotoxins contamination of food to the cases mentioned above in patients when compared to other causes of diseases. This is due to the following reasons;

1. Lack of adequate facilities and fund for mycotoxins research in teaching hospitals

2. Low technical know-how of laboratory technicians and doctors

3. Inability of patient to pay the require charges.

Atanda et al. [1] also stated that policy enforcement agencies such as the National Agency for Food and Drug Administration and Control (NAFDAC) and the Standards Organization of Nigeria (SON) which are supposed to help detect mycotoxins in foods do not allow staff of the agency to do research. This has further limit staff of these agencies from building capacity in mycotoxins research.

According to Atanda et al. [1] the major factors hindering the documentation of mycotoxin related human health cases in Nigeria, is the legislation on Medical Ethics which prohibits medical practitioners from disclosing the cases of patient. Atanda et al. [1] made several references to outbreaks recorded in literatures to include

1. The death of some children who consumed mouldy Kulikuli (Groundnut cake) in Ibadan was suspected to be due to the presence of aflatoxin in the groundnut.

2. Detection of aflatoxins in the urine of liver disease patients in Zaria, Kaduna State and also in the organs of children who died of kwashiorkor in Southern and Western Nigeria, respectively.

3. Detection of aflatoxins in human semen in Benin City.

4. Detection of aflatoxin M1 in breast milk blood of umbilical cord of babies in the country.

Uriah et al. [3] also reported on the occurrence of aflatoxin in the blood and semen of infertile men which was significantly higher in level when compared than that in fertile men.

Apart from the health challenges associated with mycotoxin contamination of food, it was also stated that Africa loses an estimated US$670 million in rejected export trade annually due to contamination by aflatoxins [4].

## 2. The socio-economic and demographic impact on mycotoxin contamination of food

Socioeconomic factors such as level of education, methods of skill acquisition, methods of food display, methods of food handling and storage, vending sites, hygienic practices and poor water supply are reported to be responsible for food contamination. In relation to mycotoxins contamination of food, Kumar and Popat [5] and Mohd Redzwan et al. [6] noted that farmers generally lack knowledge on mycotoxins contamination of food and factors contributing to this include their level of education, farm size, participation in social and extension services, market orientation, economic motivation, level of innovation, ignorant of negative health effects of consuming mycotoxins contaminated food and overall perception. According to the authors, most farmers do not consider control of mycotoxins contamination of food important because the domestic markets do not make additional payment provide for uncontaminated products.

### 2.1 Level of education and awareness

Education is positively related to awareness, knowledge and perceived benefits [7]. Dosman et al. [8] stated that people with higher educational level are likely to be better informed about the risks of mycotoxins and chemically contaminated food. This might be attributed to their ability to read and understand basic communication skills [9]. Sabran et al [10] noted that individuals with high educational status had high level of knowledge on the occurrence of fungal infections in food when compared to those with low educational status. The authors indicated that education is an important mode to disperse information and knowledge to the public and also that low level of education is likely to promote lack of appreciation for food handling practices and this factors may presents potential risk to food safety.

### 2.2 Marital status

**Studies** have showed that marital status may contribute to the level of knowledge about mycotoxins contamination of food. This is because marriage enhances couples to exchange knowledge and this has also helped to enhance diet thus promoting good health and disease prevention [11].

### 2.3 Gender

Sabran et al [10] reported that women seem to have higher knowledge of aflatoxin contamination of food. This is because women have sound knowledge and practice in regard to food safety than men and also have the strongest reaction to assessing food safety risk [12].

### 2.4 Methods of food handling and display

In developing countries, food handling and vending sites are a major challenge encouraging fungi contamination of food. Food vendors and buyers serve and select their choice of food products with bare hands which could promote contamination of food especially if the hands are not properly washed and dried. These practices are commonly noticed among fruit sellers were a particular fruit is handled severally before being purchased and eaten by the buyers. Vending sites are also characterized by flies and waste dump which served as sources of cross-contamination [13].

## 3. Indigenous methods of food processing and preservation on mycotoxins contamination of food

Indigenous knowledge refers to what indigenous people know and do, and have become good at it through series of trial and error processes [14]. According to Sundamari and Ranganathan [15], African indigenous knowledge is an unwritten body of knowledge held in different brains, languages across diverse cultures. Its application cuts across different areas such as traditional medicine, land use and management, family healthcare, breeding of food crop species, preservation of seeds and the domestication and use of wild edible plants. One major aspect that affects mycotoxins contamination of food the respects to indigenous knowledge is some of the methods of food processing and preservation.

Indigenous foods can be regarded as those foods that are obtained from the immediate environment and are made edible or processed through the application of indigenous methods of food processing. Indigenous knowledge on methods of food processing is important because its application

1. can enhance the flavor of the food.

2. removal of toxic substances, for example the conversion of cassava (*Manihot esculenta, Crantz* syn. *Manihot utilissima* Pohl) to garri significantly reduces the cyanide content to a safe level by WHO standards [16].

3. enhance preservation and digestibility of food.

4. helps to reduce anti-nutritional components.

### 3.1 Sun drying and smoke drying

Indigenous method of sun drying involves spreading the food material on bare grounds, road sides or on roof tops. According to Asogwa *et al.* [17] sun drying is a key traditional and inexpensive method for removing substantial amount of moisture from food, and some of the food items that can be sun dried include tubers, cereals, vegetables, fruits, fish, meat etc. The smoking of meat and fish during drying adds flavor and increases its shelf life [18]. These indigenous practices also help in maintaining food accessibility at all times [19].

During indigenous method of food processing, food quality parameters are mainly assessed through physical inspection and tasting. This is due to the fact that the indigenous food processors lack the technology of monitoring quality and conditions affecting the level of mycotoxins in food. After processing, the food is sometimes exposed to conditions that enhance cross-contamination. This is because indigenous food processors lack the necessary awareness.

In the case of meat, after drying, the product is stored whole or sometimes cut into smaller bits and kept in wire gauze cage for storage or displayed in the market for sale. The essence of the wire gauze cage is also to expose dried meat to air to prevent further moisture buildup. According to meat processors, the meat can be preserved for more than six months as long as it is exposed dry smoking at intervals. This method is not ideally relevant in contemporary situations today because the wire gauze cage exposes to flies and airborne pathogens which might enhance mycotoxin buildup in the stored meat.

Also, in the processing of local delicacies such as 'amala' or 'elubo' from plantain or yam undergo a series of process which begins with the peeling of the skin of plantain or yam and then slicing it into smaller thin bits before grinding it to form the powder called 'amala' or 'elubo'. Rural food processors developed the local initiative of drying the sliced thin bits of the plantain or yam under the sun for several days will reduce the moisture content and also the mixing of the powdered plantain or yam will results to a local delicacy called 'amala' or 'elubo' which becomes gary white in colour. Scientifically, the drying process under the sun can serve the purpose. But the indigenous imitative of drying on any available floor or slab exposes the raw materials to atmospheric dust, sand and airborne pathogens in which aflatoxigenic fungi are mainly associated [20]. Fungi can thrive within the substrate releasing many toxins into the food substance. Consumers feel that the preparation of the plantain powder into 'amala' which involves mixing with hot water under heat condition will destroy the accumulated toxins. Scientifically, aflatoxins are known to be heat stable and scientific methods have developed techniques for its monitoring its contents along food processing chain. The processing of pistachio nuts, heating at a temperature of 90–150 °C for 30–120 min was found to reduce its aflatoxin content by about 17–63%. While in other food products such as bread and biscuits, temperature did not have any significant effect on the ochratoxin content but significantly reduce its content in biscuits [21, 22]. Some factors affecting the level of mycotoxin content in food includes variety of the food, moisture content, temperature and time of heating [23, 24].

Indigenous food processors also lack the technology of knowing the type of mycotoxins that will be destroyed or not destroyed.

### 3.2 Leaves wrapping and packaging

Packaging equally refers to the process of design, evaluation and production of packages [25]. Packaging can also be described as a coordinated system of preparing goods for transport, warehousing, logistics and sales [26]. It is important because it serves as a physical protection for the food during transportation, distribution, handling, sales, opening, use and re-use [25]. The type of material used for packaging also serves as a source of attraction to consumers and also helps in defining the quality of the product [27].

In Nigeria and other parts of Africa, the indigenous use of plant leaves for food packaging is important because it is believed that such leaves posses natural pesticides which serves as pest control while others believe that it adds natural aroma and flavor to the packaged food. Examples of some plant leaves for food preservation include *Dorax* sp., *Alchornea laxiflora* (Esin), *Costus lucanusianus* and *Spondia Mombin* (Iyeye) used in the preservation of kolanuts.

The challenges with food packaging in developing countries are that different materials such as leaves, cellophane, paper, used and discarded bottles are used for food packaging without the food handler considering the hygienic status of the packaging material, and as such, this may serve as a possible source of microbial contamination of food [28]. Hicks [29] also highlighted the benefits of food manufacturer and handlers keeping food safe from pathogenic microorganisms [29].

In the use of broad leaves for food packaging, as the leaves deteriorate, it also serves as a source of contamination to the food. Ihejirika et al. [30] stated that pathogen invades *Garcinia kola* seeds especially if the processing methods and packaging materials used have are contaminated with microbes. According to the authors, the mycotoxigenic fungi associated with *G. kola* package with leaves include *Penicillum* spp., *Aspergillus* spp. and *Diplodia* spp. Atanda et al. [31] also detected *A. flavus* and *Rhizopus arrhizus* in kola nuts together with aflatoxin level of 2 μg/kg.

Adejumo and Ola [32] stated that the disadvantages of using local methods to preserve food include

1. Most of the packaging materials used originally held other manufactured products such as beer, soft drinks container that have been discarded and in most cases they are not properly washed etc.

2. Some of the packaging materials used are mainly collected from refuse dump without considering even if they have minor defect such as absent of cover or heavily dirty

3. Attitude of reusing the packaging materials as long as they remain undamaged

4. Food package/displayed in glass slides are handled many times by different customers for inspection before purchase, such practice provide avenues for contamination

5. Leaves used for food packaging are often dirty and are kept in the open with little or no provision for washing before use

6. Paper such as newspapers and magazine used for food packaging is not properly stored and cannot be clean even when dirty

7. Cellophane use for food packaging sometimes contain moisture condensation which enhances mould growth on the food

These disadvantages served as possible sources of mycotoxingenic contamination of the packaged food as against the reversal in scientific approach where these methods are not employed and even if the methods are to be used, the materials used be free from microbes and sources of cross-contamination [13].

### 3.3 Fermentation

Indigenous methods of food fermentation began more than 7000 years ago [33]. According to the authors fermented foods are important in that they enhances digestion, flavour, aroma, preservation, shelf-life and detoxification of anti-nutrient presents in food. Food fermentation involves mainly the activities of microbes that contribute towards enhancing the quality of the food.

In indigenous food fermentation, local food processor have learnt from experience and continuous practices the number of days to ferment a food and also access the quality of the fermented food formed without applying science. Esiegbuya [34] noted that indigenous method of food processing is not completely irrelevant in modern methods of food processing however it has some disadvantages such as

1. The unhygienic condition of the processing environment, utensils and food processors which can contaminate the fermented food.

2. Use of any available materials for processing and food packaging.

3. Lack of knowledge on the activities and role of the fermenting organisms

4. Inconsistency of the use of processing materials

5. Unhygienic condition of keeping used and unused processing materials

6. Poor method of waste disposal

7. The processed food only satisfies a small segment of the society

The overall effects of some of the poor processing practices by indigenous food processors is the continuous contamination of the processing equipments/utensils, raw materials and finished products by vectors such as insects, rodents and domestic animals. These vectors are known carriers of diseases and other contaminants (urea) from animal droppings. The overall effect of these is possibly mycotoxins contamination of the processed products [34].

In the fermentation of sorghum beer (*bil bil*) from sorghum, Darman [35] highlighted seven points of possible mycotoxin contamination along the processing chain. According to the authors, these points include the stage of soaking, germination, drying, decoction, cooking, mixing of clarified wort and starter culture and fermentation. The reason stated by the author was that some of these stages such as soaking of the sorghum at high temperature reduces the growth of yeast and thus increase the risk of mould growth which can enhance mycotoxins contamination of the fermented product. With the application of modern approach, this process can be monitored when compared in the natural fermentation of maize dough for *doklu* production, it was found that fermentation significantly reduce the amount of aflatoxins. According to Lillehoj et al. [36], aflatoxin was not detected in distilled alcohol but accumulated mainly in spent grains. Toxins such as fumonisins B1 and B2 and ochratoxin A were also found to be stable during beer fermentation [37]. Zearalenone was also found to be stable during the fermentation of corn by *S. uvarum* [38].

Scientific approach also shown that the activities of some microbial enzymes during fermentation process according to Wolf-Hall and Schwarz [39] may transform mycotoxins into non-toxic products but no microbial strain has been recommended so far as a processing aid targeting mycotoxins [40].

## 4. The policies and actions that enhance the use of indigenous knowledge in food industry

Currently in Nigeria and in some other African countries, there are no known policies or actions for the production of indigenous food and as such the market is free for all without any regulation.

Some of the factors enhancing the application of indigenous knowledge in the food industry include

1. Poor implementation of government policies towards food security

2. Mycotoxins mitigating measures are routinely not applied in Nigeria.

3. Lack of adequate storage system for locally produced food

4. Poor storage facilities as a result of poor power supply have further enhanced the application of indigenous knowledge to preserve food

5. High patronage of products due to availability and low cost

6. Its simplicity

7. Serves as a survival strategy for income generation

8. Lack of awareness on the side of the producers and buyers

9. Lack of set out agenda on the impact of poor food processing practices on food quality

## 5. Tackling mycotoxins contamination of indigenous food through government policies

In Nigeria, more than 50% of the foods displayed in market places are locally produced using indigenous knowledge and as such are possibly expose to contamination by microorganisms. Udomkun et al. [41] stated that the problem of food insecurity occurs mainly in developing countries and the major factors leading to food insecurity are the methods of food production and postharvest losses.

Presently, emphasis on assessment of imported and exported foods has increased considerably. But not much emphasis has been on the risk assessment of indigenously processed foods which are not exported but consumed locally. This is important because the wellbeing of any population is important for national development. According to a report by Abt associates [42], in collaboration with the Mycotoxicology Society of Nigeria (MYCOTOXSON) and Nigeria's National Agency for Food and Drug Administration and Control (NAFDAC) on the risk assessment of aflatoxin on human health, they found out that despite the rise in the awareness of aflatoxin contamination of foods, unpackaged foods and foods destined for domestic consumption are not regulated. This is so with indigenously processed food consumed locally. The lack of regulation for foods destined for domestic consumption can enhance mycotoxins contamination of indigenously processed food. To address this challenge, there is the need proper regulations which will involved risk analyses (risk assessment, risk management and risk communication) of indigenously processed food.

Food and Agricultural Organization (FAO) stated that up to 25% of the world's food crops are estimated to be contaminated with mycotoxins (Eskola, [43]). The consumption of mycotoxins contaminated food leads to chronic mycotoxicoses and death [44]. Therefore as the global occurrence and importance of mycotoxins cannot be overemphasized, there is the need for improved risk management and communication strategies especially for indigenously processed food in developing countries. This is because there is no stand out policy regulating the activities of indigenous food processors thus any person to get involved in it either for household or commercial purpose.

Omojokun [45] stated that many health problems encountered today arose as a result of consuming unsafe food and that health problems associated with unsafe food are not new as they date far back in history. Indigenous methods of food processing serve as one major source of unsafe food that not much attention has been given to its application. This is not to say that the use of indigenous knowledge of food production be neglected because it has a lot of socio-economic benefits towards national development which includes

1. Serving as a source of livelihood improvements for mostly rural women who are involved in it.

2. Enhancing the sustainability of indigenous food, and

3. Eradication of food waste.

In order to effectively harness these benefits and conserve the use of knowledge indigenous for future generations, there is the need for proper policy assessment to include the following.

1. Government at the federal level should set up a body or assign to any of its agencies to carry out a proper risk assessment and implement management strategies for all food produced indigenously using local knowledge within her country and also profer solutions on how the risk associated with the documented food can be tackled through food safety policies such as establishment of locally acceptable guidelines for mycotoxins control of indigenously processed food.

2. Staff of agencies assigned to monitor the activities of food processors using indigenous knowledge should be those with academic qualifications in such areas and also should be empowered to undergo constant training so as to enhance their capacity on how to coordinate, monitor and audit the activities of food processors. Agencies should be empowered through the provision of laboratory support to vet the quality of products

3. Issuance of license of operation to anyone involved or interested in food processing using indigenous methods especially at commercial level after such individuals must have been made to undergo basic training on area of interest.

4. Routine inspection and enforcement such as routine market surveillance, investigative inspection and compliance investigation and defaulters should be sanctioned with measures such as holding of products, rejecting of products, recalling of products, seal up and prosecution

5. Government agencies should network with academic societies such as the Mycotoxicological Society of Nigeria, Mycological society of Nigeria, Botanical society of Nigeria, Universities and Research institutions who are knowledgeable in the areas of mycotoxins research to help in the training of staff of the monitoring agencies and indigenous food processors on basic Sanitary and Phytosanitory Standards (SPS), Hazard Analysis and Critical Control Points (HACCP) and Good Processing Practices (GPP), risk assessment and management and food packaging techniques and also develop effective risk communication strategy

## 6. Conclusion

The application of indigenous knowledge for food processing is important for socioeconomic development and empowerment however, methods of application enhance mycotoxigenic fungi contamination of the processed food. In order for **its** benefits to be adequately harnessed for national development, there is the need for government of developing countries to develop a legal framework for monitoring and managing the activities of indigenous food processors so as to enhance food safety.

### Conflict of interests

There are no conflicts of interest.

## Author details

Esiegbuya Daniel Ofeoritse* and Ojieabu Amarachi
Nigerian Institute for Oil Palm Research, Plant Pathology Division,
Benin City, Edo State, Nigeria

*Address all correspondence to: esiegbuya@gmail.com

## References

[1] Atanda, O., Makun, A.H., Ogara, I.M., Edema, M., Idahor, O.K., Eshiett, M.E. and Bosede F. O (2013). In: Makun, A.H, editor. Mycotoxin and Food Safety in Developing Countries: Janeza Trdine 9, 51000 Rijeka, Croatia; 2013. P. 3-38

[2] Darwish, W. S., Ikenaka, Y., Nakayama, S. M .M and Ishizuka, M. (2014) An Overview on Mycotoxin Contamination of Foods in Africa Journal of Veterinary Medical Science. 76(6): 789-797.

[3] Uriah, N., Ibeh, I. N. and Oluwafemi, F. 2001. A study of the impact of aflatoxin on human reproduction. African Journal of Reproductive Health 5: 106-110.

[4] Bankole, S.A, and Adebanjo A (2003). Mycotoxins in food in West Africa: current situation and possibilities of controlling it. African Journal of Biotechnology 2:254-263

[5] Kumar, G. D. S., and Popat, M. N. (2010). Farmers' perceptions knowledge and management of aflatoxins in groundnuts (*Arachis hypogaea* L.) In India Crop Protection, 29:1534-1541

[6] Mohd Redzwan, S., Rosita, J., Mohd Sokhini, A. M., & Nurul'Aqilah, A. R. (2012). Socio-demographic and socio-economic determinants of adults' knowledge on fungal and aflatoxin contamination in the diets. Asian Pacific Journal of Tropical Biomedicine, S1835-S1841.

[7] Jolly, C.M., Bayard, B., Awuah, R.T., Fialor, S.C. and Williams, J.T. (2009). Examining the structure of awareness and perceptions of groundnuts aflatoxin among Ghanaian health and agricultural professionals and its influence on their actions. Journal of Socioeconomics; 38: 280-287.

[8] Dosman, D.M., Adamowiez, W. L, Hrudey, S.E (2001). Socioeconomic determinants of health- and food safety-related risk perceptions. Risk Analysis 21: 307-317.

[9] Baker, G.A. (2003) Food safety and fear: Factors affecting consumer response to food safety risk. International Food for Agribusiness Manager Revision 6: 1

[10] Sabran, Mohd Redzwan; Jamaluddin, Rosita*; Abdul Mutalib, Mohd Sokhini; Abdul Rahman, Nurul 'Aqilah (2012) Socio-demographic and socio-economic determinants of adults' knowledge on fungal and aflatoxin contamination in the diets Asian Pacific Journal of Tropical Biomedicine S1835-S1841

[11] Kawada, T. and Suzuki S. (2011) Marital status and self-rated health in rural inhabitants in Japan: A cross sectional study. Journal of Divorce and Remarriage 52: 48-54.

[12] Osaili TM, Obeidat BA, Jomous DOA, Bawadi HA. Food safety knowledge and practices among female college students in north Jordan. Food Control 2011; 22: 269-276.

[13] Esiegbuya, O. D. Okungbowa, F. I., Okogbenin O.B., Omoregie, K.O. and Koloche, I. M. (2015) Microbiological analysis of Shea butter sold in markets in Nigeria. Nigerian Journal of Mycology.7: 33-43

[14] Melchias, G, Biodiversity and Conservation. Science Publishers, Inc., Enfield, 2001

[15] Sundamari, M. and Ranganathan T.T, (2003). Indigenous agricultural practices for sustainable farming. Agrobios (India). Jodhpur, India.

[16] FAO/WHO, Joint FAO/WHO (1991) Food Standards Programme.

Codex Alimentarius Commission XII, Supplement 4, Food and Agriculture Organization of the United States, Rome.

[17] Asogwa I.S., Okoye, J.I. and Oni, K (2017) Promotion of Indigenous Food Preservation and Processing Knowledge and the Challenge of Food Security in Africa Journal of Food Security, 5(3): 75-87

[18] Walingo M.K, (2008) Indigenous Food Processing Methods that Improve Nutrient Bioavailability in Plant-based Diets of the Kenyan Population: the Example of Zinc. In: Robertson, G.L. and Lupien, J.R. (Eds), Using Food Science and Technology to Improve Nutrition and Promote National Development.1-9.

[19] Kamwendo, G. and Kamwendo, J. (2014) Indigenous Knowledge-Systems and Food Security: Some Examples from Malawi. Journal of Human Ecology. 48(1). 97-101.

[20] Osho A., Mabekoje O. O. and Bello O. O. (2010) Comparative study on the microbial load of Gari, Eluboisu and Iru in Nigeria African Journal of Food Science 4(10):646-649

[21] Hetmanski M.T and Leonard, C.T. (1996) The effects of milling and processing on wheat contaminated with ochratoxin A. Food Additives and Contaminants 13(2):141-153.

[22] Subirade I. (1996) Fate of Ochratoxin A during breadmaking. Food Additives and Contaminants 13:25-26

[23] Romani, S., Pinnavaia G.G and Rosa, M.D. (2003) Influence of roasting levels on ochratoxin A content in coffee. Journal of Agricultural and Food Chemistry 51(17):5168-5171.

[24] Yazdanpanah, H., Mohammadi, T., Abouhossain, G. and Cheraghali, A.M. (2005) Effect of roasting on degradation of aflatoxins in contaminated pistachio nuts. Food and Chemical Toxicology : 43(7):1135-1139

[25] Robertson, (2005), "Consumer and their brands: developing relationship theory in consumer research", Journal of Consumer Research, 24 (4):343-373

[26] Fieider, (1995), Packaging as an Effective Marketing Tool, Pira International, Surrey

[27] Institute of Food Technologists (1991). Guiding Principles for Optimum food safety oversight and regulation in the United States Food Technology 52(5):30

[28] Faseyi C O (1996): Effect of Processing, Packaging Materials and Storage Period on the Customer Acceptability of Akara. Nigerian Food Journal 1(14):40-51.

[29] Hicks PA (2003): The Principles of Food Packaging. Chagrin Publisher, Asia, 3rd edition, Pg 12-25.

[30] Ihejirika, G. O., Nwufo, M. I., Ibeawuchi, I. I., Obilo, O. P., Ofor, M. O., Ogbedeh, K. O., Okoli, N. A., Mbuka, C. O., Agu, G. N., Ojiako, F. O., Akalazu, N. and Emenike H. I.. (2015) Effect of Processing and Packaging Materials on the Storability and Microorganisms Associated with Garcinia kola (Bitter kola). Agriculture, Forestry and Fisheries. Special Issue: Environment and Applied Science Management in a Changing Global Climate. 4(3-1)51-58.

[31] Atanda, O.O., Olutayo, A., Mokwunye, F.C., Oyebanji, A. O. and Adegunwa, M. O. (2011) The quality of Nigerian kola nuts African Journal of Food Science 5(17):904-909

[32] Adejumo B.A. and Ola F.A. (2018) The Appraisal of Local Food Packaging Materials in Nigeria Continental Journal of Engineering Sciences 3:13-20

[33] Egwim, E., Amanabo, M., Yahaya, A. and Bello M. In: Makun, A.H, editor. Mycotoxin and Food Safety in Developing Countries: Janeza Trdine 9, 51000 Rijeka, Croatia; 2013. P. 153-180

[34] Esiegbuya O. D. (2015) *Effect of Fungal and Bacterial Contamination on the Quality of Shea Butter and Identification of Sources of Contamination During Processing.* PhD thesis, University of Benin, Nigeria

[35] Darman R.D (2013) Sustainability and Effectiveness of Artisanal Approach to Control Mycotoxins Associated with Sorghum Grains and Sorghum Based Food in Sahelian Zone of Cameroon In: Makun, A.H, editor. Mycotoxin and Food Safety in Developing Countries: Janeza Trdine 9, 51000 Rijeka, Croatia; 2013. P. 137-152

[36] Lillehoj, E.B., Lagoda, A. and Maisch, W.F. (1979) The fate of aflatoxin in naturally contaminated corn during the ethanol fermentation. Canadian Journal of Microbiology 25(8):911-914.

[37] Scott, P.M., Kanhere, S.R., Lawrence, G.A., Daley EF, Farber J.M (1995) Fermentation of wort containing added ochratoxin A and fumonisins B1 and B2. Food Additives and Contaminants 12(1):31-40.

[38] Bennett, G.A, Lagoda, A.A, Shotwell, O.L. and Hesseltine, C.W. (1981) Utilization of zearalenone contaminated corn for ethanol production. Journal of the American Oil Chemists' Society 58(11):974-976.

[39] Wolf-Hall CE, Schwarz PB (2002) Mycotoxins and fermentation—beer production. In: DeVries JW, Trucksess MW, Jackson LS (eds) Mycotoxins and food safety. Springer, New York, pp. 217-226

[40] Karlovsky, P., Suman, M., Berthiller, F., De Meester, J., Eisenbrand, G., Perrin., I., Isabelle P. Oswald., Speijers, G., Alessandro Chiodini., A., Recker., T. and Dussort, P (2016) Impact of food processing and detoxification treatments on mycotoxin contamination Mycotoxin Research 32:179-205

[41] Udomkun, P., Wiredu, A.N., Nagle, M., Bandyopadhyay, R., Müller, J. and Vanlauwe. B (2016) Mycotoxins in Sub-Saharan Africa: Present situation, socio-economic impact, awareness, and outlook Food Control 72:110-122

[42] Abt associates Inc (2012) Aflatoxin Contamination and Potential Solutions for Its Control in Nigeria (internet) available from https://pdfs.semanticscholar.org/7ea0/fc926408dc7a90e46cbc464427de613e5cef.pdf

[43] Eskola, M., Kos, G., Elliott, C. T., Hajšlová, J., Mayar, S., and Krska, R. (2019). Worldwide contamination of food- crops with mycotoxins: Validity of the widely cited 'FAO estimate' of 25%. Critical Reviews in Food Science and Nutrition. https://doi.org/10.1080/10408398.2019.1658570

[44] Bathnagar, D. and Garcia, S. (2001). *Aspergillus.* In: Guide to Foodborne Pathogens, Labbe, R.G. and Garcia, S. (Eds), John Wiley and Sons, New York, pp. 35-49.

[45] Omojokun, J,. : Makun A.H, editor. Mycotoxin and Food Safety in Developing Countries: Janeza Trdine 9, 51000 Rijeka, Croatia; 2013. P. 3-38

Chapter 4

# Influence of Indigenous Processing Methods on Aflatoxin Occurrence in Africa

*Abdul Rashid Hudu, Mahunu Gustav Komla and Nelson Opoku*

## Abstract

Aflatoxin is a major mycotoxin naturally produced in plants. Various postharvest treatments such as drying, storage materials and storage conditions have shown to influence the accumulation of this toxin in food crops. Beside indigenous processing methods including fermentation, roasting, and cooking have contributed to the reduction in aflatoxin expression. Although these methods are not used in exclusion, each stage has an inherent impact on the levels of aflatoxin in the final products. This chapter reviewed studies on the use of indigenous processing methods in African against aflatoxin occurrences in traditional foods and beverages.

**Keywords:** aflatoxin, *Aspergillus* species, postharvest, indigenous processing methods, Africa

## 1. Introduction

*Aspergillus* species and its derivative mycotoxins are involved in numerous postharvest losses and health threaten conditions in plants and human. Among *Aspergillus* toxins, aflatoxin is known to carry the most potent carcinogenic activity as a natural product. The isomers aflatoxin B1 (AFB1), aflatoxin B2 (AFB2), aflatoxin G1 (AFG1) and aflatoxin G2 (AFG2) are curial for their varied biological activities [1–3], whereas the transcriptional regulators climate, soil properties, genotype of crops, and daily net evaporation exert their occurrences in food crops [3, 4]. Globally, their negative impact on health, social life and economy are more pronounced in developing countries. Consequently, it has been estimated that more than 5 billion people in developing countries are exposed to aflatoxin-associated diseases [5, 6].

Because aflatoxins are xenobiotic to animals and humans, they must consume diet with contaminated aflatoxins. Cereals, spices, oilseeds, tree nuts, and dried fruits exhibits greater susceptibility to aflatoxin contamination with maize and groundnuts being the widely consumed staple foods throughout Africa [7, 8]. Contaminations are influenced by many factors and can occur at any stage of food production (preharvest, harvest, and postharvest storage).

To protect consumers from the harmful effects of aflatoxins, a number of nations and International recognized organizations have established regulations for aflatoxins in food and animal feed. In United States and European Union, the Food and Drug Administration has established maximum limits of 20 μg/kg and 4 μg/kg respectively. At the moment few regulations on aflatoxin exit in Africa, as a result majority of these countries live on the Joint FAO/WHO Expert Committee on Food Additive (JECFA) recommendation of 2 μg/kg body-weight per day [9, 10].

Processing methods and conditions, which are heavily influenced by multitudinous intrinsic and extrinsic factors are supposed to be involved in degrading and reducing aflatoxins levels in foods and beverage to safe and standards levels. Therefore, this review focuses on advances in the elucidation of activities of aflatoxin by indigenous processing methods. Furthermore, it summarizes the impact of variations in indigenous processing conditions in aflatoxins degradation [10, 11].

## 2. Postharvest factors affecting *Aspergillus* and aflatoxin production in grain

### 2.1 Water activity and temperature

Fungal growth and their corresponding mycotoxin production are controlled by several factors including temperature, water availability, pH, light and nature of substrate, which vary among species to species and isolated strains. Although it has become difficult to describe a set of optimum conditions for growth and production of mycotoxins, it has generally been agreed that adequate amount of moisture and temperature are crucial for aflatoxin biosynthesis in cereal and legumes during storage [12].

Reports on minimum and optimum water activity levels required for aflatoxin production differs among authors, but are within the range of 0.78 to 0.84 for *Aspergillus flavus*; and 0.81 to 0.82 for *Aspergillus parasiticus*, with 0.95 to 0.99 optimum for both strains [10–15]. Regarding to temperature, data suggest aflatoxin production occur at a range of 28 °C to 35 °C [15].

### 2.2 Storage methods on aflatoxin occurrence

It is well documented that storage systems and the length of storage increase fungal infestation of grains and their subsequent production of mycotoxins [14, 15]. Despite the suggestion that there is a limited increase in aflatoxin contamination of grain from field to storage [16], it has been argued that more than 6 months storage length assures efficient growth of *Aspergillus* species and significant production of Aflatoxin in maize under Africa's storage methods through increase moisture level [17, 18].

Although it is arguable that the increased aflatoxin occurrence in stored grains is simply due to the increased favorable environmental conditions for *Aspergillus* activities, it has clearly been shown that storage structure and material types affects *Aspergillus* species activities and aflatoxin occurrence (**Figure 1**). Conventional to most traders and rural households in Africa, grains are stored in jute sack or plastic sack. *Aspergillus flavus* prevalence was 51% and 56% higher in maize stored in plastic sack (18%) or hanging shed (13%) compared to those stored in jute sacks [19]. Consequently in Ghana, aflatoxin occurrence in maize grains stored in jute sack was higher (about 55%) compared to grains stored in polyethylene sack [20]. This was also indicated for groundnut stored in jute sacks for 2 months that demonstrate a higher aflatoxin occurrences (148.21 ppb) than their counterpart stored in interlaced polyethylene jute sack [21]. Another study conducted in Tanzania to determine the occurrence of *Aspergillus* species and aflatoxin in maize stored in room (n = 32) and sacks (n = 8) showed that aflatoxin concentration was high in maize stored in room (334.33 μg/kg) than their counterpart stored in sacks (305.76 μg/kg) though the difference was not significant [22].

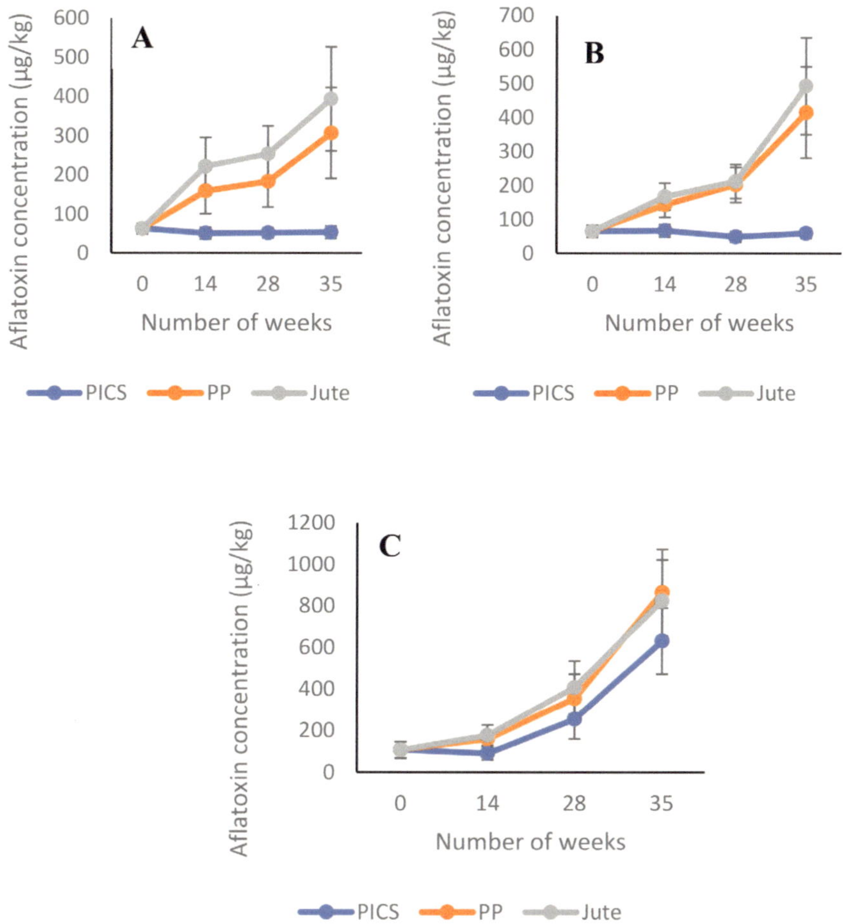


**Figure 1.**
*Total aflatoxin concentration (µg/kg) of maize grain stored in triple layer hermetic bags (PICS), polypropylene (PP) and jute sack for 35 weeks. A = moisture level < 13%, n = 7; B = moisture level between 13% and 14%, n = 13; C = moisture level > 14%, n = 7. Source: Ng'ang'a et al. [17].*

Another study conducted by Ng'ang'a et al. [17] to determine the impact of three storage materials on aflatoxin levels under three moisture levels (moisture level < 13%, n = 7; moisture level between 13% and 14%, n = 13; and moisture level > 14%, n = 7) showed that jute sacks and polyethene promoted aflatoxin production in grains stored for 35 weeks under all the moisture levels (**Figure 1**). Similarly, total mold counts in the maize grain was higher in maize grain stored in jute sack and polypropylene sacks [17].

In contrast, a study conducted by Worku et al. [23] did not find significant increased aflatoxin in maize (n = 149) stored in mud mix with teff straw, (13.1 ± 2.3–14.7 ± 2.8 ng/g; n = 33), polypropylene bag (13.7 ± 3.4 ng/g; n = 116). Similar to this distribution of aflatoxin in storage structure, it was shown that highest aflatoxin levels were found in maize stored in polypropylene and nylon sacks compared to those stored in granaries [24].

## 3. Effect of processing methods on aflatoxin reduction in food

A variety of indigenous processing methods have shown to influence aflatoxin content in food and feed. These methods could be physical (cleaning and segregation; roasting; boiling; and milling), chemical or biological (fermentation). Although these methods are not used in exclusion, each stage have an inherent impact on the levels of aflatoxin in the final products [25–28].

### 3.1 Postharvest drying methods on aflatoxin occurrences

Drying methods affects aflatoxin status in grain and is possibly the most important factor that determine subsequent fungal contamination and production of aflatoxin in grain under storage [21, 29]. Regardless of the moisture levels of harvested grains and source of drying energy, the level and rate of production of mycotoxin would partly be influence by drying methods. Indigenous dry methods used in Africa are broadly categories into three main groups; in-field drying, on-platform drying and on-ground drying. In sub-Saharan Africa especial in West Africa, the tradition on-field drying methods where maize cobs and other cereal grains are allowed to dry on the maize plants before harvest has resulted in significant increased fungal infestation, insect damage and aflatoxin concentration [30].

Despite the suggestion that groundnuts dried on clean tarpaulin could reduce aflatoxin concentration compared to the traditional on-ground drying [21], it was recently shown that tarpaulin increased aflatoxin levels of three different varieties of groundnut during dried at two different locations in Ghana [31].

### 3.2 Physical separation

Physical separation (cleaning, and sorting) affects aflatoxin status in processed or raw kernels. Hand picking coupled with floating and density techniques are the most widely home-based indigenous separation methods employed in Africa to remove unwanted and mycotoxin contaminated kernels, while willowing is involved in removing dust and fine particles. The efficacy of these methods varies, depending on the level of contamination of raw materials, maturity of grains and on the percentage of removed grains [26–30, 32, 33]. Physical cleaning and separation procedures, where mycotoxin contaminated kernels are removed from good kernel, can result in 40–80% reduction in aflatoxin levels [26]. Immature shrivelled kernels and dehulled shrivelled immature kernels if not removed can increase total aflatoxin, AFG1, AFB2 and AFB1 levels in processed peanuts kernels by up to 67%, 92%, 94% and 57% respectively [33]. Similarly, Phillips et al. [31] after separating denser peanuts from less dense ones using tap water mentioned that less dense peanuts contain higher aflatoxin contents (21 out of 29 samples) and may increase total aflatoxin levels of processed kernels by 95% (mean aflatoxin concentration decreased from 301 to 20 μg/kg).

Though time consuming, the study of Matumba et al. [34] indicated that hand sorting of maize kernel had greater positive impact on the removal of aflatoxin (97.9%) than separation using the floatation technique (63.4%). Galvea et al. [35] also revealed that blanching of peanuts at 140 °C for 25 minutes facilitated the manual sorting process of aflatoxin-contaminated kernels (86%; discolored and broken kernels) after dehulling. Also it was reported that manual sorting of raw peanuts with baseline aflatoxin content of 300 μg/kg resulting in peanut kernels with no detectable concentration (< 15 μg/kg) [35].

### 3.3 Roasting

Roasting, mainly as dry or oil, are the main types employ in Africa by rural households and communities. Studies have established that initial aflatoxin concentration has a correlational link to aflatoxin reduction during roasting [36]. The results of Martins et al. [37] showed that aflatoxin degradation of roasted groundnut was 81%, 64% and 55% when the baseline aflatoxin concentration was 695 μg/kg, 332 μg/kg and 35 μg/kg respectively. Arzandeh and Jinap [38] observed similar trend in groundnuts with initial aflatoxin concentration of 237 ng/g (% reduction = 78.4), 215 ng/g (% reduction = 73.9%), 68 ng/g (% reduction = 57.3%). This was also indicated for soybeans that malted and roasted aflatoxin contaminated soybeans with initial AFG1 concentrations of 56 μg/g, 45 μg/g and 38 μg/g reduced by 73%, 62% and 61% respectively [39].

Information on the effect of indigenous roasting methods on mycotoxin occurrence is limited in Africa. However, there are some studies on final food products mainly from cereal and legumes processed using indigenous roasting methods. In Sudan, traditionally prepared peanuts better was reported to have $AFB_1$ concentrations ranging from 54.5–101 μg/kg, followed by peanut better from retail stores (14.5 μg/g) and then laboratory prepared peanut butter of 3.3 μg/g [40]. Aflatoxins in Nigerian dry-roasted peanuts sampled from markets, retail shops and street hawkers at different locations exhibited high $AFB_1$ (5–165 μg/g), AFG2 (6–26 μg/g) and AFG1 (2–20 μg/g) [41].

More importantly, Lee et al. [36] pointed out that there is no significant effects in degrading aflatoxins in contaminated grains either by dry roasting or oil roasting as the two method produced uniform effect. Therefore, irrespective of the dominance of a roasting method in a particular locality, consumption of these contaminated food may be minimal.

### 3.4 Boiling, parboiling and bran removal

Kpodo et al. [42] examined aflatoxin reduction among cooked kenkey made from aflatoxin fermented corn dough. Ga kenkey (a sourdough dumpling from Ga and Fante-inhabited regions of West Africa) degrade about 80% and AFB2 and 35% of AFG2 after 30 minutes of cooking. Mtega et al. [43] reported 68.12%, 51.48% and 85.21% reduction in cooked porridge from un-dehulled maize flour, dehulled maize flour and maize meal (*kande*) respectively.

Aflatoxin expression in parboiled samples, mostly rice, have been studied under different experimental condition with resulting conflicting data. Aflatoxin level were reported to be higher in parboiled rice than in raw milled rice, with AFB1 (185 μg/kg) and AFG1 (963 μg/kg) recording higher occurrence rate. With regard to the migration of aflatoxins from the outer layer to the inner layer of rice during parboiling, it was demonstrated that AFB1, AFB2, AFG1 and AFG2 may be transferred from the outer layer into the starchy endosperm of rice [44, 45]. Therefore, there is some indication that soaking time and temperature of soaking promote movement of mycotoxins from one define region to another. More importantly slow heat during parboiling process might enhance the availability of aflatoxins in foods. **Table 1** present data on the influence of boiling, parboiling and bran removal on aflatoxin (μg/kg) occurrence in indigenous African foods.

### 3.5 Effect of fermentation on aflatoxin occurrence

Majority of Africa fermented foods and beverages are obtained through spontaneous fermentation, with varied degree of aflatoxin levels. Assohoun et al. [27] screened for AFB1 (initial level; 2.52 μg/kg); AFG1 (initial level; 2.52 μg/kg); and AFG2 (initial level; 0.33 μg/kg) in raw maize and after fermenting maize for 72 hours. The authors reported aflatoxin levels below detectable limited in all the three aflatoxin variants after 24, 48 and 72 hours of fermentation. Another study conducted by Adelekan and Nnamah [49] to assess the effect of fermentation on aflatoxin content of moldy maize showed 65% reduction in total aflatoxin content

| | | Cooking condition | | | |
|---|---|---|---|---|---|
| **Treatment** | **Product** | **Time (temp °C)** | **Before** | **After** | **Ref** |
| Un-dehulled maize flour | Stiff porridge | - (90) | 4.36 | 1.39 | [43] |
| Dehulled maize flour | | | 1.01 | 0.49 | |
| Maize meal | | | 4.26 | 0.63 | |
| Rice cooker | Plain rice | -(–) | 1.49 | 1.12 | [46] |
| Local method | | 1 h:10 min | 1.49 | 1.23 | |
| Ordinary cooked rice | Plain rice | 20 min (160 °C) | 2.37 | 1.63 | [47] |
| Pressure cooked rice | | | 2.37 | 0.31 | |
| Parboiled with bran | | — | — | 70000 | [48] |
| Polished without bran | | — | — | 39000 | |
| Raw milled with bran | | — | — | 21000 | |
| Polished without bran | | — | — | Trace | |

*—; not reported.*

**Table 1.**
*Influence of boiling, parboiling and bran removal on aflatoxin (μg/kg) occurrence in indigenous African foods.*

| Aflatoxin | Detoxifying microorganism | Strain origin | Place of fermentation | Reduction (%) | Ref |
|---|---|---|---|---|---|
| AFB1 | Indigenous microbial communities | Ogi | Ogi | 40–60.8 | [52] |
| | | Maize meal | Maize meal | 27.5 | |
| | *Lactobacillus brevis* | Kutukutu | kutukutu | 63 | |
| | *Lactobacillus bucheneri* | Kutukutu | Kutukutu | 64.2 | |
| | *Lactobacillus rhamnosus, Saccharomyces thermophilus* | Commercial strain | Kwete | 92–100 | [52] |
| | *Sacharromyces lactis and Lactobacillus delbrueckii* | Commercial strain | Maize meal | 75 | [50] |
| AFB2 | *Indigenous microbial communities* | Ogi | Ogi | 68–82.8 | [50] |
| | *Lactobacillus rhamnosus, Saccharomyces thermophilus* | Commercial strain | Kwete | 91.8–100 | [52] |
| AFG1 | *Lactobacillus brevis* | Milk | — | 33–53 | [53] |
| | *Lactobacillus acidophilus* | Food Research Institute, Canada | Milk | 33–53 | |
| AFG2 | *Lactobacillus acidophilus* | Food Research Institute, Canada | — | 46–68 | [53] |
| | *Lactobacillus casei* | Lab strain | — | 46–68 | |

| Aflatoxin | Detoxifying microorganism | Strain origin | Place of fermentation | Reduction (%) | Ref |
|---|---|---|---|---|---|
| Total aflatoxin | *Indigenous microbial communities* | Mawe | Mawe | >92 | [54, 55] |
| | | Ogi | Ogi | 80 | [51] |
| | *Lactobacillus acidophilus* | Ogi | Maize | 37.5 | [51] |
| | *Lactobacillus brevis* | Ogi | Maize | 75 | [51] |
| | *Lactobacillus casei* | Ogi | Maize | 62.5 | [51] |
| | *Lactobacillus delbrueckii* | Ogi | Maize | 56.3 | [51] |
| | *Lactobacillus plantarum* | Ogi | Maize | 95 | [51] |

*Ref; Reference.*

**Table 2.**
*Binding capacity of Lactobacillus spp. and yeast to aflatoxins during fermentation.*

| Treatment | Product | Aflatoxin type and levels (μg/kg) | | | | | Ref |
|---|---|---|---|---|---|---|---|
| | | AFB1 | AFB2 | AFG1 | AFG2 | Total | |
| No fermentation | Raw maize kernel | 2.25 | ND | 2.25 | 0.33 | 0.77–4.59 | [27] |
| 24 hours fermentation | Dough | ND | ND | ND | ND | 0.5 | |
| 48 hours fermentation | Dough | ND | ND | ND | ND | ND | |
| 72 hours fermentation | Dough | ND | ND | ND | ND | ND | |
| No fermentation | Raw maize kernels | 69.80 | 4.5 | — | — | — | [42] |
| 24 hours fermentation | Steeped kernel, wet milled | 117 | 11.50 | — | — | — | |
| 24 hours fermentation | Fermented Dough (Lab fermentation) | 206 | 18.90 | — | — | — | |
| 48 hours fermentation | Fermented Dough (Lab fermentation) | 270 | 22.20 | — | — | — | |
| 72 hours fermentation | Fermented Dough (Lab fermentation) | 290 | 25.50 | — | — | — | |
| 24 hours fermentation | Fermented dough (sample from processing site) | 106.1 | 6.7 | 21.7 | 2.4 | 135.4 | |
| No treatment | Raw sorghum | — | — | — | — | 1.70–3.0 | [25] |
| | Malted sorghum for *thobwa* | — | — | — | — | 6.10–54.6 | |
| | *Thobwa* | — | — | — | — | 2.1–7.1 | |

| Treatment | Product | Aflatoxin type and levels (μg/kg) | | | | | Ref |
|---|---|---|---|---|---|---|---|
| | | AFB1 | AFB2 | AFG1 | AFG2 | Total | |
| | Malted sorghum for beer | — | — | — | — | 4.3–1138.8 | |
| | Beer | — | — | — | — | 8.8–34.5 | |
| No spike, no starter | *Kwete* | 0 | 0 | 0 | 0 | 0 | [50] |
| No spike, starter | *Kwete* | 0 | 0 | 0 | 0 | 0 | |
| Spike, no starter | *Kwete* | 2.40 | 1.10 | 2.4 | 1.1 | 7 | |
| Spike, starter, no fermentation | *Kwete* | 2.40 | 1.20 | 2.40 | 0.90 | 6.90 | |
| Spike, starter, 12 hours fermentation | *Kwete* | 0.20 | 0.10 | 0.20 | 0.10 | 0.60 | |
| Spike, starter, 24 hours fermentation | *Kwete* | 0 | 0 | 0 | 0 | 0 | |

*ND; not detected, --; not analyzed, Ref.; reference.*

**Table 3.**
*Summary of studies on aflatoxin levels as influenced by fermentation.*

after 24 hours of fermentation, subsequent fermentation (48 and 72 hours) yield levels below detectable limits. On the other hand, Kpodo et al. [42] reported 40.3% and 60.9% increase in AFB1 and AFB2 contents respectively, in maize dough after 24 hours of fermentation. Subsequent fermentation of this 24-hour fermented dough also led to increase AFB1 and AFB2.

In recent times, the use of starter cultures aimed at reducing aflatoxin concentrations in indigenous fermented foods and beverage have been investigated. Since these cultures could exclusively bind to specific toxins [39, 40], *Lactobacillus rhamnosus* have shown to have as high as 83% binding affinity for AFB1, resulting significant reduction of AFB1, AFB2, AFG1 and AFG2 in *kwete* [50]. Chaves-López et al. [51] reviewed several studies that have isolated various microbial populations from indigenous fermented foods and beverages, majority of which belong to *Saccharomyces* and *Lactobacillus* species. **Table 2** present summary of binding capacities of *Lactobacillus* spp. and yeast commonly isolated from indigenous foods to aflatoxins during fermentation.

Aflatoxin detoxification during fermentation is achieved through microbial binding and/or biotransformation of aflatoxin into less toxic substances. This binding capacity of microbial consortium to aflatoxins are influenced by acidic medium (optimum pH of 6) and temperature (30 °C) associated with noncovalent binding of aflatoxins to cell wall of bacteria and yeast [56]. Aflatoxin degradation and/or biotransformation of aflatoxin during fermentation of indigenous food and beverages have been reported and summarized in **Table 3**.

## 4. Conclusions

There are many indigenous approaches to reduce aflatoxins occurrence in food, feed and beverage. If prevention techniques during postharvest treatments do not fully avoid aflatoxins contamination, indigenous decontamination methods such as cleaning, milling, roasting, cooking, dehulling and fermentation can help remove significant part of aflatoxins. Microbial fermentation is the most promising technology as it enhances consumer acceptability and limit nutrients losses. This chapter has highlighted the link between diverse indigenous processing methods used by rural households and communities with aflatoxin degradation and reduction of toxicity in processed foods and beverages.

## Conflict of interest

The authors declare no conflict of interest.

## Author details

Abdul Rashid Hudu[1]*, Mahunu Gustav Komla[2] and Nelson Opoku[1]

1 Faculty of Biosciences, Department of Biotechnology, University for Development Studies, Tamale, Ghana

2 Faculty of Agriculture, Food and Consumer Sciences, Department of Food Science and Technology, University for Development Studies, Tamale, Ghana

*Address all correspondence to: abdul.hudu@uds.edu.gh

## References

[1] N. K. Kortei, A. A. Agyekum, F. Akuamoa, V. K. Baffour, and H. W. Alidu, "Risk assessment and exposure to levels of naturally occurring aflatoxins in some packaged cereals and cereal based foods consumed in Accra, Ghana," Toxicol. Reports, vol. 6, pp. 34-41, 2019, doi: 10.1016/j.toxrep.2018.11.012.

[2] J. W. Bennett, M. Klich, and M. Mycotoxins, "Mycotoxins," Clin. Microbiol. Rev., vol. 16, no. 3, pp. 497-516, 2003, doi: 10.1128/CMR.16.3.497.

[3] WHO/FAO, "Codex general standard for contaminants and toxins in food and feed," Codex Stand., vol. 193, pp. 1-48, 1995.

[4] M. A. Achaglinkame, N. Opoku, and F. K. Amagloh, "Aflatoxin contamination in cereals and legumes to reconsider usage as complementary food ingredients for Ghanaian infants: A review," *J. Nutr. Intermed. Metab.*, vol. 10, pp. 1-7, 2017, doi: 10.1016/j.jnim.2017.09.001.

[5] H. Strosnider *et al.*, "Workgroup report: Public health strategies for reducing aflatoxin exposure in developing countries," *Environ. Health Perspect.*, vol. 114, no. 12, pp. 1898-1903, 2006, doi: 10.1289/ehp.9302.

[6] J. H. Williams, "Human aflatoxicosis in developing countries_ a review of toxicology, exposure, potential health consequences, and interventions _ The American Journal of Clinical Nutrition _ Oxford Academic," *Am. J. Clin. Nutr.*, vol. 80, no. 5, pp. 1106-1122, 2004.

[7] N. Ali, N. H. Hashim, and N. S. Shuib, "Natural occurrence of aflatoxins and ochratoxin A in processed spices marketed in Malaysia," *Food Addit. Contam. - Part A Chem. Anal. Control. Expo. Risk Assess.*, vol. 32, no. 4, pp. 518-532, 2015, doi: 10.1080/19440049.2015.1011712

[8] M. Rezaei *et al.*, "An Empirical Study on Aflatoxin Occurrence in Nuts Consumed in Tehran, Iran 2013," *Health (Irvine. Calif).*, vol. 06, no. 08, pp. 649-653, 2014, doi: 10.4236/health.2014.68084.

[9] EFSA, "Opinion of the Scientific Panel on Contaminants in the Food Chain on a request from the commission related to the potential increase of consumer health risk by a possible increase of the existing maximum levels for aflatoxin in almonds, and pistachios and," *EFSA J.*, vol. 446, pp. 1-127, 2007

[10] J. Akello *et al.*, "Prevalence of Aflatoxin- and Fumonisin-Producing Fungi Associated with Cereal Crops Grown in Zimbabwe and Their Associated Risks in a Climate Change Scenario," *Foods*, vol. 10, no. 287, pp. 1-18, 2021.

[11] N. Opoku, M. A. Achaglinkame, and F. K. Amagloh, "Aflatoxin content in cereal-legume blends on the Ghanaian market far exceeds the permissible limit," *Food Secur.*, vol. 10, no. 6, pp. 1539-1545, 2018, doi: 10.1007/s12571-018-0849-5.

[12] K. Hell and C. Mutegi, "Aflatoxin control and prevention strategies in key crops of Sub-Saharan Africa.," *African J. Microbiol. Res.*, vol. 5, no. 5, pp. 459-466, 2011, doi: 10.5897/AJMR10.009.

[13] F. Fleurat-lessard, "Integrated management of the risks of stored grain spoilage by seedborne fungi and contamination by storage mould mycotoxins e An update," *J. Stored Prod. Res.*, vol. 71, pp. 22-40, 2017, doi: 10.1016/j.jspr.2016.10.002.

[14] W. G. Sorenson, C. W. Hesseltine, and O. L. Shotwell, "Effect of temperature on production of aflatoxin on rice by Aspergillus flavus," Mycopathol Mycol., vol. 33, pp. 49-55, 1966.

[15] M. Mannaa and K. D. Kim, "Mycobiology Influence of Temperature and Water Activity on Deleterious Fungi and Mycotoxin Production during Grain Storage," *Mycobiology*, vol. 45, no. 4, pp. 240-254, 2017, doi: 10.5941/MYCO.2017.45.4.240.

[16] A. Seetha *et al.*, "Occurrence of aflatoxins and its management in diverse cropping systems of central Tanzania," *Mycotoxin Res.*, vol. 33, no. 4, pp. 323-331, 2017, doi: 10.1007/s12550-017-0286-x.

[17] J. Ng'ang'a, C. Mutungi, S. Imathiu, and H. Affognon, "Effect of triple-layer hermetic bagging on mould infection and aflatoxin contamination of maize during multi-month on-farm storage in Kenya," *J. Stored Prod. Res.*, vol. 69, pp. 119-128, 2016, doi: 10.1016/j.jspr.2016.07.005.

[18] A. N. Kaaya and W. Kyamuhangire, "The effect of storage time and agroecological zone on mould incidence and aflatoxin contamination of maize from traders in Uganda," *Int. J. Food Microbiol.*, vol. 110, no. 3, pp. 217-223, 2006, doi: 10.1016/j.ijfoodmicro.2006.04.004.

[19] E. N. K. Sowley, F. Kankam, and E. Tawiah, "Comparative Study on the Incidence of Aspergillus flavus in Farmer's Field and Stored Maize (Zea mays) Seed in Northern Region of Ghana," *Asian Plant Res. J.*, no. January 2020, pp. 1-7, 2018, doi: 10.9734/aprj/2018/v1i226269.

[20] E. N. K. Sowley, F. Kankam, and P. Ahenkan, "Preliminary study on aflatoxin contamination of maize (Zea mays ) grains in two districts of Northern Region of Ghana Elias Nortaa Kunedeb Sowley, Frederick Kankam, Ahenkan Pious" *Ghana J. Hortic.*, vol. 14, no. 1, pp. 48-55, 2019.

[21] K. Ahiakpa, A. Yeboah, and L. D. Board, "Aflatoxin levels in seeds of commonly grown groundnut varieties ( Arachis hypogaea L .) in Ghana as influenced by storage method," *African J. Food, Agric. Nutr. Dev.*, vol. 20, no. 1, pp. 15402-15414, 2020, doi: 10.18697/ajfand.89.18335.

[22] R. Mboya, P. Tongoona, K. S. Yobo, J. Derera, M. Mudhara, and A. Langyintuo, "The quality of maize stored using roof and sack storage methods in Katumba Ward, Rungwe District, Tanzania: Implications on household food security," *J. Stored Prod. Postharvest Res.*, vol. 2, no. 9, pp. 189-199, 2011.

[23] A. F. Worku, M. Abera, and K. K. Kalsa, "Occurrence of Mycotoxins in Stored Maize in Ethiopia," *Ethiop. J. Agric. Sci.*, vol. 29, no. 2, pp. 31-43, 2019.

[24] M. Mohamed, "Factor influencing aflatoxin contamination in maize at harvest and during storage in Kongwa district, Tanzania," Sokoine University of Agriculture, 2017.

[25] L. Matumba, M. Monjerezi, E. B. Khonga, and D. D. Lakudzala, "Aflatoxins in sorghum , sorghum malt and traditional opaque beer in southern Malaw," *Food Control*, vol. 22, no. 2, pp. 266-268, 2011, doi: 10.1016/j.foodcont.2010.07.008.

[26] D. L. Park, "Effect of processing on aflatoxin," *Adv. Exp. Med. Biol.*, vol. 504, pp. 173-179, 2002.

[27] M. C. N. Assohoun, T. N. Djeni, M. Koussémon-camara, and K. Brou, "Effect of Fermentation Process on Nutritional Composition and Aflatoxins Concentration of Doklu , a Fermented Maize Based Food," *Food Nutr. Sci.*, vol. 4, pp. 1120-1127, 2013.

[28] D. Jordan *et al.*, "Evaluating Improved Management Practices to Minimize Aflatoxin Contamination in the Field, During Drying, and in Storage in Ghana," *Peanut Sci.*, vol. 47, pp. 72-80, 2020, doi: 10.3146/ps20-3.1.

[29] K. Hell, K. F. Cardwell, M. Setamou, and H. M. Poehling, "The influence of storage practices on aflatoxin contamination in maize in four agroecological zones of Benin, West Africa," *J. Stored Prod. Res.*, vol. 36, no. 4, pp. 365-382, 2000, doi: 10.1016/S0022-474X(99)00056-9.

[30] A. N. Kaaya, H. L. Warren, S. Kyamanywa, and W. Kyamuhangire, "The effect of delayed harvest on moisture content , insect damage , moulds and aflatoxin contamination of maize in Mayuge district of Uganda," *J. Sci. Food Agric.*, vol. 85, pp. 2595-2599, 2005, doi: 10.1002/jsfa.2313.

[31] T. D. Phillips, B. A. Clement, and D. L. Park, Approaches to Reduction of Aflatoxins in Foods and Feeds. ACADEMIC PRESS, INC., 1994.

[32] E. Zuza, A. Muitia, M. I. V. Amane, R. L. Brandenburg, A. Emmott, and A. M. Mondjana, "Effect of Harvesting Time and Drying Methods on Effect of Harvesting Time and Drying Methods on Aflatoxin Contamination in Groundnut in Mozambique Aflatoxin Contamination in Groundnut in Mozambique," in *Mycotoxins-Impact and Management Strategies*, Intech Open Access Publisher: Rijeka, Croatia., 2018, pp. 26-39.

[33] G. Anyebuno, "Effect of manual sorting on Aflatoxins content in peanuts (Arachis Hypogaea, L.) from a Ghanaian market," *Ghana J. Agric. Sci.*, vol. 52, no. 1, pp. 5-15, 2018.

[34] L. Matumba, C. Van Poucke, E. Njumbe Ediage, B. Jacobs, and S. De Saeger, "Effectiveness of hand sorting, flotation/washing, dehulling and combinations thereof on the decontamination of mycotoxin-contaminated white maize," *Food Addit. Contam. - Part A*, vol. 32, no. 6, pp. 960-969, 2015, doi: 10.1080/19440049.2015.1029535.

[35] F. C. F. Galvez, M. L. D. L. Francisco, B. J. Villarino, A. O. Lustre, and A. V. A. Resurreccion, "Manual Sorting to Eliminate Aflatoxin from Peanuts," *J. Food Prot.*, vol. 66, no. 10, pp. 1879-1884, 2003, doi: 10.4315/0362-028X-66.10.1879.

[36] L. S. Lee, A. F. Cucullu, A. O. Franz, and W. A. Pons, "Destruction of Aflatoxins on Peanuts," *J. Food Prot.*, vol. 50, no. 6, pp. 504-508, 1987.

[37] L. M. Martins, A. S. Sant'Ana, B. T. Iamanaka, M. I. Berto, J. I. Pitt, and M. H. Taniwaki, "Kinetics of aflatoxin degradation during peanut roasting," *Food Res. Int.*, vol. 97, pp. 178-183, 2017, doi: 10.1016/j.foodres.2017.03.052.

[38] S. Arzandeh and S. Jinap, "Effect of initial aflatoxin concentration, heating time and roasting temperature on aflatoxin reduction in contaminated peanuts and process optimization using response surface modeling.," *Int. J. Food Sci. Technol.*, vol. 46, pp. 485-491, 2011.

[39] A. S. Hamada and E. Megalla, "Effect of malting and roasting on reduction of aflatoxin in contaminated soybeans," *MycopathologiaMycopathologia*, vol. 79, no. 1, pp. 3-6, 1982, doi: 10.1007/BF00636174.

[40] S. Z. B. Elshafie, A. ElMubarak, S. A. F. El-Nagerabi, and A. E. Elshafie, "Aflatoxin B 1 Contamination of Traditionally Processed Peanuts Butter for Human Consumption in Sudan," *Mycopathologia*, 2010, doi: 10.1007/s11046-010-9378-2.

[41] S. A. Bankole and D. A. Eseigbe, "Aflatoxins in Nigerian dry-roasted groundnuts," *Nutr. Food Res.*, vol. 34, no. 6, pp. 268-271, 2004, doi: 10.1108/00346650410568336.

[42] K. Kpodo, A. K. Serensenb, and M. Jakobsen, "The occurrence of mycotoxins in fermented maize

products," *Food Chem.*, vol. 56, no. 2, pp. 147-153, 1996.

[43] M. Mtega, C. A. Mgina, E. Kaale, J. Sempombe, and K. F. Kilulya, "Occurrence of Aflatoxins in Maize and Maize Products from Selected Locations of Tanzania and the Effects of Cooking Preparation Processes on Toxin Levels," *Tanzania J. Sci.*, vol. 2, no. 46, pp. 407-418, 2020.

[44] C. S. Coelho and T. L. Almeida, "Mycotoxin Migration During the Parboiling of Rice," *Brazilian J. Food Technol.*, vol. 2, no. 12, pp. 39-44, 1999.

[45] G. C. Dors, L. Antônio de Almeida Pinto, and E. Badiale-Furlong, "Migration of mycotoxins into rice starchy endosperm during the parboiling process," *LWT - Food Sci. Technol.*, vol. 42, no. 1, pp. 433-437, 2009, doi: 10.1016/j.lwt.2008.03.012.

[46] A. M. Sani, Q. Branch, E. A. Salehi, and Q. Branch, "Reduction of aflatoxin in rice by different cooking methods," *Toxicol. Ind. Health*, vol. 30, no. 6, pp. 546-550, 2012, doi: 10.1177/0748233712462466.

[47] W. P. Je and Y. B. Kim, "Effect of pressure cooking on aflatoxin B1 in rice," *J. Agric. Food Chem.*, vol. 54, no. 6, pp. 2431-2435, 2006, doi: 10.1021/jf053007e.

[48] J. M. R. S. Bandara, A. K. Vithanege, and G. A. Bean, "Effect of parboiling and bran removal on aflatoxin levels in Sri Lankan rice," *Mycopathologia*, vol. 115, pp. 31-35, 1991, doi: 10.4018/978-1-4666-6252-0.ch006.

[49] A. O. Adelekan and N. C. Nnamah, "Effect of Fermentation on Aflatoxin Content of Ogi Produced from Mouldy," *J. Food Process. Technol.*, vol. 10, no. 3, pp. 1-3, 2019, doi: 10.4172/2157-7110.1000783.

[50] A. P. Wacoo *et al.*, "Probiotic enrichment and reduction of aflatoxins in a traditional african maize-based fermented food," *Nutrients*, vol. 11, no. 2, pp. 1-15, 2019, doi: 10.3390/nu11020265.

[51] F. Oluwafemi and F. a Da-Silva, "Removal of aflatoxins by viable and heat-killed Lactobacillus species isolated from fermented maize," *J. Appl. Biosci.*, vol. 16, pp. 871-876, 2009.

[52] C. Chaves-López, C. Rossi, F. Maggio, A. Paparella, and A. Serio, "Changes Occurring in Spontaneous Maize Fermentation: An Overview," *Fermentation*, vol. 6, no. 1, 2020, doi: 10.3390/FERMENTATION6010036.

[53] J. R. Byun and Y. H. Yoon, "Binding of Aflatoxin G1, G2 and B2 by Probiotic Lactobacillus spp.," *Asian-Australasian J. Anim. Sci.*, vol. 16, no. 11, pp. 1686-1689, 2003, doi: 10.5713/ajas.2003.1686.

[54] S. Shukla, H. K. Park, J. S. Lee, J. K. Kim, and M. Kim, "Reduction of biogenic amines and aflatoxins in Doenjang samples fermented with various Meju as starter cultures," *Food Control*, vol. 42, pp. 181-187, 2014, doi: 10.1016/j.foodcont.2014.02.006.

[55] P. Fandohan, D. Zoumenou, D. J. Hounhouigan, W. F. O. Marasas, M. J. Wingfield, and K. Hell, "Fate of aflatoxins and fumonisins during the processing of maize into food products in Benin," *Int. J. Food Microbiol.*, vol. 98, no. 3, pp. 249-259, 2005, doi: 10.1016/j.ijfoodmicro.2004.07.007.

[56] M. Eshelli, L. Harvey, R. Edrada-Ebel, and B. McNeil, "Metabolomics of the bio-degradation process of aflatoxin B1 by actinomycetes at an initial pH of 6.0," *Toxins (Basel).*, vol. 7, no. 2, pp. 439-456, 2015, doi: 10.3390/toxins7020439.

Chapter 5

# Aflatoxins in Mozambican Online Mainstream Press

*Edgar Cambaza, Alberto Sineque, Edson Mongo, Aline Gatambire, Edirsse Mateonane and Raquel Chissumba*

## Abstract

Aflatoxins gained increased recognition in Mozambique due to their negative impact on health, food security, and trade. Most contamination occurs in peanuts, maize, and their products. Nevertheless, there is little awareness, probably because the press and mass media do not disseminate enough information. This study analyzed the quantity and quality of information on aflatoxins in Mozambique's leading online newspapers between 2009 and 2018. After analyzing articles using Atlas.ti, the information was synthesized and compared to scholarly sources. Mozambique requires more press and media coverage of aflatoxin research and development activities. Awareness campaigns should be reinforced, distribute information to multiple organizations, and use multiple means, including online mainstream press, spreading information to reach a broad range of people, given the diversity of cultures and villages' remoteness. Organizations providing information, including universities, need to translate the highly technical information published in scientific journals to help reporters understand the research's implications. Furthermore, there is a need to identify groups that do not receive messages from current campaigns and appropriate methods for reaching those populations.

**Keywords:** aflatoxin, awareness, online, newspapers, Mozambique

## 1. Introduction

In July 2005, experts from the Centers for Disease Control and Prevention (CDC) and the World Health Organization (WHO) created a workgroup to design strategies to minimize aflatoxin exposure in developing countries [1]. They proposed combining activities, some ongoing, grouped into three major categories: preparedness, surveillance, and response. The first category includes education materials and awareness promotion, which shows how important information is to prevent outbreaks of aflatoxicosis. Furthermore, communication favors smooth coordination between the different sectors involved in the mitigation of aflatoxins.

Aflatoxigenic *Aspergillus* spp. are endemic in Mozambique [2]. Aflatoxins have been found in local groundnuts [3], several other commodities [4], and even in chicken giblets [5]. Aflatoxins caused a 2004 outbreak in Eastern Kenya [6–8]. Also, an influential study correlated aflatoxin exposure and hepatocellular carcinoma in southern Mozambique [9]. Thus, people have to be aware of their risk every day by consuming cereals and other grains. Nevertheless, such awareness seems low outside academic circles and even among some scholars [4]. There should be more effort to disseminate information on aflatoxins in Mozambique [10].



IntechOpen

One could argue that nowadays, there is enough scholarly information on aflatoxins in Mozambique, covering aspects such as how widely spread they are, the volume of research, or what to do to control them. There is some truth in that [3–5, 10–12]. However, it is essential to consider that: (1) most scholarly literature is written in English, but the average Mozambican citizen barely understands this language; (2) most Mozambicans have low educational degrees, and they can hardly understand technical terms frequent in academic publications; (3) access to such publications is limited; and (4) it is necessary awareness on aflatoxin to search for information about them in the first place.

The advent of inexpensive online resources and information technologies is unquestionably providing access to information at an unprecedented scale in volume and novelty. Such access is critical in developing countries, where many people can hardly afford printed sources regularly. Mozambique is not an exception, as people actively use mobile phones and other platforms to access online newspapers [13–15]. It will not be surprising if some studies demonstrate wider consumption of online press concerning the printed counterpart. According to Chichava and Pohlmann [16], the social impact of the internet in Mozambique as a source of information increased exponentially. Such impact requires responsibility, and it is essential to know how much effort internet sources, particularly online newspapers, inform citizens in public health matters. This manuscript discusses how much the Mozambican online mainstream press contributes to disseminating citizens' awareness about aflatoxins. Articles related to aflatoxins from major online newspapers were selected and synthesized into a consistent theoretical knowledge body and then compared with scholarly literature.

## 2. Study area

Mozambique (**Figure 1**) is a tropical Southern African country in the region's eastern coastline (Indian Ocean). The country shares its border with Tanzania, Malawi (north), Zambia (northwest), Zimbabwe (west), South Africa, and Eswatini (southwest) [18]. The area is 801,590 $km^{2,}$ and the population 27,909,798 inhabitants, according to the 2017 census [19]. Approximately 68% of the population lives in rural areas [20].

The country's official language is Portuguese, but there are at least 23 local languages. The National Educational System (SNE) is almost entirely in Portuguese [21], with few exceptions, such as the international schools to accommodate international students and basic English and French studies in the secondary and higher education programs. Moreover, the government and the civil society also use Portuguese for all official affairs, including the mainstream press and media.

In Mozambique, the media, associated with Information and Communication Technologies (ICTs), play various roles in society. The Mozambican journalistic landscape includes press, radio, TV, the internet, a community media subsector, community radios and TVs, and the Community Multimedia Center (CMC) [22]. The internet is a significant driver of social change in Mozambique due to communication and information sources [23]. For instance, a daily newspaper costs approximately US $0.34, a price considerably high as the country had 48.4% of people under the poverty line (US $1.90) [24], which worsened after the subsequent economic crisis. Furthermore, the press hardly reaches rural areas, where mobile technologies are gaining stage. Thus, one must expect that rural communities are more reliant on online press than physical.

Another critical feature in Mozambique is its predominantly agricultural economy. Most people in Mozambique live in rural areas, and agriculture plays a crucial

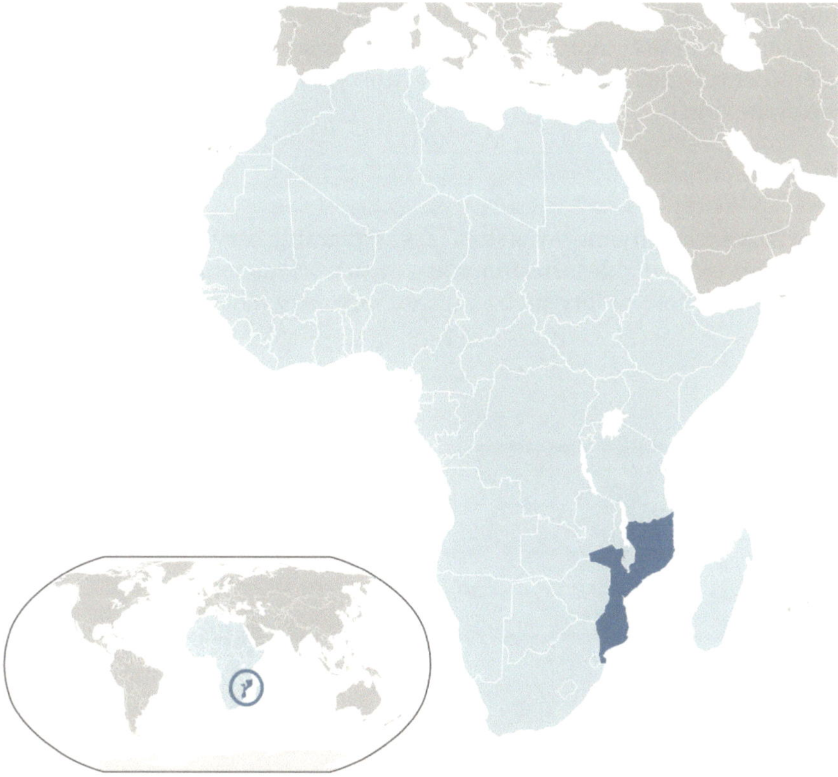

**Figure 1.**
*Location of Mozambique in Africa and the world. Source: Alvaro1984 18 [17], under public domain worldwide.*

role in the Mozambican economy as a source of food for most of the population and a source of income for about 70% of the population [25]. Some cash crops are groundnuts and maize, both susceptible to aflatoxin contamination [4]. According to Abbas [26], food insecurity is more significant in rural areas compared to urban areas due to some factors that occur in cities such as (1) obtaining higher monetary income, (2) subsidized prices of essential goods, (3) greater availability of food due to imports, and (4) more diverse diets. With limited research output and capacity to screen food for aflatoxins, Mozambique should at least spread awareness. The online mainstream press and media are perhaps a good alternative for the highly costly traditional awareness campaigns.

### 2.1 Search strategy

On 11 June 2019, the term "*jornais online de Moçambique*" [Portuguese: online newspapers of Mozambique] was introduced on Google Search™, as **Figure 2** shows, and the resulting links were consulted. Ten consecutive pages of the search were analyzed, and sources matching this research's scope were included, regardless of how many would appear.

#### *2.1.1 Inclusion criteria*

The sources selected were websites belonging to significant publishing entities recognized in Mozambique as such. They could be non-Mozambican, but they had to be written in Portuguese or any national language and have traceable

Mozambican authors or sources, regardless if they were individual or corporate. Bilingual sources were acceptable as long as if at least one of the languages was among mother tongues recognized in the country. The articles included should mention aflatoxins.

### *2.1.2 Exclusion criteria*

The search excluded non-press sites (e.g., streaming services, personal blogs, or social media), unreliable, sensationalist, or suspicious sources due to lack of elements of evidence traceability such as author's identity (corporate were included),

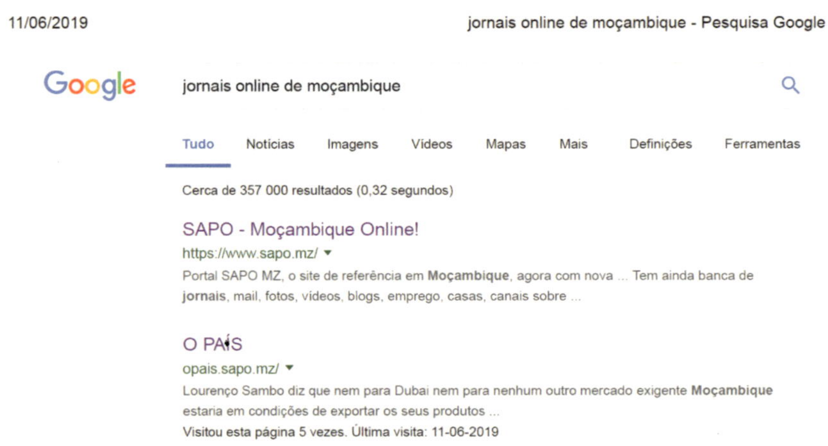
11/06/2019
jornais online de moçambique - Pesquisa Google
Google
jornais online de moçambique
Tudo
Notícias
Imagens
Vídeos
Mapas
Mais
Definições
Ferramentas
Cerca de 357 000 resultados (0,32 segundos)
SAPO - Moçambique Online!
https://www.sapo.mz/
Portal SAPO MZ, o site de referência em Moçambique, agora com nova ... Tem ainda banca de jornais, mail, fotos, vídeos, blogs, emprego, casas, canais sobre ...
O PAÍS
opais.sapo.mz/
Lourenço Sambo diz que nem para Dubai nem para nenhum outro mercado exigente Moçambique estaria em condições de exportar os seus produtos ...
Visitou esta página 5 vezes. Última visita: 11-06-2019

**Figure 2.**
*Google search page showing results for* "jornais online de Moçambique."

| Year | Newspaper | Author | Title* |
|---|---|---|---|
| 2009 | *@Verdade* | @Verdade [27] | Laboratory starts tests with corn and beans |
| 2009 | *@Verdade* | @Verdade [28] | PMA helps to build 300 improved barns |
| 2012 | *@Verdade* | @Verdade [29] | After a strong draught, corn flow is changed in the US |
| 2013 | *Sapo Notícias* | Lusa [30] | Mozambique will produce biocontrol products to reduce toxins and post-harvest losses |
| 2013 | *Notícias* | Notícias [31] | Post-harvest losses: Mozambique starts producing biocontrol products |
| 2015 | *@Verdade* | @Verdade [32] | Approximately 420.000 people die yearly due to unhealthy food |
| 2015 | *Notícias* | Notícias [33] | Africa: Mozambican woman receives a scholarship for agricultural research |
| 2017 | *@Verdade* | Caldeira [34] | |
| 2018 | *Sapo Notícias* | Lusa [35] | US study aflatoxin exposure and undernutrition in Mozambique |
| 2018 | *Notícias* | Notícias [36] | Mozambique launches a study on aflatoxin and chronic undernutrition |

**Titles are translated from Portuguese.*

**Table 1.**
*List of online newspapers with publications mentioning aflatoxins in Mozambique.*

year of publication, titles, name of the publisher and contact. Sites with unidentified sources or no evidence that the information was collected from Mozambican primary sources and article duplicates were also excluded.

### 2.2 Data extraction

Several websites matched the general search, but only 15 were considered online newspapers according to the criteria considered for this study. Among them, only 3 had articles mentioning aflatoxins and, again, fulfilling the criteria (**Table 1**). After that, the software Atlas.ti 8.1 was used to summarize the general information related to aflatoxins in the selected articles. Quotes were codified as etiology and contaminated food, epidemiology and susceptible groups, detection and control, impact, resources, and regulation. The information was reorganized and written as a coherent synthesis using the "code forest" tool.

It is essential to clarify that the synthesis is written for academic purposes. The way its information is organized does not correspond to the chronological order in which the newspaper contents were presented. Some reinterpretation was necessary for the sake of scientific rigor and coherence of the synthesis. Furthermore, the information was translated from Portuguese, implying that the language's idioms and other peculiarities were adapted for English-speaking readers. However, there was an effort to be as faithful as possible to the sources.

## 3. Synthesis

### 3.1 Etiology and sources of contamination

Filamentous molds of the genus *Aspergillus* produce aflatoxins when they grow in food [29, 31, 32, 34]. Aflatoxins can be found in foods like groundnuts, some varieties of maize [27, 34], in cassava [36], beans, and can also be found in cereals like sesame [28].

### 3.2 Geographical distribution and susceptible groups

According to Notícias [31], there are at least 10 African countries where aflatoxins are significant health and agricultural burden: Mozambique, Nigeria, Senegal, Uganda, South Sudan, Burkina Faso, Zambia, Tanzania, Rwanda, and Kenya. The same newspaper added that they all developed biocontrol products for toxigenic *Aspergillus*. The only Mozambican area reported on the online mainstream press was Nampula province [27].

The people most affected by aflatoxins are farmers, either directly consuming contaminated food or indirectly through a deficit in their sales. The market is becoming more demanding in terms of quality and safety [27, 30]. The toxins can also cause livestock losses [29].

### 3.3 Detection and control

Dr. Carla Menezes of the Faculty of Veterinary, Eduardo Mondlane University recommended the citizens to use organoleptic approaches to detect contaminated groundnuts [34] since Mozambique still lacks resources for routine analysis of aflatoxins.

The University of Lúrio (UniLúrio), in Nampula Province, has one laboratory for aflatoxin analyses in maize, beans, and other grains [27]. The World Food Program funded improved barns to local farmers to support production, and perhaps most samples now analyzed at UniLúrio come from the barns and are meant for export [28].

In 2013, Lusa [30] and Notícias [31] reported that Mozambique would start producing and commercializing biocontrol for aflatoxins in 2015. The same sources stated that each country has to develop its biocontrol products, as they are specific for the geographical area. The price is around US $10 per hectare [31].

### 3.4 Risk and impact

Aflatoxins are among the significant foodborne toxicants in the world [32]. However, a recent analysis based on maize at UniLúrio presented low contamination levels [27], suggesting that the toxins do not pose a significant risk for public health in Mozambique and this product. The newspaper, known as @Verdade [27], did not specify such levels. According to Dr. Charity Mutegi, researcher of the Institute of Agricultural Research in Kenya, aflatoxins' actual problem is the widespread lack of awareness among the population [30].

Chronic exposition to subcritical aflatoxin levels does not seem to be a significant concern. However, it increases hepatocellular carcinoma risk [30, 34, 35] and aggravates undernutrition by reducing nutrient absorption, consequently retarding fetal growth [30, 36]. Acute cases include liver damage such as necrosis, hepatic cirrhosis, or edema, sometimes with fatal consequences [30, 31].

Aflatoxins reduce the local market's safe food, compromises export, and such reduction devalues the farmers' efforts throughout Africa [30, 31]. For instance, in 2000, Malawi could not export peanuts to the European markets because the grains had levels above the limit required [31]. With the introduction of the biocontrol product, the farmers are expected to reduce post-harvest losses, thus increasing their income [30].

### 3.5 Resources

In 2018, Lusa [35] reported a joint study about the impact of aflatoxins on food security, conducted by the American Laboratory of Nutritional Innovation of the universities of Tufts and Georgia, and the Mozambican UniLúrio, National Institute of Health and the Association for Nutrition and Food Security. Notícias [36] added that the study was mainly conducted in Nampula City, but it also involved the districts of Angoche, Larde, Malema, Meconta, Mecuburi, Mogovolas, Moma, Monapo, Murrupula, and Rapale.

Very little was said about experts working directly with aflatoxins, although all examples mentioned so far about laboratories and other projects engaged in aflatoxin control [27, 30, 31, 35, 36] imply the involvement of multidisciplinary teams, probably including scholars, researchers, farmers, and possibly government administrative entities. Notícias [33] mentioned the scholarship "African Women in Agricultural Research and Development AWARD 2015", in which 70 scientists working on agriculture were selected to research on several subjects, including aflatoxins. The only expert directly mentioned was Charity Mutegi, from Kenya [31].

### 3.6 Levels and regulation

In Nampula, the World Food Program supports the farmers, but the organization demands the farmers to comply with international requirements to export their maize, groundnuts, and other commodities [28]. Aflatoxin analyses are among such demands, and the results are sent abroad to the clients, who approve and purchase the products.

## 4. Discussion

The number of articles is minimal compared to how frequently these newspapers publish their issues and how long they have been publishing. Their presence in online platforms is recent compared to internationally well-known publications such as The Guardian or New York Times. However, it is hard to explain why the mainstream press barely mentions contaminants in Mozambique's main cash crops. More should be expected in an endemic area for toxigenic *Aspergillus* spp. and "hotspot" of aflatoxin exposure [4, 10]. When compiled, the information seems highly informative and perhaps enough for the ordinary citizen if one regularly reads all these sources. The attentive reader can find high-quality scientific information simplified in a very comprehensive fashion. However, we have to assume that the reader has to "connect the dots" every time he reads about *Aspergillus* spp. and aflatoxins.

### 4.1 Etiology and epidemiological considerations

The most crucial information about etiology and contamination is stated: what causes, which kind of organism it is, and some food where it can be found. They even emphasize groundnuts and maize (two sources mentioning them), which are, in fact, the essential sources as significant staple food and cash crops [4]. Foods like Cassava, beans, sesame, and other cereals have not received a significant concern. However, a survey carried in the country during the 1980s detected aflatoxins in the products mentioned and sorghum, most with levels at least above 4 μg/kg [37]. In this study, cassava flour (12 samples) presented an average aflatoxin level of 28 μg/kg and the median of 40 μg/kg. It should be a serious concern if the post-harvest techniques have not improved.

Regarding the geographical distribution, there is an acceptable degree of accuracy in regards to the countries mentioned are precisely the places where aflatoxins have been reported the most [38, 39], and it is understandable the lack of depth in the information considering the media and their priorities, directed to the general public. It likewise makes sense that Nampula (**Figure 3**) is the only area reported because most export groundnuts are produced there [4].

Nevertheless, it is somewhat misleading for the ordinary citizen because the person might think that aflatoxins occur only in that area. However, aflatoxins have also been found in several types of food from the southern area. There was indeed research by Van Rensburg et al. [32] demonstrating the relationship between aflatoxin exposure and hepatocellular carcinoma in their pioneering research. Furthermore, recent studies by Sineque et al. [5] and Hlashwayo [3] demonstrated that aflatoxins also occur in Maputo, including groundnuts. The evidence so far, and even the common sense, suggest that aflatoxins occur everywhere in Mozambique and the countries around [43]. In any case, Nampula might not be the only area where aflatoxins contaminate groundnuts. However, it still holds a higher significance, considering its relative volume of groundnut production.

The current Mozambican literature does not mention farmers as the primary group exposed to aflatoxins, as two recent reviews discussed [4, 11]. However, it can be deduced since they are the primary food handlers, in contact with the commodities from production until sale in the market, and sometimes they sell

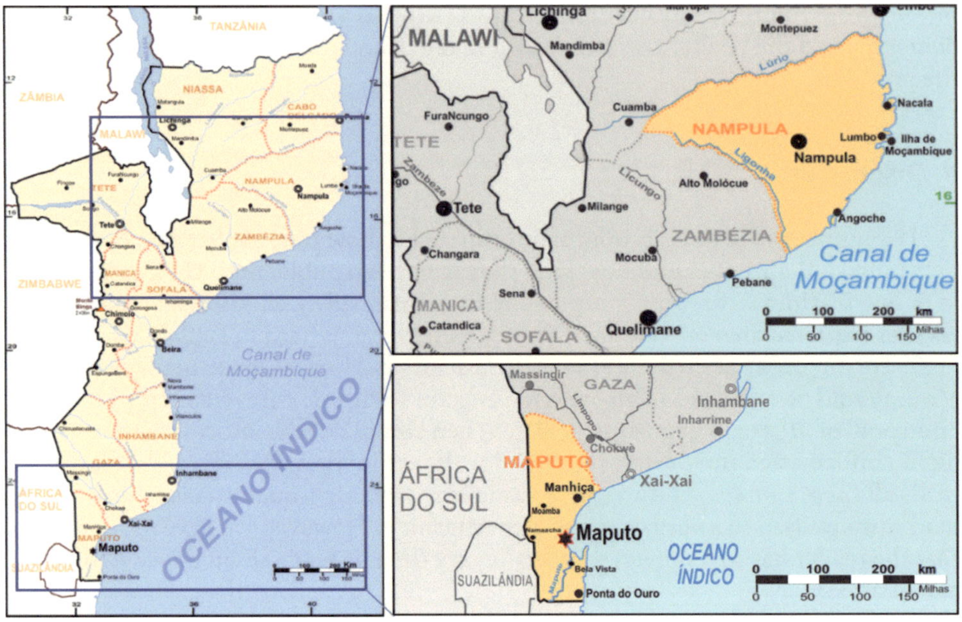


**Figure 3.**
*Draft of the Mozambican map highlighting Nampula province and part of the southern area, where aflatoxin contamination in food has been reported. Adapted from Koehne [40], Koehne [41], and Koehne [42].*

themselves. Furthermore, the market pressure for high quality and safe products, combined with maximized harnessing, leads the farmers to deliver their best product and keep the less safe for themselves or feed their livestock. Such a scenario results in a very high risk for their health and animal production. Indeed, aflatoxins' impact on husbandry cannot be underestimated, as the pioneering study of turkey X disease showed [44], followed by an overwhelming body of evidence [45].

## 4.2 Detection and control

Concerning detection, Dr. Carla Menezes stated in an article from the newspaper @Verdade [34] that the citizens could recognize aflatoxin-contaminated groundnuts when they present "that rancid taste" [in Portuguese]. Visual sorting of damaged grains can help reduce cases of extreme contamination, but Dr. Menezes' recommendation not scientifically sound for the following reasons: (1) there is no evidence that aflatoxins can be detected by testing food; (2) tasting food is not a right approach for toxicological analysis because it compromises the person's safety; (3) groundnut rancidity usually results from hydrolysis or autoxidation of fats into aldehydes and ketones [46, 47], and these processes do not require the presence of *Aspergillus*. However, people still need to avoid rancid groundnuts because they are indicators of spoilage and even safety issues. High moisture (for hydrolysis) and oxidation often result from exposure to water and air, and respectively such media can be sources of contamination or facilitate the process.

Another topic, still related to detection, is Mozambique's increased capacity to detect aflatoxins in food. The aflatoxin analysis laboratory is still the only one certified for aflatoxin analysis in the entire country. However, other laboratories can now perform aflatoxin analysis, and there have been efforts to improve the situation. Cambaza et al. [10] described a few other laboratories with capacity for aflatoxin analysis: National Laboratory for Water and Food Hygiene (LNHAA), also certified, Directorate of Animal Sciences from the Mozambican Institute for Agricultural Research (IIAM), International Institute for Tropical Agriculture (IITA) and Tertiary Polytechnic Institute of Manica (ISPM). IIAM, together with Eduardo Mondlane University (UEM) and the Italian International Cooperation for Development, organized the Workshop for Food Quality Control and Laboratory Accreditation (WQCA) on 28 and 29 November 2019. There were representatives of companies that use quality control services, quality control providers, central laboratories, and technical support providers for accreditation. The Department of Chemistry of the Faculty of Sciences (UEM) also revealed their capacity for aflatoxin analysis, with methods including high-performance liquid chromatography (HPLC) and enzyme-linked immunoassay (ELISA), among others. However, none is accredited by the International Standardization Organization (ISO). Among the significant barriers for accreditation of methods in Mozambique there is a lack of financial means, little support from authorities, and lack of consistent regulation for food quality, safety, and nutrition.

There have been initiatives to control aflatoxins, especially in cash crops destined for foreign markets. The barns of the World Food Organization, reported by the newspaper @Verdade [28], is an example. Such initiatives aim to respond to increasing demands from influential entities such as the European Union. Most limits throughout the world are within the range of 4–20 μg/kg [10], and they do not seem likely to become less demanding in the future. Thus, the most reasonable option is the adoption of sustainable methods to control and mitigate the aflatoxins. Another aspect to consider, often overshadowed by the urge to improve export products, is Mozambique's public health. Indeed, this issue was raised during the WQCA. According to Cambaza et al. [11], early aflatoxin studies were focused on public health due to the internationally very influential study, conducted by Van Rensburg et al. [9] and published in 1985, demonstrating a strong association between aflatoxin intake and hepatocellular carcinoma, in large part based on data collected in southern Mozambique. After that, there was a minimal follow-up in the country, but aflatoxins remained nearly known as a significant public health issue for approximately 15 years until van Wyk et al. [48] drew attention to a new problem: South African companies were no longer purchasing groundnuts from Nampula province because the high aflatoxin content led Europeans to refuse the products. From that moment on, aflatoxin research became mostly motivated by the need to meet international standards rather than a public health issue. In any case, aflatoxin research intensified as a worldwide concern after the 2004 outbreak of aflatoxicosis in Kenya [6], both as a public health matter and a global trade issue. Since most newspapers are directed to the ordinary citizen, it is perhaps for them to prioritize the dissemination of information on aflatoxins related to public health.

Regarding the introduction of the biocontrol agent marketed as Aflasafe™, the coverage seems reasonable. Newspapers Lusa [30] and Notícias [31] covered the information somewhat, indicating the price, benefits, and where to find the product. Furthermore, the US Embassy website in Mozambique also published information about this product in English and Portuguese, making the information more accessible to ordinary citizens. However, very few Mozambican citizens are likely to visit the website, except to search for scholarships and opportunities. Even though there is no direct competition and the commercialization of Aflasafe™ could be technically considered a monopoly, it is a social business, and the benefits of the product to farmers outweigh the fact that these newspapers are freely advertising it in favor of IITA and the US Department of Agriculture (USDA), the investors. Indeed, the product should be further promoted, as it is currently sold in Nampula [49], but aflatoxins' problem is countrywide.

### 4.3 Risk and impact

The extent of aflatoxin's impact on health, economy, and society in Mozambique is unknown, although Cambaza et al. [10] considerably discussed the matter in their recent review. In any case, it seems understandable why there is very little information throughout the mainstream press. It is challenging even for scholars and researchers. Knowledge of the impact requires context-specific information about biological, socio-cultural, and economic variables, and these are different in rural and urban settings. However, the risk is quite well-known among academics, and the same principles are applicable worldwide, requiring only knowledge about acceptable food safety practices throughout the value chain. Local press agents can easily find information about the risk of aflatoxin contamination and its management, even at very comprehensive levels for the ordinary citizen. Thus, Dr. Charity Mutegi was right when she stated that lack of awareness is the major problem in Africa [30]. The authorities should encourage any activities facilitating the dissemination of knowledge about the risk of exposure to aflatoxins.

In one article, @Verdade [32] defined aflatoxins as major foodborne toxicants in the world. This sort of necessary explanation, perhaps slightly more elaborated, is essential and should be part of all newspapers' articles on Mozambique's toxins because there is very little awareness. People should be well aware of the risk, although the press should be careful not to cause panic. Indeed, the fear of panic is possibly among the reasons why aflatoxins have never been considerably mediatized in the country, but not disseminating such important information might lead to the risk of an ill-managed outbreak of acute aflatoxicosis, with people not even knowing about the cause or nature of the disease. Surprisingly, Mozambique shares several natural and cultural features with Kenya, but the 2004 outbreak in Eastern Kenya was bare to non-covered by the Mozambican press. In truth, acute aflatoxicosis cases might be quite common in Mozambique, but the primary symptoms, such as anorexia, malaise, fever, vomiting and abdominal pain [8] indicate several other more common diseases. Even resulting in jaundice and consequent death [6, 8] can result from well-known cases of hepatitis, some endemic, and as frequent in Mozambique [9]. Doctors need skills and tools for differential diagnoses, but this is still a challenge in developing countries.

The newspapers presented specific consequences of aflatoxin contamination in foods and intake [30, 34, 35], and they deserve praise for this reason. They even distinguished clearly features associated with chronic and acute cases in very realistic explanations. They are described in a very comprehensive way, yet using precisely the terminology that even experts would use to explain the general public. The association between aflatoxin intake and undernutrition is still under research in Mozambique, and it is a concern in neighboring countries like Zambia [50]. However, even this information was clearly explained in Notícias [36] newspaper. Furthermore, they described the farmers' socioeconomic consequences as the international market rejects their products. These are two sides of aflatoxin concern already discussed in the previous section (public health and trade issues), seemingly well-covered by the Mozambican online mainstream press.

### 4.4 Resources and regulation

Some online newspapers revealed synergies between Mozambican and foreign organizations for aflatoxin control, some implying large investments enough open laboratories [27], building barns [28], research [35], business [30, 31], and other initiatives. Indeed, in Mozambique, aflatoxins have been gaining interest from academia, researchers, and the industry. Cambaza et al. [11] identified the four major driving forces of aflatoxin research: cancer studies, academic curiosity, international trade, and opportunities (or foreign incentives), the latter two more influential. Unfortunately, the major driving forces come from foreign sources, resulting in very little local control. During the Workshop for Food Quality Control and Laboratory Accreditation, Dr. Ricardo Velho, representative of INSITE (accreditation mediating firm), called for more active involvement of local leaders in the improvement of laboratories in order to properly respond to current challenges. One reason is the lack of a legal framework and a consistent strategy to address food safety issues. It results in clustered information distributed through sporadic, scarcely related reports, and the resulting low awareness outside academic circles [4], and sometimes within such circles. This would be a good point where newspapers could contribute substantially by spreading awareness and sensitizing authorities to take action. One has to understand that leaders have many issues to address, and the less aware they are about some problem, the less likely are they to take any adequate measure.

As it was already mentioned, the newspapers indirectly revealed specialists working on aflatoxin research and other sectors where they are relevant by mentioning organizations contributing to aflatoxin mitigation: Eduardo Mondlane University, UniLúrio and other institutions of tertiary education, the National Institute of Health, Association for Nutrition and Food Security and a few more. Institutions for tertiary education are critical because they annually increase the number of people with knowledge and skills for aflatoxin research. There is no doubt about personnel ready to research aflatoxins in Mozambique [9]. The only problem is the shortage of incentives. Local researchers doing remarkable work on aflatoxins include Anjos et al. [12], Sineque et al. [5], Hlashwayo [3], and others [4, 10, 11, 51]. Some researchers publish their monographs locally and end up not indexing their works in major international databases. Mozambique's major problem is the lack of science writers, people with interest and skills to approach researchers and scholars and comprehensively translate their information to the general public.

The only regulations affecting aflatoxins mentioned in the newspapers were international [28], and they were mentioned indirectly, with little detail. They mentioned the major commodities affected (groundnuts and maize) and how the World Food Program helps enforce such demands. They did not mention that such demands come from the European Union, the United States, other countries and are recommended by Codex Alimentarius [10]. However, this information might not be crucial for the general public, in part because most locals reach these markets through South African companies [48], and it means that farmers only need to deal with these firms' demands. It makes sense that local regulations are not mentioned in the newspapers because, so far, there are no specific Mozambican laws or standards for aflatoxins. This situation could be a good opportunity for the online mainstream press to raise the issue and influence the competent authorities to consider a bill to establish limits for aflatoxins in food. It seems inevitable soon if Mozambique is planning to continue exporting maize, groundnuts, and other grains.

## 5. Conclusion

Mozambique requires more press and media coverage of aflatoxin research. The most relevant features of aflatoxin sources, exposure, intake, control, and consequences seem covered, but the publications should be more frequent and widespread. First, farmers, the most affected people, have very restricted access to the internet. When they do, which are the odds of finding such sporadically published information, assuming they are interested in the periodicals mentioned? The question remains, even if the core target readers are city dwellers concerned with food safety. To a certain extent, the lack of information on Mozambique's aflatoxin situation reflects its limited research. However, there is also little coordination between academia, researchers, industry, and the press. Because the number of students who graduated from tertiary education in 2016 alone was 18,244 [52] and that the great majority writes a research dissertation as a partial requirement for graduation, there is undoubtedly an abysmal disparity between the country's scientific production and the mediatization of the significant findings for the general public, regardless of how significant they are. Thus, scholars, businesspeople, researchers, and journalists should reach out to each other and start a harmonized effort to inform the general public about its scientific progress, significant findings, and events related to aflatoxin research and management.

## Conflicts of interest

The authors declare no conflict of interest.

## Author details

Edgar Cambaza[1*], Alberto Sineque[2], Edson Mongo[3], Aline Gatambire[4], Edirsse Mateonane[4] and Raquel Chissumba[3]

1 Faculty of Health Sciences, ISCED Open University, City of Beira, Mozambique

2 DREAM Sant'Egídio Molecular Laboratory, Comunity of Sant'Egídio, Maputo City, Mozambique

3 Centro de Investigação e Treino em Saúde da Polana Caniço (CISPOC), Rua do Costa do Sol, Maputo, Mozambique

4 Independent Scientist, Mozambique

*Address all correspondence to: ecambaza@isced.ac.mz

## References

[1] Strosnider H, Azziz-Baumgartner E, Banziger M, Bhat RV, Breiman R, Brune MN, et al. Workgroup report: public health strategies for reducing aflatoxin exposure in developing countries. Environ Health Perspect. 2006;114(12): 1898-903.

[2] Augusto J, Atehnkeng J, Akello J, Cotty P, Bandyopadhyay R. Prevalence and distribution of *Aspergillus* section Flavi in maize and groundnut fields and aflatoxin contamination in Mozambique. 2014 APS-CPS Joint Meeting; Minneapolis, Minnesota: The American Phytopathological Society; 2014.

[3] Hlashwayo DF. Aflatoxin B1 contamination in raw peanuts sold in Maputo City, Mozambique and associated factors. Journal of Stored Products. 2018;9(6):58-67.

[4] Cambaza E, Koseki S, Kawamura S. Aflatoxins in Mozambique: Etiology, Epidemiology and Control. Agriculture. 2018;8(7):87.

[5] Sineque AR, Macuamule CL, Dos Anjos FR. Aflatoxin B1 Contamination in Chicken Livers and Gizzards from Industrial and Small Abattoirs, Measured by ELISA Technique in Maputo, Mozambique. Int J Environ Res Public Health. 2017;14(9).

[6] Gieseker KE. Outbreak of Aflatoxin Poisoning - Eastern and Central Provinces, Kenya, January–July 2004. 2004.

[7] Probst C, Njapau H, Cotty PJ. Outbreak of an acute aflatoxicosis in Kenya in 2004: identification of the causal agent. Appl Environ Microbiol. 2007;73(8):2762-4.

[8] Azziz-Baumgartner E, Lindblade K, Gieseker K, Rogers HS, Kieszak S, Njapau H, et al. Case-control study of an acute aflatoxicosis outbreak, Kenya, 2004. Environ Health Perspect. 2005;113(12):1779-83.

[9] Van Rensburg SJ, Cook-Mozaffari P, Van Schalkwyk DJ, Van der Watt JJ, Vincent TJ, Purchase IF. Hepatocellular carcinoma and dietary aflatoxin in Mozambique and Transkei. Br J Cancer. 1985;51(5):713-26.

[10] Cambaza E, Koseki S, Kawamura S. Aflatoxins in Mozambique: Impact and Potential for Intervention. Agriculture. 2018;8(7):100.

[11] Cambaza E, Koseki S, Kawamura S. A Glance at Aflatoxin Research in Mozambique. Int J Environ Res Public Health. 2018;15(8):1673.

[12] Anjos FRD, Ledoux DR, Rottinghaus GE, Chimonyo M. Efficacy of Mozambican bentonite and diatomaceous earth in reducing the toxic effects of aflatoxins in chicks. World Mycotoxin Journal. 2016;9(1): 63-72.

[13] Aker JC, Collier P, Vicente PC. Is Information Power? Using Mobile Phones and Free Newspapers during an Election in Mozambique. The Review of Economics and Statistics. 2017;99(2):185-200.

[14] Mare A. New Media Technologies and Internal Newsroom Creativity in Mozambique. Digital Journalism. 2013;2(1):12-28.

[15] Paterson C, Doctors S. Participatory journalism in Mozambique. Ecquid Novi: African Journalism Studies. 2013;34(1):107-14.

[16] Chichava S, Pohlmann J. Uma breve análise da imprensa moçambicana. In: Brito Ld, Castel-Branco CN, Chichava S, Francisco A, editors. Desafios para Moçambique, 2010. Maputo,

Mozambique: Instituto de Estudos Sociais e Económicos; 2009. p. 127-38.

[17] Alvaro1984 18. File:Location Mozambique AU Africa.svg San Francisco, California: Wikimedia Foundation Inc; 2009 [Available from: https://commons.wikimedia.org/wiki/File:Location_Mozambique_AU_Africa.svg.

[18] Cambaza EM, Mongo E, Anapakala E, Nhambire R, Singo J, Machava E. An Update on Cholera Studies in Mozambique. In: Bacha U, Rozman U, Turk SŠ, editors. Healthcare Access - Regional Overviews. London, UK: IntechOpen Limited; 2020. p. 1-20.

[19] Cambaza EM, Viegas GC, Cambaza CM. Potential impact of temperature and atmospheric pressure on the number of cases of COVID-19 in Mozambique, Southern Africa. Journal of Public Health and Epidemiology. 2020;12(3):246-60.

[20] Cambaza E. A glance at Mozambican dairy research. African Journal of Agricultural Research. 2018;13(53):2945-56.

[21] Lemos AFFC. Língua e cultura em contexto multilingue: um olhar sobre o sistema educativo em Moçambique. Educar em Revista. 2018;34(69):17-32.

[22] Sekelekani. Comunicação e TIC's Maputo, Mozambique: Sekelekani; 2020 [Available from: https://www.sekelekani.org.mz/?page_id=51.

[23] Tsandzana D. Juventude urbana e redes sociais em Moçambique: a participação política dos conectados desamparados. Comunicação e Sociedade. 2018(34):235-50.

[24] World Bank Group. Mozambique Poverty Assessment: "Strong but not Broadly Shared Growth". Washington, D.C., USA: World Bank Group; 2018.

[25] Abbas M. Segurança alimentar. Auto-suficiência alimentar: mito ou verdade? Maputo, Mozambique: Observatório do Meio Rural (OMR); 2017.

[26] Abbas MJRN. (In) segurança alimentar e território em Moçambique: discursos políticos e práticas. 2017;20(38).

[27] @Verdade. Laboratório inicia com testes em milho e feijões Nampula, Mozambique: @Verdade; 2009 [Available from: www.verdade.co.mz/tecnologias/5257-laboratorio-inicia-com-testes-em-milho-e-feijoes.

[28] @Verdade. PMA apoia construção de 300 celeiros melhorados Nampula, Mozambique: @Verdade; 2009 [Available from: www.verdade.co.mz/nacional/5211-pma-apoia-construcao-de-300-celeiros-melhorados.

[29] @Verdade. Depois de uma forte seca, o fluxo do milho é alterado nos EUA Nampula, Mozambique: @Verdade; 2012 [Available from: www.verdade.co.mz/ambiente/31705-depois-de-uma-forte-seca-o-fluxo-do-milho-e-alterado-nos-eua.

[30] Lusa. Moçambique vai produzir biocontrolos para reduzir toxinas e perdas pós colheita: SAPO Notícias; 2013 [Available from: https://noticias.sapo.mz/actualidade/artigos/mocambique-vai-produzir-biocontrolos-para-reduzir-toxinas-e-perdas-pos-colheita.

[31] Notícias. Redução de perdas pós-colheitas: Moçambique passa a produzir biocontrolos Nampula, Mozambique: Sociedade Notícias; 2013 [Available from: www.jornalnoticias.co.mz/index.php/ciencia-e-ambiente/2466-reducao-de-perdas-pos-colheitas-mocambique-passa-a-produzir-biocontrolos.html.

[32] @Verdade. Cerca de 420 mil pessoas morrem por ano por ingerir

alimentos não saudáveis Nampula, Mozambique: @Verdade; 2015 [Available from: www.verdade.co.mz/saude-e-bem-estar/55985-cerca-de-420-mil-pessoas-morrem-por-ano-por-ingerir-alimentos-nao-saudaveis.

[33] Notícias. África: Moçambicana ganha bolsa para investigação agrária Maputo, Mozambique: Sociedade Notícias; 2015 [

[34] Caldeira A. Amendoim tem de ser testado pois pode ter "aflatoxinas que têm potencial cancerígeno" Nampula, Mozambique: @Verdade; 2017 [Available from: http://www.verdade.co.mz/saude-e-bem-estar/61888-amendoim-tem-de-ser-testado-pois-pode-ter-aflatoxinas-que-tem-potencial-cancerigeno.

[35] Lusa. Estados Unidos estudam exposição à aflatoxina e desnutrição em Moçambique: Sapo Notícias; 2018 [Available from: https://noticias.sapo.mz/sociedade/artigos/estados-unidos-estudam-exposicao-a-aflatoxina-e-desnutricao-em-mocambique.

[36] Notícias. Moçambique lança estudo sobre aflatoxinas e desnutrição crónica Maputo, Mozambique: Sociedade Notícias; 2018 [Available from: https://www.jornalnoticias.co.mz/index.php/tecnologias/83102-mocambique-lanca-estudo-sobre-aflatoxinas-e-desnutricao-cronica.

[37] Casadei E. Moçambique: Águas, Alimentos e Ambiente. Rome, Italy: MOLISV; 1980.

[38] Bankole S, Schollenberger M, Drochner W. Mycotoxins in food systems in Sub Saharan Africa: A review. Mycotoxin Res. 2006;22(3):163-9.

[39] Sibanda L, Marovatsanga LT, Pestka JJ. Review of mycotoxin work in sub-Saharan Africa. Food Control. 1997;8(1):21-9.

[40] Koehne A. File:Mozambique map cities.png San Francisco, California, United States: Wikimedia Foundation Inc.; 2007 [Available from: https://commons.wikimedia.org/wiki/File:Mozambique_map_cities.png.

[41] Koehne A. File:Moçambique Nampula map.png San Francisco, California, United States: Wikimedia Foundation; 2007 [Available from: https://commons.wikimedia.org/wiki/File:Mo%C3%A7ambique_Nampula_map.png.

[42] Koehne A. File:Moçambique Maputo.gif San Francisco, California, United States: Wikimedia Foundation; 2006 [Available from: https://commons.wikimedia.org/wiki/File:Mo%C3%A7ambique_Maputo.gif.

[43] Misihairabgwi J, Ezekiel C, Sulyok M, Shephard G, Krska RJCrifs, nutrition. Mycotoxin contamination of foods in Southern Africa: A 10-year review (2007-2016). 2019;59(1):43-58.

[44] Van Der Zijden ASM, Koelensmid WAAB, Boldingh J, Barrett CB, Ord WO, Philp J. Aspergillus Flavus and Turkey X Disease: Isolation in Crystalline Form of a Toxin responsible for Turkey X Disease. Nature. 1962;195(4846):1060-2.

[45] Atherstone C. Assessing the impact of aflatoxin consumption on animal health and productivity. African Journal of Food, Agriculture, Nutrition and Development. 2016;16(03):10949-66.

[46] MatÉ JI, Saltveit ME, Krochta JM. Peanut and Walnut Rancidity: Effects of Oxygen Concentration and Relative Humidity. Journal of Food Science. 1996;61(2):465-9.

[47] Maté JI, Frankel EN, Krochta JM. Whey Protein Isolate Edible Coatings: Effect on the Rancidity Process of Dry Roasted Peanuts. Journal of

Agricultural and Food Chemistry. 1996;44(7):1736-40.

[48] van Wyk P, Van der Merwe P, Subrahmanyam P, Boughton D. Aflatoxin contamination of groundnuts in Mozambique. International Arachis Newsletter. 1999;19:25-7.

[49] U.S. Embassy in Mozambique. Inauguration of IITA's new facilities in the celebration of its 50th year anniversary 2017 [Available from: https://mz.usembassy.gov/inauguration-iitas-new-facilities-celebration-50th-year-anniversary/.

[50] Ismail S, Shindano J, Nyirenda DB, Bandyopadhyay R, Akello J. Does Exposure to Aflatoxin Constrain Efforts to Reduce Stunting in Zambia. 2014.

[51] Cambaza EM, Koseki S, Kawamura S. Aflatoxinas em Moçambique: Impacto e Potencial para Intervenção. Conference: 3° Congresso de Controlo da Qualidade Laboratorial para Países de Língua Portuguesa, (CCQL–PLP), 27 a 31 de Maio de 2019; Maputo, Mozambique: National Health Institute (INS); 2019.

[52] Sociedade Notícias. Multiplica população de graduados universitários em Moçambique Maputo, Mozambique: Sociedade Notícias S. A.; 2018 [Available from: https://www.jornalnoticias.co.mz/index.php/tecnologias/81501-multiplica-populacao-de-graduados-universitarios-em-mocambique.

Section 2

# Aflatoxin Detoxification and Analysis

Chapter 6

# Promising Detoxification Approaches to Mitigate Aflatoxins in Foods and Feeds

*Vishakha Pandey*


## Abstract

Aflatoxins are a group of naturally occurring carcinogenic mycotoxins produced by certain *Aspergillus* species in nuts, grains, oilseeds and vegetables. Ingestion of aflatoxin contaminated food and feed has extremely negative health implications in humans and livestocks. Additionally, exporting countries face the trade barrier due to strict regulations in international market to maintain food quality. This led to huge economic losses to global exporters. Therefore, there is an urgent need for development of effective methods for detoxification of aflatoxins from food and feed to ensure food security. Till date, numerous methods for detoxification of aflatoxins from foods have been employed. Physical, chemical and biological treatment are the novel promising approaches for partial/complete detoxification of aflatoxins from the foodstuffs. In this chapter, we will address the efficacy and shortcomings of each methods in with respect to economic importance, human health and food security.


**Keywords:** Aflatoxin, mycotoxin, carcinogenic, detoxification, food security

## 1. Introduction

Aflatoxins are toxic secondary metabolites, mainly produced by many species of *Aspergillus*, namely *Aspergillus parasiticus, A. flavus, A. nomius,* A. astellatus [1, 2]. They contaminate various crops (wheat, maize, cotton), dried fruits, spices, meat and milk products [3, 4]. Aflatoxins were first discovered as a causative agent of Turkey X disease in early 1960s, led to the death of numerous turkey in England [5]. Generally, *A. flavus* specifically produces B-type aflatoxins while *A. parasiticus* produce B- as well as G-type aflatoxins [6]. Among these four aflatoxins, AFB1 being most dangerous, accounts for more than 75% of all food and feed related aflatoxin contamination [7]. Cytochrome P450 mediated metabolism of AFB1 in liver, resulting in its epoxidation to AFB1-exo-8, 9-epoxide and AFB1-endo-8, 9-epoxide, demethylation to aflatoxin P1 (AFP1) and hydroxylation to aflatoxin Q1 (AFQ1) and aflatoxin M1 (AFM1) [8]. The International Agency for Research on Cancer (IARC) has classified aflatoxin type B and G as Group 1 carcinogen and AF-M1 as Group 2B [9]. Derived from polyketides, consumption of aflatoxin contaminated food and feed cause a range of serious health complications in humans and animals, together named as aflatoxicosis [10, 11]. Short term exposure to high dose of aflatoxins results in jaundice, hemorrhage, liver damage and subsequent death



IntechOpen

and long term exposure to sublethal levels of aflatoxins cause nutritional disorders, immunosuppression, cancer [12].

The challenges related to aflatoxins can be overcome by adopting innovative and novel strategies. The risk of aflatoxins can be reduced by preventing the contamination of foods from aflatoxins at the pre-harvest stage and removing/eliminating the aflatoxins from aflatoxin contaminated food at the post-harvest stage. Prevention strategies, including the use of pesticides, fertilizers, maintaining optimum temperature and moisture for storage, right harvesting time, are only partly responsible for achieving aflatoxin-free food and feed. In order to eliminate aflatoxin completely, post-harvest strategies are followed. The post-harvest strategies include cleaning, sorting, milling and dehulling [13], treatment at temperature between 237 and 306°C [14], mineral binders such as, montmorillonite, zeolite, aluminosilicate, bentonite that bind aflatoxins. Such binders may partially or completely conteract the toxicity of dietary aflatoxins [15]. Elliott et al. [16] have reported the cytotoxic effects induced by mineral binders like DNA damage, reduced cell viability, apoptosis, oxidative stress.

## 2. Novel strategies for aflatoxin degradation

In the past decades, numerous promising novel strategies for aflatoxin mitigation have been developed. They are broadly categorized as physical, chemical and biological approaches. Physical strategies involve the utilization of radiations and cold plasma for the fast aflatoxin degradation [17]. Chemical methods include the treatment with electrolyzed oxidizing water, organic acids, ozone and natural plant extracts. These are methods have been widely used in several countries such as USA and China [18]. Microbial and enzymatic based conversion of highly toxic aflatoxins into less toxic or non-toxic metabolites are included in biological methods [19]. In this chapter, we will address each of these novel technologies for aflatoxin degradation in detail.

### 2.1 Physical treatment for aflatoxins degradation

#### *2.1.1 Irradiation*

In the recent times, ionizing irradiation (viz. electron beam, gamma and ultraviolet rays) and nonionizing irradiation (viz. infrared waves, radio waves, visible light waves and microwaves) has been employed extensively for the degradation of aflatoxin present in the food and feed (**Table 1**).

Electron beam irradiation (EBI) technology has great potential for aflatoxin degradation. EBI technology offers the advantage of high effectiveness, low equipment cost, dosage control, short processing time, low heat generation, few variables and in-line processing [36]. EBI technology has been applied for degradation of aflatoxins in coconut agar [37]. Efficiency of EBI technology for degradation of aflatoxin is lesser than that of γ radiation. Assuncao et al. [20] found that EBI at doses of 10 and 5 kGy decreased the content of AFB1 in Brazilnuts by 65.7 and 53.3%, respectively, whereas γ irradiation at same doses led to reduction in AFB1 by 84.2 and 70.6%, respectively. Liu et al. [21] used EBI dose of 300 kGy for reduction of AFB1 by 70%. As the selected dose was ten times of the maximum permissible dosage allowed by FDA, so this method is not highly efficient and preferable in AFB1 degradation in peanut meal.

Gamma (γ) rays has been the most preferred radiation source for the food owing to its high penetrability and reactivity. Treatment of food by gamma rays of

| Physical Degradation method | Food product treated | Aflatoxin ($\mu g\ kg^{-1}$ or $\mu g\ L^{-1}$) | Degradation Percentage | Parameters for treatment | Reference |
|---|---|---|---|---|---|
| **Electron beam** | Brazil nut | AFB1 (4.8) | 65.7 | 300 kGy | [20] |
| | Peanut | AFB1 (1000) | 70.0 | 300 kGy | [21] |
| **$^{60}$Co gamma Irradiation** | Red chili | AFB1 (11–35) | 86–98 | 6 kGy | [22] |
| | Cattle feed | AFB1 (50) | 85 | 10 kGy | [23] |
| | Corn | AFB1 (57–1210) | 85.6–98.6 | 10 kGy | [23] |
| | Brazil nut | AFB1 (4.8) | 84.2 | 10 kGy | [20] |
| | Peanut | AFB1 (300) | 43 | 9 kGy | [24] |
| | White pepper | AFB1 (60), AFB2 (18), AFG1 (60) and AFG2 (18) | 50.6, 35.2, 47.7 and 42.9 | 30 kGy | [25] |
| | Almond | AFB1 (20), AFB2 (20), AFG1 (20) and AFG2 (20) | 19.3, 11.0, 21.1and 16.6 | 15 kGy | [26] |
| **UV irradiation** | Peanut | AFB1 (2000) | 100 | 220–400 nm at 0.8 mW $cm^{-2}$ for 80 min | [21] |
| | Peanut | AFB1 (350) | 99.1 | 254 nm for 10 h | [27] |
| | Peanut oil | AFB1 (128) | 96 | 365 nm at 55–60 mW $cm^{-2}$ for 20 min | [28] |
| | Peanut oil | AFB1 (52.0) | 86.1 | 365 nm at 6.4 mW $cm^{-2}$ for 10 min | [29] |
| | Peanut oil | AFB1 (2000) | 100 | 220–400 nm at 0.8 mW $cm^{-2}$ for 30 min | [30] |
| | Red chili powder | AFB1 (1872) | 87.8 | 365 nm for 60 min | [31] |
| **Pulsed light** | Rice bran | AFB1 (36) and AFB2 (4.4) | 90.3 and 86.7 | 0.52 J $cm^{-1}$ per pulse for 15 s | |
| | Rough rice | AFB1 (132) and AFB2 (45) | 75.0 and 39.2 | 0.52 J $cm^{-1}$ per pulse for 80 s | [32] |
| **Microwave heating** | Peanut | AFB1 (5–183) and AFB2 (7–46.7) | 50–60 and 100 | Heating in microwave oven at 92°C for 5 min | [33] |
| | Corn flour | AFB1 (100) | 67.7 | Heating in microwave oven for 10 min | [34] |
| | Alkalized corn | AFB1 (22.5) and AFB2 (69.6) | 36 and 58 | 1650 W | [35] |

**Table 1.**
*Physical methods for aflatoxin degradation in food and feed.*

upto 10 kGy has no toxicological, or microbiological hazards [38]. Additionally, γ irradiation results in the interaction of high energy of γ rays with the water present in the food products. This produces highly reactive free radicals such as superoxide radical ($O2\bullet^-$), hydrogen ($H\bullet$) radical and hydroxyl ion ($OH^-$) that in turn destroy aflatoxins and also attack DNA of pathogenic microbes [14, 39]. Markov *et al.* [23] have used high-energy photons from cobalt-60 (gamma source) for destruction of pathogenic microbes by directly damaging DNA of microbial cells.

Many studies in the literature showed that treatment of food commodities with γ rays ranging from 5 to 10 kGy led to degradation of significant amount of aflatoxins. For instance, irradiation with γ rays at low dose of upto 6 kGy has reduced Aflatoxin B1 ($AFB_1$) level in red chillies and fruits for around 90% [22, 40]. The $AFB_1$ level reduced for about 95% in maize seed samples with γ irradiation dose of 10 kGy [23]. AFB1 in Brazil nuts can be eliminated upto 84.2% by irradiation of γ rays at 5 to 10 kGy [20]. Likewise, γ irradiation at dose of 10 kGy decreased ochratoxin A (OTA) in coffee beans and dry-cured meat for almost 100% and 22.5% respectively [41, 42]. Nevertheless, few studies in the literature concluded that γ irradiation could not effectively eliminate aflatoxins in food. For e.g. irradiation of black and white pepper with γ rays at 10 kGy dose has no significant effect on its aflatoxins content [25]. Gamma irradiation of poultry feed at 15 kGy dose resulted in 13.6, 11.0, 21.1, 18.2% decrease in AFG2, AFB2, AFG1 and AFB1, respectively [43]. However, the efficiency of γ rays - mediated aflatoxin degradation depends on numerous factors such as concentration of mycotoxin, dose of radiation, content of water, air humidity, composition of food and type and number of fungal strains [25, 39].

The advantage γ irradiation offers is high capacity for microbial inactivation that reduces the microbial load and increases shelf life of food. Gamma irradiation technology has been approved by more than 55 countries such as Japan, USA, European countries, China for food processing [44]. This technology is not preferable with high vitamin and lipid content because polyunsaturated fatty acids undergo extensive peroxidation in unsaturated bonds, leading to increased oxidative rancidity [45].

Apart from being an economical non-thermal technology for Alfatoxin decontamination, Ultraviolet (UV) irradiation is also highly cost effective and eco-friendly [46]. Treatment of food products with moderate doses of UV rays has no negative impact on its sensory and physicochemical properties [47]. Though UV rays can efficiently penetrate into transparent or clear liquids, its penetration efficiency through solids is limited. Therefore, granular or opaque foods has to be in the form of thin layer for decontamination by UV rays [48]. UV light effectively removed of Patulin (PAT) from apple cider and juice. Zhu et al. [49] have used different wavelengths of UVC for PAT reduction in apple juice. They found UVC of 222 nm wavelength was most effective. Exposure to UV affected the taste of apple cider and juice. Intensity and duration of UV irradiation are important factors that affect the elimination efficiency of aflatoxins elimination efficiency Irradiation with short wavelenght (254 nm) and long wavelength (362 nm) UV rays for 30 minutes resulted in complete elimination of AF-B1 and AF-G1 in wheat grains, whereas exposure to same dose of short and long wavelength of UV rays for 2 hours reduced AF-B2 in wheat grains by 50 and 74% respectively [50]. Exposure of pistachio, almond and groundnut with UVC at 265 nm for 15 minutes led to 100% removal of AF-G2 from all the nut samples and complete degradation of AF-G1 in pistachio and almond. UV-C irradiation at 265 nm for 45 minutes showed 97% degradation of AF-B1 [51]. Treatment with UV-A and UV-B rays can also be used for reduction of mycotoxins produced from *A. parasiticus* and *A. carbonarius* in pistachio and grape media [52].

Non-thermal Pulsed light (PL) technology has been used for degradation of aflatoxins in food and feed. This FDA-approved technology generates short, high-intensity flashes of broad spectrum light (100–1100 nm) including UV, visible and IR radiation that destroy the nucleic acid and cell wall structure of microbes within few seconds [53]. Eight PL flashes of 1 J $cm^{-2}$ during 300 ms flash resulted in degradation of AFB1 in water by 92.7% [54]. In another study, PL at 0.52 J $cm^{-1}$ per pulse was applied for 80 seconds and 15 seconds to treat rough rice and bran, respectively. It was observed that on 15 seconds of PL treatment AFB1 and AFB2 in rice bran reduced by 90.3 and 86.7% respectively, while on 80 seconds of treatment AFB1 and AFB2 in rough rice reduced by 75.0 and 39.2% respectively [32]. PL treatment also inactivated the mutagenicity and cytotoxicity of these aflatoxins. Abuagela et al. [55] treated dehulled peanuts with PL at 0.4 J cm-1 per pulse. No significant variation in the chemical properties including acidity value, fatty acid content and peroxide value of oil obtained from PL treated peanuts. Aflatoxins levels significantly decreased by 91% in PL treated dehulled peanuts. For large industrial scale application of PL technology would require the development of cost- effective equipment for PL treatment.

Microwave heating generates a high temperature (130°C or higher) that is required for aflatoxin reduction in peanut and corn [56, 57]. Aflatoxin contaminated corn was microwave heated at 1650 W power for 5.5 minutes, resulted in reduction in AFB1, AFB2 by 36 and 58%, respectively [35]. Mobeen et al. [33] microwave cooked peanut and its products and reported reduction in AFB1 level by 50–60%, while level of AFB2 reduced to non-detectable limits. Treatment of corn flour by microwave heat for 10 minutes duration led to decrease in AFB1 content up to 67.7% [34]. Major drawback of aflatoxin decontamination by this method is the uneven distribution of temperature during microwave heating. This results in the generation of hot and cold spots in the treated food product [58]. Overheating in the hot spot may lead to loss of nutritional value and quality whereas lesser temperature in cold spot may not be sufficient for degradation of aflatoxins. In view of this, aflatoxin detoxification using microwave heating method has moderate success and limited application.

#### *2.1.2 Cold plasma*

The fourth state of matter, plasma predominantly consists of UV rays, ions, electrons, reactive nitrogen species (RNS), reactive oxygen species (ROS) [59]. Based on its temperature, plasma can be categorized into thermal and non-thermal (cold) plasma. Cold plasma is generated through electrical discharges in gases at temperature between 30 and 60°C and atmospheric pressure [60]. Cold plasma technology has been employed for aflatoxin degradation at ambient pressure and temperature [61, 62]. Ouf et al. [63] used argon cold plasma at atmospheric pressure for 9 minutes on *Aspergillus niger* spore and mycotoxin production in palm fruits. Authors found that mycotoxin fumonisin B2, OTA content reduced from 6 and 25 μg/100 $mm^2$ respectively and all the spores were killed. Another study used dielectric barrier discharge nitrogen plasma (1150 W) for detoxification of aflatoxin inoculated dehulled hazelnuts. Authors demonstrated that after 12 minutes treatment around 70% of AFB1 was detoxified. They also showed that AFB1 and AFG1 were more sensitive whereas AFB2 and AFG2 was less sensitive to nitrogen plasma treatment [64]. Treatment with corona discharge plasma jet (CDPJ) for 30 minutes on AFB1 spiked rice and wheat samples and AFB1 on glass slides reduced the AFB1 concentration by 56.6, 45.7, 95% respectively [65]. Authors suggested the inconsistency in detoxification of AFB1 is due to possible chemical interaction of toxin with the food matrix. The effectiveness of cold plasma technology for aflatoxin degradation depends on the type of food commodities, kind of plasma system, operating parameters used (energy input, moisture, working gas) and the time of plasma exposure [60]. This novel technology has great potential for detoxification of aflatoxin in food and feed. However, it is still in its infancy and there is a need to standardize conditions for plasma treatment suitable to decontaminate various foods. Further research is required to study the effect of plasma on the nutritional quality and organoleptic characteristics of food.

## 2.2 Chemical detoxification of aflatoxins

### *2.2.1 Electrolyzed oxidizing water*

Electrolyzed oxidizing water (EOW) or electro-activated water is produced by the electrolysis of water containing 1% sodium chloride (NaCl). The resulting water is an electrolyzed one that can be used as a disinfectant. EOW can be categorized into two major types according to its pH and oxidation–reduction potential (ORP): a) neutral electrolyzed oxidizing water (NEOW) with pH of 5.0–6.5, ORP of 800–900 mV; b) acidic electrolyzed oxidizing water (AEOW) with pH of less than 3.0, ORP of more than 1000 mV [66]. Major advantage of EOW is that it turns to ordinary water after use that has no potential threat to animals and environment. Treatment of aflatoxin contaminated corn with NEOW at room temperature for 15 minutes, resulted in significant reduction in the genotoxicity and cytotoxicity of aflatoxins in HepG2 cells [67]. Gomez- Espinosa et al. [68] further confirmed that NEOW treatment of aflatoxin contaminated corn significantly reduces the aflatoxicosis in turkey.

### *2.2.2 Organic acids*

Organic acids have been widely used for aflatoxin degradation in food industry. AFB1 contaminated soyabean soaked in 1.0 N tartaric acid, lactic acid and citric acid,, and at room temperature for 18 hours, resulted in reduction in AFB1 level by 95.1, 92.7 and 94.1%, respectively [69]. Acidulation with lemon juice for 60 minutes at 120°C for decontamination of AFB1 in roasted pistachio nuts, reduced the AFB1content by 50.2% [70]. Acidulation can be combined with other decontamination technologies for better results. For instance, acidulation coupled with pulsed light technique led to aflatoxin degradation in peanuts up to 98.3%. On the other hand, pulsed light and citric acid treatment separately decreased aflatoxins by 78.1 and 20.2%, respectively [71]. Organic acid treatment results in leaching of nutrients such as water-soluble proteins, starch, minerals. However, it has several health benefits on livestocks. The only drawback of this method is the high cost of organic acids.

### *2.2.3 Ozone*

Ozone (O3), a most powerful oxidizing, antimicrobial and disinfecting agent, can be used directly for decontaminating various food products [72]. FDA has granted ozone as Generally Recognized As Safe (GRAS) status for water and food industry [73]. Ozone cause the progressive oxidation of sulfhydryl group of amino acids of proteins, peptides and enzymes or polyunsaturated fatty acids into shorter molecular fragments. Ozone also result in degradation of unsaturated lipids in cell wall envelope, disruption and leakage of microbial cellular contents [74]. Ozone degrade aflatoxins AF-B1 and AF-G1 through an electrophilic attack on C8-C9 double bond of difuran ring, resulting in ozonide formation. This is followed by rearrangement into molozonide derivatives like organic acids, ketones and aldehydes [75]. On the contrary, AF-B2 and AF-G2 are more resistant to ozonisation as they lack C8-C9 double bond in their structure [76]. Ozone treatment of groundnut samples increased the rate of aflatoxin detoxification and has no effect on the peroxide, resveratrol, acids and polyphenol content [77]. Treatment of AFB1- contaminated maize with ozone resulted in decreased toxicity of the treated samples [78].

Major advantages of using ozone as aflatoxin detoxification method are (i) ozone can be applied in gaseous as well as liquid forms (ii) no leftover residue after contact and no hazardous disposal (iii) easy on-site generation of ozone [72, 79]. Till date several studies have been conducted on ozonation at laboratory scale. There is a need to develop efficient eqipments to scale up the process for successful commercial application of this technology for detoxification of aflatoxin contaminated food and feed.

#### *2.2.4 Plant extracts*

Natural plant extracts are considered as food additives by food industry worldwide. They are well known for their anti-inflammatory and anti-microbial properties. Incubation of AFB1 with *Rosmarinus officinalis* aqueous leave extracts at different time intervals showed 60.3% reduction in AFB1 after 48 hours of incubation [80]. Iram, *et al.* [81, 82] studied the effectiveness of aqueous extracts of *Corymbia citriodora* and *Trachyspermum ammi* for detoxification in AFB1 and AFB2 spiked corn. After treatment with *C. citriodora* leaf extract, AFB1 and AFB2 levels were reduced to to 91.7 and 88.8%, respectively. AFB1 and AFB2 were degraded by 89.6 and 86.5%, respectively, following *T. ammi* seeds extract treatment. These results were in consistent with the findings of Velazhahan *et al.* [83]. In another study, authors tested the aqueous extracts from 31 medicinal plants for their AFB1 detoxifying ability. *Adhatoda vasica* Nees leaf extract showed the highest AFB1 degradation ability (98%) at 24 hours after incubation at 37°C [84]. The same group found that *Adhatoda vasica* Nees leaf extract contained the partially purified alkaloids that was responsible for its strong AFB1 detoxification ability. Brinda *et al.* [85] fed rats with spraydried formulation of *Adhatoda vasica* Nees leaf extract and exposed them to AFB1. They found that such pre-fed rats counteracted hepatotoxicity induced by AFB1 exposure. To date, there is a meager knowledge on the active compounds present in the plant extracts that is responsible for their aflatoxins detoxification ability. Further research is needed to gain insights into the aflatoxin detoxifying compounds, their mode of action and complex interaction with the food matrices.

### **2.3 Biological decontamination of aflatoxins**

Biological degradation of aflatoxins involves microorganism or enzyme based detoxification of aflatoxins into less toxic or non-toxic metabolites. This method has emerged as an efficient and eco-friendly strategy for degradation of aflatoxins.

#### *2.3.1 Microbial degradation*

Various microorganisms isolated from different sources can degrade afltatoxins present in food and feed. Risa *et al.* [86] investigated the effectiveness of 42 *Rhodococcus* strains for detoxification of AFB1 and zearalenone (ZON). 18 *Rhodococcus* strains were capable of degrading more than 90% of AFB1 and 15 strains could cease the genotoxicity in 72 hours. Only one of these strains, namely *R. percolatus JCM 10087 T* was capable of detoxifying ZON by more than 90% and decreasing the oestrogenicity by 70%. Another group studied the role of *R. pyridinivorans* K408 strain in detoxification of AFB1 in corn based stillage and revealed that the level of AFB1in liquid and solid phases of whole stillage was degraded by 75 and 63%, respectively [87]. A number of *Bacillus* strains such as *B. subtilis* ANSB060 [88], *B. subtilis* UTBSP1 [89], *B. subtilis* JSW-1 [90], *B. licheniformis* CFR1 [91], *B. licheniformis* BL010 [92], *B. velezensis* DY3108 [93] and *Bacillus* sp. TUBF1 [94] have been reported to degrade aflatoxins. *B. subtilis* has been approved as Generally Recognized As Safe (GRAS) strains of bacteria that is safe for commercial pharmaceutical and nutritional purpose.

Adebo *et al.* [95] used the lysates of bacterial strains (*Staphylococcus* sp. VGF2, *Pseudomonas fluorescens* and *Pseudomonas anguilliseptica* VGF1) isolated from goldmine aquifer to study the degradation of AFB1. It was found that *Staphylococcus* sp. VGF2 lysate showed the highest AFB1 degradation capacity of 100% while *P. fluorescens* and *P. anguilliseptica* VGF1 reduced the AFB1 by 63 and 66.5%, respectively. About 124 *Streptomyces* strains were examined for AFB1 degradation capability. It was found that 55% of the *Streptomyces* strains could degrade AFB1 [96]. Eshelli *et al.*, [97] demonstrated that *S. lividans* TK 24 was capable of degrading AFB1 by 88% in liquid culture upon 24 hour incubation. *E. coli* CG1061, AFB1 detoxifying bacterium, was isolated from chicken cecum and found to degrade AFB1 by 93.7% following 72 hours of incubation. It resulted in formation of degradation products of lower molecular weight [98]. The non-toxigenic strains of *Aspergillus niger* with aflatoxin detoxification capability have been used in the food industry. *A. niger* FS-UV1 strain, derived from *A. niger* FS-Z1 wild strain following UV irradiation showed superior AFB1 detoxification capability up to 95.3% and significantly decreased mutagenic activity [99]. A novel thermophilic microbial consortium TADC7 was constructed for efficient, specific and stable $AFB_1$ degradation. Microbial consortium TADC7 showed the degradation of AFB1 by more than 95% of the toxin after 72 hours of incubation in the temperature range between 50 and 60°C. 16S rRNA sequencing revealed that *Tepidimicrobium* and *Geobacillus* may play a major role in AFB1 degradation [100].

### *2.3.2 Enzymatic degradation*

Recently, the reports on isolation, identification and purification of aflatoxin-degrading enzymes from microorganisms have increased significantly. Various enzymes such as oxidases, peroxidases, reductases and laccases are capable of degrading aflatoxins. Laccases represent a class of multicopper oxidase enzymes widely present in fungi, plants, bacteria and insects. They catalyze oxidation of various phenolic and non-phenolic compounds coupled to reduction of molecular oxygen in water. Alberts *et al.* [101] first proposed the role of fungal laccases in decontamination of AFB1. Enzyme laccase (Lac2) produced and purified from *Pleurotus pulmonarius* showed AFB1 degradation up to 90% with mediator acetoseringone present in the medium [102]. Verheecke *et al.* [103] documented purified enzymes effective for AFB1 detoxification. Guo *et al.* [104] summarized the reaction mechanisms of aflatoxin-degrading enzymes responsible for AFB1 detoxification in the review. Alberts *et al.* [101] purified laccase from *Trametes versicolor* and produced recombinant laccase using *A. niger*. The laccase from *T. versicolor* resulted in reduction in AFB1 pro-oxidative properties by 59% and genotoxicity by 100% [105]. Compared to fungal laccases, bacterial laccases are excellent candidates for xenobiotics degradation because they are extremely thermostable, tolerant to alkaline conditions, wider range of pH and substrate spectrum [106]. Enzyme CotA laccase from *B. licheniformis* catalyze the C3-hydroxylation of AFB1 and transformed toxic AFB1 into products epi-aflatoxin Q1 and aflatoxin Q1 that are non-toxic human liver L-02 cells. Laccase CotA was found to be highly thermostable with the half life of 1 hour. It was capable of degrading AFB1 in the temperature range between 60 and 80°C by more than 70% in a period of 30 minutes [107].

Peroxidases are a class of oxidoreductases that catalyze oxidation of substrates with the use of hydrogen peroxide or organic peroxide. They are mainly heme- proteins with contain iron (III) protoporphyrin IX as the prosthetic group. Peroxidases are widespread in nature, found in both prokaryotes and eukaryotes. Researchers have achieved 65 and 97% reduction in AFM1 and AFB1, respectively in milk with horse radish peroxidase (HRP) treatment at 30°C following 8 hours of incubation [108]. Another group used manganese peroxidase (MnP) isolated from *Phanerochaete sordida* YK-624 for AFB1 degradation. MnP reduced the AFB1 level by 86.0% and mutagenicity by 69.2% [109]. Type B dye decolorizing peroxidase (Rh_DypB) was isolated and purified from *Rhodococcus jostii* and tested for AFB1 degradation. Authors achieved 96% degradation of AFB1 in the sodium malonate buffer [110].

Scientists are working constantly towards identification, isolation and purification of novel aflatoxin detoxifying enzymes from wide variety of organisms. For instance, an extracellular enzyme MADE was purified from *Myxococcus fulvus* ANSM068 from a culture supernatant. At the temperature of 35°C and pH 6.0, degraded AFB1 by 71.89% following 48 hours of incubation. The purified MADE also degraded AFM1 and AFG1 by 96 and 97%, respectively [111]. Xu *et al.* [112] purified enzyme MADE from *Bacillus shackletonii* that resulted in degradation of AFB1 by 48% with 72 hours of incubation at 70°C. BADE was found to be extremely thermostable, even at 100°C for 10 minutes. Nine F420H2- dependent reductases (FDRs) were identified and characterized from *Mycobacterium smegmatis*. FDRs catalyze the α, β-unsaturated ester reduction in aflatoxins, using deazaflavin as cofactor. They are categorized into two classes, namely FDR-A and FDR-B with FDR-A class of enzymes being 100 times more active against aflatoxins than FDA-B [113].

The main advantage of cell free enzyme based aflatoxin degradation is that it has no negative impact on the degradation ability and organoleptic properties of food products [95]. Although cell free aflatoxin degradation enzymes are extremely effective, however their application in food and feed industry is still limited due to certain shortcomings. Firstly, the low yield of aflatoxin-degrading enzymes in the native hosts. This can be solved by the intervention of recombinant DNA technology. Secondly, food processing generally requires the use of solvents, extreme temperature and pH conditions. This can effect the catalytic efficiency and stability of the wild type enzymes. The use of enzyme engineering technologies such as random or site directed mutagenesis could address these issues [114].

In comparison to natural enzymes, nanozymes are more robustness, cost effective, stabile and durable. Nanozymes are the nanomaterials with intrinsic enzyme like properties that catalyze the substrates of natural enzymes following the same catalytic mechanisms and kinetics under physiological conditions [115]. The laccase-mimicking nanozyme was prepared by coordinating guanosine monophosphate (GMP) with $Cu^{2+}$ at room temperature. This led to formation of amorphous metal–organic framework (MOF) nanomaterial. Cu/GMP nanozyme has the same catalytic efficiency as the natural laccase but it is 2400-fold more cost-effective and more robust against extreme temperature, pH salt and storage conditions [116]. Nanozymes with peroxidase-like activity such as $CuMnO_2$ nanoflakes [117], $FeMnO_3$ nanoparticle-filled polypyrrole nanotubes [118], FePt nanoparticle-decorated graphene oxide nanosheets [119], $Pt_{74}Ag_{26}$ nanoparticle-decorated ultrathin $MoS_2$ nanosheets [120] have been prepared. The recent technological advancements will open the gate for the development and application of nanozymes to aflatoxin detoxification in food and feed industry.

## 3. Conclusion

Contamination caused by aflatoxins in food and feed poses a great threat to human and animal health and result in considerable economic loss to the agriculture production of the country. To produce healthy, high quality, aflatoxin free food products is the worldwide concern. Researchers have been working continuously for the development of effective aflatoxin decontamination strategies since decades. Despite all the efforts, there still a need to come up with an efficient decontamination technology that meets all these criteria for industrial commercialization: (i) Retain/enhance the nutritional quality of the food (ii) Efficiently reduce aflatoxins to the safe limits without leaving toxic residues (iii) cost effective and eco-friendly. So far, no aflatoxin decontamination strategy has been developed that meet all the mentioned criteria. For instance, physical and chemical methods may change the organoleptic properties and chemical composition of food and feed. Biological approaches are more specific, effective with more control over the generated bio-products of aflatoxin detoxification. Use of pure enzyme for aflatoxin degradation has no negative impact on the degradation efficiency, chemical composition and organoleptic properties of food products. Further, adoption of enzyme engineering technology would provide highly efficient and specific aflatoxin detoxifying enzymes in the near future.

## Acknowledgements

Author is grateful to University of Hyderabad for providing necessary facilities.

## Conflict of interest

Authors have no competing interests.

## Author details

Vishakha Pandey
University of Hyderabad, Hyderabad, India

*Address all correspondence to: vishakhapandey2@gmail.com

## References

[1] Reiter E, Zentek J, Razzazi E. Review on sample preparation strategies and methods used for the analysis of aflatoxins in food and feed. Molecular Nutrition and Food Research. 2009;53:508-524. DOI: 10.1002/mnfr.200800145.

[2] Payne GA and Brown MP. Genetics and physiology of aflatoxin biosynthesis. Annual Review of Phytopathology. 1998;36:329-362. DOI: 10.1146/annurev. phyto.36.1.329.

[3] Perrone G, Haidukowski M, Stea G, Epifani F, Bandyopadhyay R, Leslie JF, et al. Population structure and Aflatoxin production by Aspergillus Sect. Flavi from maize in Nigeria and Ghana. Food Microbiology. 2014. 41, 52e59. DOI: 10.1016/j.fm.2013.12.005.

[4] Iqbal SZ, Jinap S, Pirouz AA and Ahmad Faizal AR . Aflatoxin M1 in milk and dairy products, occurrence and recent challenges: A review. Trends in Food Science and Technology. 2015;46:110e119. DOI:10.1016/J. TIFS.2015.08.005.

[5] Blount WP. Turkey “X” disease. In the Proceeding of Turkeys. 1961;9:52-77.

[6] Zinedine A and Manes J. Occurrence and legislation of mycotoxins in food and feed from Morocco. Food Control. 2009;20:334e344. DOI: 10.1016/j. foodcont.2008.07.002.

[7] My A and Sachan D. Dietary factors affecting aflatoxin Bi carcinogenicity. Malaysian Journal of Nutrition. 1997;3:161-179. DOI: 10.1.1.581.8466.

[8] Bbosa GS, Kitya D, Odda J and Ogwal-Okeng J. Aflatoxins metabolism, effects on epigenetic mechanisms and their role in carcinogenesis. Health. 2013; 05:14-34. DOI: 10.4236/health.2013.510A1003.

[9] Baan R, Grosse Y, Straif K, Secretan B, El Ghissassi F, Bouvard V, Benbrahim-Tallaa L, Guha N, Freeman C, Galichet L, Cogliano V. WHO International Agency for Research on Cancer Monograph Working Group. A review of human carcinogens-Part F: chemical agents and related occupations. Lancet Oncology. 2009;12:1143-1144. DOI: 10.1016/s1470-2045(09)70358-4.

[10] Roze LV, Hong SY and Linz JE. Aflatoxin biosynthesis: current frontiers. Annual Review of Food Science and Technology. 2013;4: 293-311. DOI: 10.1146/annurev-food-083012-123702.

[11] Kensler TW, Roebuck BD, Wogan GN and Groopman JD. Aflatoxin: A 50-year Odyssey of mechanistic and translational toxicology. Toxicological Sciences. 2011;120:28-48. DOI: 10.1093/toxsci/kfq283.

[12] Marchese S, Polo A, Ariano A, Velotto S, Costantini S and Severino L. Aflatoxin B1 and M1: Biological properties and their involvement in cancer development. Toxins. 2018;10:214-233. DOI: 10.3390/toxins10060214.

[13] Karlovsky P, Suman M, Berthiller F, De Meester J, Eisenbrand G, Perrin I, … Dussort P. Impact of food processing and detoxification treatments on mycotoxin contamination. Mycotoxin Research. 2016;32: 179-205. DOI:10.1007/s12550-016-0257-7.

[14] Rustom IYS. Aflatoxin in food and feed: Occurrence, legislation and inactivation by physical methods. Food Chemistry. 1997;59:57-67. DOI: 10.1016/S0308-8146(96)00096-9.

[15] Vekiru E, Fruhauf S, Rodrigues I, Ottner F, Krska R, Schatzmayr G. … Bermudez AJ. *In vitro* binding

assessment and *in vivo* efficacy of several adsorbents against aflatoxin B1. World Mycotoxin Journal. 2015.;8:477-488. DOI: 10.3920/WMJ2014.1800.

[16] Elliott CT, Connolly L and Kolawole O. Potential adverse effects on animal health and performance caused by the addition of mineral adsorbents to feeds to reduce mycotoxin exposure. Mycotoxin Research. 2019;36:115-126. DOI: 10.1007/s12550-019-00375-7.

[17] Gavahian M and Cullen PJ. Cold plasma as an emerging technique for mycotoxin-free food: Efficacy, mechanisms and trends. Food Reviews International. 2019;36:1-22. DOI: 10.1080/87559129.2019.1630638.

[18] Loi M, Paciolla C, Logrieco AF and Mule G. Plant bioactive compounds in pre-and postharvest management for aflatoxins reduction. Frontiers in Microbiology. 2020; 11:243-259. DOI:10.3389/fmicb.2020.00243.

[19] Kumar P, Mahato DK, Kamle M, Mohanta TK, Kang SG. Aflatoxins: A Global Concern for Food Safety, Human Health and Their Management. Frontiers in Microbiology. 2017;7:2170-2180. DOI: 10.3389/fmicb.2016.02170.

[20] Assuncao E, Reis TA, Baquiao AC, Correa B. Effects of Gamma and Electron Beam Radiation on Brazil Nuts Artificially Inoculated with *Aspergillus flavus*. Journal of Food Protection. 2015;78:1397-1401. DOI: 10.4315/0362-028X.JFP-14-595. PMID: 26197295.

[21] Liu R, Lu M, Wang R, Wang S, Chang M, Jin Q and Wang X. Degradation of aflatoxin B1 in peanut meal by electron beam irradiation. International Journal of Food Properties. 2018;21:892-901. DOI: 10.1080/10942912.2018.1466321.

[22] Iqbal SZ, Bhatti IA, Asi M R, Zuber M, Shahid M, Parveen I. Effect of γ irradiation on fungal load and aflatoxins reduction in red chillies. Radiation Physics and Chemistry. 2013;82:80-84. DOI: 10.1016/j.radphyschem.2012.09.015.

[23] Markov K, Mihaljevic, B, Domijan AM, Pleadin J, Delas F and Frece J. Inactivation of aflatoxigenic fungi and the reduction of aflatoxin B1 in vitro and in situ using gamma irradiation. Food Control. 2015;54:79-85. DOI: 10.1016/j.foodcont.2015.01.036.

[24] Patil H, Shah NG, Hajare SN, Gautam S and Kumar G. Combination of microwave and gamma irradiation for reduction of aflatoxin B1 and microbiological contamination in peanuts (*Arachis hypogaea L.*). World Mycotoxin Journal. 2019;12:269-280. DOI: 10.3920/WMJ2018.2384.

[25] Jalili M, Jinap S and Noranizan A. Aflatoxins and ochratoxin a reduction in black and white pepper by gamma radiation. Radiation Physics and Chemistry. 2012;81:1786e1788. DOI: 10.1016/j.radphyschem.2012.06.001.

[26] Vita DS, Rosa P and Giuseppe A. Effect of gamma irradiation on aflatoxins and ochratoxin A reduction in almond samples. Journal of Food Research. 2014;3:113-118. DOI: 10.5539/jfr.v3n4p113.

[27] Garg N, Aggarwal M, Javed S and Khandal RK. Studies for optimization of conditions for reducing aflatoxin contamination in peanuts using ultraviolet radiations. International Journal of Drug Development and Research. 2013; 5: 408-424.

[28] Mao J, He B, Zhang L,... Zhang W. A Structure Identification and Toxicity Assessment of the Degradation Products of Aflatoxin $B_1$ in Peanut Oil under UV Irradiation. *Toxins (Basel)*. 2016;8:332. DOI: 10.3390/toxins8110332.

[29] Diao E, Shen X, Zhang Z, Ji N, Ma W and Dong H. Safety evaluation of aflatoxin B1 in peanut oil after

ultraviolet irradiation detoxification in a photodegradation reactor. International Journal of Food Science & Technology. 2015;50:41-47. DOI: 10.1111/ijfs.12648.

[30] Liu R, Jin Q, Huang J, Liu Y, Wang X, Mao W and Wang S. Photodegradation of aflatoxin B1 in peanut oil. European Food Research and Technology. 2011;232: 843-849. DOI: 10.1007/s00217-011-1452-6.

[31] Tripathi S, Mishra HN. Enzymatic coupled with UV degradation of aflatoxin B1 in red chili powder Journal of Food Quality. 2010;33:186-203. DOI: 10.1111/j.1745-4557.2010.00334.x.

[32] Wang B, Mahoney NE, Pan Z, Khir R, Wu B, Ma H and Zhao L. Effectiveness of pulsed light treatment for degradation and detoxification of aflatoxin B1 and B2 in rough rice and rice bran. Food Control. 2016;59:461-467. DOI: 10.1016/j.foodcont.2015.06.030.

[33] Mobeen, AK, Aftab A, Asif A and Zuzzer AS. Aflatoxins B1 and B2 contamination of peanut and peanut products and subsequent microwave detoxification. Journal of Pharmacy and Nutrition Sciences. 2011;1:1-3. DOI: 10.6000/1927-5951.2011.01.01.01.

[34] Alkadi, H and Altal J. Effect of microwave oven processing treatments on reduction of aflatoxin B1 and ochratoxin A in maize flour. European Journal of Chemistry. 2019;10:224-227. DOI: 10.5155/eurjchem.10.3.224-227.1840.

[35] Perez-Flores GC, Moreno-Martinez E, Mendez-Albores A. Effect of microwave heating during alkaline-cooking of aflatoxin contaminated maize. Journal of Food Sciences. 2011;76:T48–T52. DOI: 10.1111/j.1750-3841.2010.01980.x.

[36] Kim HJ, Jung S, Yong HI, Bae YS, Kang SN, Kim IS, Jo C. Improvement of Microbiological Safety and Sensorial Quality of Pork Jerky by Electron Beam Irradiation and by Addition of Onion Peel Extract and Barbecue Flavor. Radiation Physics and Chemistry. 2014;98:22-28. DOI: 10.1016/j.radphyschem.2014.01.003.

[37] Rogovschi, V. D.; Aquino, S.; Nunes, T. C. F.; Gonçalez, E.; Corrêa, B. Villavicencio A L.C.H. Use Of Electron Beam On Aflatoxins Degradation In Coconut Agar. In: Proceedings of the International Nuclear Atlantic Conference; 2009.

[38] WHO. High-dose irradiation: wholesomeness of food irradiated with doses above 10 kGy. Report of a joint FAO/IAEA/WHO study group. World Health Organization technical report series. 1999;890:1-197.

[39] Da Silva Aquino KA. Sterilization by gamma irradiation. In F. Adrovic (Ed.), Gamma radiation (pp. 171e206). Vienna, Austria: InTech. 2012. DOI: 10.5772/34901

[40] Aziz NH, Moussa LA. A. Influence of gamma-radiation on mycotoxin producing moulds and mycotoxins in fruits. Food Control. 2002;13:281-288. DOI: 10.1016/S0956-7135(02)00028-2.

[41] Kumar S, Kunwar, A, Gautam, S, Sharma, A. Inactivation of *A. ochraceus* spores and detoxification of ochratoxin A in coffee beans by gamma irradiation. Journal of Food Sciences. 2012;77:44-51. DOI: 10.1111/j.1750-3841.2011.02572.x.

[42] Domijan AM, Pleadin J, Mihaljevic B, Vahcic N, Frece J, Markov K. Reduction of ochratoxin A in dry-cured meat products using gamma-irradiation. . Food Additives and Contaminants: Part A Chemistry Analysis Control Exposure and Risk Assess. 2015;32:1185-1191. DOI: 10.1080/19440049.2015.1049219.

[43] Di Stefano V, Pitonzo R, Cicero N, D'Oca MC. Mycotoxin contamination of

animal feedingstuff: detoxification by gamma-irradiation and reduction of aflatoxins and ochratoxin A concentrations. Food Additives and Contaminants Part A: Chemical Analysis Control Exposure and Risk Assessment. 2014;31:2034-2039. DOI: 10.1080/19440049.2014.968882.

[44] Priyadarshini A, Rajauria G, O'Donnell CP and Tiwari BK. Emerging food processing technologies and factors impacting their industrial adoption. Critical Reviews in Food Science and Nutrition. 2019; 59: 3082-3101. DOI: 10.1080/10408398. 2018.1483890.

[45] Caulfield CD, Cassidy JP and Kelly JP. Effects of gamma irradiation and pasteurization on the nutritive composition of commercially available animal diets. Journal of the American Association for Laboratory Animal Science. 2008;47:61-66. PMID: 19049256.

[46] Gayan E, Condon S and Alvarez I. Biological aspects in food preservation by ultraviolet light: A review. Food and Bioprocess Technology. 2014;7:1-20. DOI: 10.1007/s11947-013-1168-7.

[47] Delorme, M. M., Guimar˜aes, J. T., Coutinho, N. M., Balthazar, C. F., Rocha, R. S., Silva, R., ... Cruz, A. G. Ultraviolet radiation: An interesting technology to preserve quality and safety of milk and dairy foods. Trends in Food Science and Technology. 2020;102;146-154. DOI: 10.1016/j. tifs.2020.06.001.

[48] Diao E, Li X, Zhang Z, Ma W, Ji N and Dong H. Ultraviolet irradiation detoxification of aflatoxins. Trends in Food Science and Technology. 2015;42:64-69. DOI: 10.1016/j. tifs.2014.12.001.

[49] Zhu Y, Koutchma T, Warrinner K, Zhou T. Reduction of patulin in apple juice products by UV light of different wavelengths in the UVC range. Journal of Food Protection. 2014;77:963-967. DOI: 10.4315/0362-028X.JFP-13-429.

[50] Atalla, MM, Hassanein NM, El-Beih AA and Youssef YA. Effect of fluorescent and UV light on mycotoxin production under different relative humidities in wheat grains. International Journal of Agriculture and Biology. 2004;6:1006-1012. DOI: 1006e1012

[51] Jubeen F, Bhatti IA, Khan MZ, Hassan ZU and Shahid M. Effect of UVC irradiation on aflatoxins in ground nut (*Arachis hypogea*) and tree nuts (*Juglans regia, Prunus duclus* and *Pistachio vera*). Journal of the Chemical Society of Pakistan. 2012; 34:1366-1374. DOI: 1366e1374.

[52] Garcia-Cela E, Marin S, Sanchis V, Crespo-Sempere A and Ramos AJ. Effect of ultraviolet radiation A and B on growth and mycotoxin production by *Aspergillus carbonarius* and *Aspergillus paraciticus* in grape and pistachio media. Fungal Biology. 2015;119:67e78. DOI: 10.1016/j.funbio.2014.11.004.

[53] Oms-Oliu G, Martin-Belloso O and Soliva-Fortuny R. Pulsed light treatments for food preservation. A review. Food and Bioprocess Technology. 2010;3:13-23. DOI: doi. org/10.1007/s11947-008-0147-x.

[54] Moreau M, Lescure G, Agoulon A, Svinareff P, Orange N, Feuilloley M. Application of the pulsed light technology to mycotoxin degradation and inactivation. J Appl Toxicol. 2013;33:357-363. DOI: 10.1002/jat.1749.

[55] Abuagela MO, Iqdiam BM, Mostafa H, Gu L, Smith ME and Sarnoski PJ. Assessing pulsed light treatment on the reduction of aflatoxins in peanuts with and without skin. International Journal of Food Science and Technology. 2018;53:2567-2575. DOI: 10.1111/ijfs.13851.

[56] Pluyer HR, Ahmed EM, Wei CI. Destruction of Aflatoxins on Peanuts by Oven- and Microwave-Roasting. Journal of Food Protection. 1987;50:504-508. DOI: 10.4315/0362-028X-50.6.504. PMID: 30965437.

[57] Farag RS, Rashed MM, Abo Hgger AA. Aflatoxin destruction by microwave heating. International Journal of Food Science and Nutrition. 1996;47:197-208. DOI: 10.3109/09637489609012581.

[58] Menon A, Stojceska V and Tassou SA. A systematic review on the recent advances of the energy efficiency improvements in non-conventional food drying technologies. Trends in Food Science and Technology. 2020;100:67-76. DOI: 10.1016/j.tifs.2020.03.014.

[59] Kogelschatz U. Atmospheric-pressure plasma technology. Plasma Physics and Controlled Fusion. 2004;46:B63–B75. DOI: 10.1088/0741-3335/46/12B/006.

[60] Hertwig C, Meneses N and Mathys A. Cold atmospheric pressure plasma and low energy electron beam as alternative nonthermal decontamination technologies for dry food surfaces: A review. Trends in Food Science and Technology. 2018;77:131-142. DOI: 10.1016/j.tifs.2018.05.011

[61] Gavahian M and Cullen PJ. Cold plasma as an emerging technique for mycotoxin-free food: Efficacy, mechanisms, and trends. Food Reviews International. 2019;36:1-22. DOI: 10.1080/87559129.2019.1630638.

[62] Misra NN, Yadav B, Roopesh MS and Jo C. Cold plasma for effective fungal and mycotoxin control in foods: Mechanisms, inactivation effects, and applications. Comprehensive Reviews in Food Science and Food Safety. 2019;18:106-120. DOI: 10.1111/1541-4337.12398.

[63] Ouf SA, Basher AH, Mohamed AA. Inhibitory effect of double atmospheric pressure argon cold plasma on spores and mycotoxin production of *Aspergillus niger* contaminating date palm fruits. Journal of Science and Food Agriculture. 2015;95:3204-3210. DOI: 10.1002/jsfa.7060.

[64] Siciliano I, Spadaro D, Prelle A, Vallauri D, Cavallero MC, Garibaldi A. and Gullino ML. Use of cold atmospheric plasma to detoxify hazelnuts from aflatoxins. Toxins. 2016;8:125. DOI: 10.3390/toxins8050125.

[65] Puligundla P, Lee T and Mok C. Effect of corona discharge plasma jet treatment on the degradation of aflatoxin B1 on glass slides and in spiked food commodities. Lwt-Food Science and Technology. 2019;124:108333. DOI: 10.1016/j.lwt.2019.108333.

[66] Huang YR., Hung YC, Hsu SY, Huang YW and Hwang DF. Application of electrolyzed water in the food industry. Food Control. 2008;19:329-345. DOI: 10.1016/j.foodcont.2007.08.012.

[67] Jardon-Xicotencatl S, Diaz-Torres R, Marroquin-Cardona A, Villarreal-Barajas T, Mendez-Albores A. Detoxification of Aflatoxin-Contaminated Maize by Neutral Electrolyzed Oxidizing Water. Toxins (Basel). 2015;23;7:4294-4314. DOI: 10.3390/toxins7104294.

[68] Gomez-Espinosa D, Cervantes-Aguilar FJ, Del Río-Garcia JC, Villarreal-Barajas T, Vazquez-Duran A, Mendez-Albores A. Ameliorative Effects of Neutral Electrolyzed Water on Growth Performance, Biochemical Constituents, and Histopathological Changes in Turkey Poults during Aflatoxicosis. Toxins *(Basel)*. 2017;9: 104-119. DOI:10.3390/toxins903010.

[69] Lee J, Her JY, Lee KG. Reduction of aflatoxins ($B_1$, $B_2$, $G_1$, and $G_2$) in soybean-based model systems. Food

Chemistry. 2015;189:45-51. DOI: 10.1016/j.foodchem.2015.02.013.

[70] Rastegar H, Shoeibi S, Yazdanpanah H, Amirahmadi M, Khaneghah AM, Campagnollo FB and S Sant Ana, A. Removal of aflatoxin B1 by roasting with lemon juice and/or citric acid in contaminated pistachio nuts. Food Control. 2017; 71:279-284. DOI: 10.1016/j.foodcont.2016.06.045.

[71] Abuagela MO, Iqdiam BM, Mostafa H, Marshall SM, Yagiz Y, Marshall MR, ... Sarnoski P. Combined effects of citric acid and pulsed light treatments to degrade B-aflatoxins in peanut. Food and Bioproducts Processing. 2019; 117:396-403. ISSN : 0960-3085.

[72] Pandiselvam R, Subhashini, S, Banuu Priya EP, Kothakota A, Ramesh SV and Shahir S. Ozone based food preservation: A promising green technology for enhanced food safety. Ozone: Science & Engineering. 2019;41:17-34. DOI: 10.1080/01919512.2018.1490636.

[73] Food and Drug Administration (FDA). Secondary direct food additives permitted in food for human consumption. Federal Register. 2001;66:33829-33830.

[74] Das E, Gurakan GC and Bayindirli A. Effect of controlled atmosphere storage, modified atmosphere packaging and gaseous ozone treatment on survival of *Salmonella Enteridis* on cherry tomatoes. Food Microbiology. 2006;23:430e438. DOI: 10.1016/j.fm.2005.08.002.

[75] Jalili, M. A review on aflatoxins reduction in food. Iranian Journal of Health, Safety and Environment. 2016;3:445-459.

[76] Agriopoulou S, Koliadima A, Karaiskakis G and Kapolos J. Kinetic study of aflatoxins' degradation in the presence of ozone. Food Control. 2016;61:221e226. DOI: 10.1016/j.foodcont.2015.09.013.

[77] Chen R, Ma F, Li PW, Zhang W, Ding XX, Zhang Q, Li M, Wang YR, Xu BC. Effect of ozone on aflatoxins detoxification and nutritional quality of peanuts. Food Chemistry. 2014;146: 284-288. DOI: 10.1016/j.foodchem.2013.09.059.

[78] Luo X, Wang R, Wang L, Li Y, Bian Y and Chen Z. Effect of ozone treatment on aflatoxin B1 and safety evaluation of ozonized corn. Food Control. 2014;37:171e176. DOI: 10.1016/j.foodcont.2013.09.043.

[79] Torres AM, Palacios SA, Yerkovich N, Palazzini JM, Battilani P, Leslie JF, ... Chulze SN. *Fusarium* head blight and mycotoxins in wheat: Prevention and control strategies across the food chain. World Mycotoxin Journal. 2019; 12:333-355. DOI: 10.3920/WMJ2019.2438.

[80] Ponzilacqua B, Rottinghaus GE, Landers BR and Oliveira CAF. Effects of medicinal herb and Brazilian traditional plant extracts on in vitro mycotoxin decontamination. Food Control. 2019;100:24-27. DOI: 10.1016/j.foodcont.2019.01.009.

[81] Iram W, Anjum T, Iqbal M, Ghaffar A and Abbas M. Mass spectrometric identification and toxicity assessment of degraded products of aflatoxin B1 and B2 by *Corymbia citriodora* aqueous extracts. Scientific Reports. 2015, 5:14672-14687. DOI: doi.org/10.1038/srep14672.

[82] Iram W, Anjum T, Iqbal M, Ghaffar A, Abbas M. Structural Elucidation and Toxicity Assessment of Degraded Products of Aflatoxin B1 and B2 by Aqueous Extracts of *Trachyspermum ammi*. Fronteirs in Microbiology. 2016;7:346-362. DOI: 10.3389/fmicb.2016.00346.

[83] Velazhahan R, Vijayanandraj S, Vijayasamundeeswari A, Paranidharan V, Samiyappan R, Iwamoto T, ... Muthukrishnan, S. Detoxification of aflatoxins by seed extracts of the medicinal plant, *Trachyspermum ammi* (L.) Sprague ex Turrill - Structural analysis and biological toxicity of degradation product of aflatoxin G1. Food Control. 2010;21:719-725. DOI: 10.1016/j.foodcont.2009.10.014.

[84] Vijayanandraj S, Brinda R, Kannan K, Adhithya R, Vinothini S, Senthil K, Chinta RR, Paranidharan V, Velazhahan R. Detoxification of aflatoxin B1 by an aqueous extract from leaves of *Adhatoda vasica Nees*. Microbiological Research. 2014;169:294-300. DOI: 10.1016/j.micres.2013.07.008.

[85] Brinda R, Vijayanandraj S, Uma D, Malathi D, Paranidharan V, Velazhahan R. Role of *Adhatoda vasica (L.) Nees* leaf extract in the prevention of aflatoxin-induced toxicity in Wistar rats. Journal of the Sciences of Food and Agriculture. 2013;93:2743-2748. DOI: 10.1002/jsfa.6093.

[86] Risa A, Krifaton C, Kukolya J, Kriszt B, Cserhati M, Tancsics A. Aflatoxin B1 and Zearalenone-Detoxifying Profile of *Rhodococcus* Type Strains. Current Microbiology. 2018;75:907-917. DOI: 10.1007/s00284-018-1465-5.

[87] Prettl Z, Desi E, Lepossa A, Kriszt B, Kukolya J and Nagy E. Biological degradation of aflatoxin B1 by a *Rhodococcus pyridinivorans* strain in by-product of bioethanol. Animal Feed Science and Technology. 2017;224: 104-114. DOI: 10.1016/j.anifeedsci.2016.12.011.

[88] Gao X, Ma Q, Zhao L, Lei Y, Shan Y and Ji C. Isolation of Bacillus subtilis: Screening for aflatoxins B1, M1, and G1 detoxification. European Food Research and Technology. 2011;232:957-962. DOI: 10.1007/s00217-011-1463-3

[89] Farzaneh M, Shi Z-Q, Ghassempour A, Sedaghat N, Ahmadzadeh M, Mirabolfathy M and Javan-Nikkhah M. Aflatoxin B1 degradation by Bacillus subtilis UTBSP1 isolated from pistachio nuts of Iran. Food Control. 2012;23:100-106 DOI: 10.1016/j.foodcont.2011.06.018.

[90] Xia X, Zhang Y, Li M, Garba B, Zhang Q, Wang Y, ... Li P. Isolation and characterization of a *Bacillus subtilis* strain with aflatoxin B1 biodegradation capability. Food Control. 2017;75:92-98. DOI: 10.1016/j.foodcont.2016.12.036.

[91] Raksha Rao K, Vipin AV, Hariprasad P, Anu Appaiah KA and Venkateswaran G. Biological detoxification of aflatoxin B1 by *Bacillus licheniformis* CFR1. Food Control. 2017;71:234-241. DOI: 10.1016/j.foodcont.2016.06.040

[92] Wang Y, Zhang H, Yan H, ... Zhang Z. Effective Biodegradation of Aflatoxin B1 Using the *Bacillus licheniformis* (BL010) Strain. Toxins (Basel). 2018;10:497-513. DOI:10.3390/toxins10120497.

[93] Shu X, Wang Y, Zhou Q, ... Wu L. Biological Degradation of Aflatoxin $B_1$ by Cell-Free Extracts of *Bacillus velezensis* DY3108 with Broad PH Stability and Excellent Thermostability. Toxins (Basel). 2018;10:330-345. DOI:10.3390/toxins10080330

[94] El-Deeb B, Altalhi A, Khiralla G, Hassan S and Gherbawy Y. Isolation and characterization of endophytic *Bacilli* bacterium from maize grains able to detoxify aflatoxin B1. Food Biotechnology. 2013;27:199-212. DOI: 10.1080/08905436.2013.811083.

[95] Adebo OA, Njobeh PB, Sidu S, Tlou MG, Mavumengwana V. Aflatoxin B1 degradation by liquid cultures and lysates of three bacterial strains. International Journal of Food Microbiology. 2016;233:11-19. DOI: 10.1016/j.ijfoodmicro.2016.06.007.

[96] Harkai P, Szabo I, Cserhati M, Krifaton C, Risa A, Rado J, ... Kriszt B. Biodegradation of aflatoxin-B1 and zearalenone by *Streptomyces* sp. collection. International Biodeterioration and Biodegradation. 2016;108:48-56. DOI: 10.1016/j.ibiod.2015.12.007.

[97] Eshelli M, Harvey L, Edrada-Ebel R, McNeil B. Metabolomics of the bio-degradation process of aflatoxin B1 by actinomycetes at an initial pH of 6.0. Toxins (Basel). 2015;7:439-456. DOI: 10.3390/toxins7020439

[98] Wang L, Wu J, Liu Z, Shi Y, Liu J, Xu X, Hao S, Mu P, Deng F, Deng Y. Aflatoxin $B_1$ Degradation and Detoxification by *Escherichia coli* CG1061 Isolated From Chicken Cecum. Frontiers in Pharmacology. 2019;9:1548-1557. doi: 10.3389/fphar.2018.01548.

[99] Sun X, Sun C, Zhang X, Zhang H, Ji J, Liu Y and Tang L. Aflatoxin B1 decontamination by UV-mutated live and immobilized *Aspergillus niger*. Food Control. 2016;61:235-242. DOI: 10.1016/j.foodcont.2015.09.017.

[100] Wang Y, Zhao C, Zhang D, Zhao M, Zheng D, Lyu Y, Cheng W, Guo P, Cui Z. Effective degradation of aflatoxin $B_1$ using a novel thermophilic microbial consortium TADC7. Bioresource Technology. 2017;224:166-173. DOI: 10.1016/j.biortech.2016.11.033.

[101] Alberts JF, Gelderblom WC, Botha A and Van Zyl WH. Degradation of aflatoxin B1 by fungal laccase enzymes. International Journal of Food Microbiology. 2009; 135:47-52. DOI: 10.1016/j.ijfoodmicro.2009.07.022.

[102] Loi M, Fanelli F, Zucca P, ... Mule G. Aflatoxin $B_1$ and $M_1$ Degradation by Lac2 from *Pleurotus pulmonarius* and Redox Mediators. *Toxins (Basel)*. 2016;8:245. DOI:10.3390/toxins8090245

[103] Verheecke C, Liboz T, Mathieu F. Microbial degradation of aflatoxin B1: Current status and future advances. International Journal of Food Microbiology. 2016;237:1-9. DOI: 10.1016/j.ijfoodmicro.2016.07.028.

[104] Guo Y, Zhao L, Ma Q, Ji C. Novel strategies for degradation of aflatoxins in food and feed: A review. Food Research International. 2020;109878: ISSN 0963-9969. DOI: 10.1016/j.foodres.2020.109878.

[105] Zeinvand-Lorestani H, Sabzevari O, Setayesh N, Amini M, Nili-Ahmadabadi A, Faramarzi MA. Comparative study of in vitro prooxidative properties and genotoxicity induced by aflatoxin B1 and its laccase-mediated detoxification products. Chemosphere. 2015;135:1-6. DOi: 10.1016/j.chemosphere.2015.03.036.

[106] Guan ZB, Luo Q, Wang HR, Chen Y, Liao XR. Bacterial laccases: Promising biological green tools for industrial applications. Cellular and Molecular Life Sciences. 2018;75:3569-3592. DOI: 10.1007/s00018-018-2883-z.

[107] Guo Y, Qin X, Tang Y, Ma Q, Zhang J and Zhao, *L. cota* laccase, a novel aflatoxin oxidase from *Bacillus licheniformis*, transforms aflatoxin B1 to aflatoxin Q1 and epi-aflatoxin Q1. Food Chemistry. 2020;325:Article 126877. DOI: 10.1016/j.foodchem.2020.126877.

[108] Marimon Sibaja, KV, de Oliveira Garcia, S, Feltrin ACP, Diaz Remedi R, Cerqueira MBR, Badiale-Furlong E and Garda-Buffon, J. Aflatoxin biotransformation by commercial peroxidase and its application in contaminated food. Journal of Chemical Technology and Biotechnology. 2018;94:1187-1194. DOI: 0.1002/jctb.5865.

[109] Wang J, Ogata M, Hirai H, Kawagishi H. Detoxification of aflatoxin

B1 by manganese peroxidase from the white-rot fungus *Phanerochaete sordida* YK-624. FEMS Microbiology Letters. 2011;314:164-169. doi: 10.1111/j.1574-6968.2010.02158.x.

[110] Loi M, Renaud JB, Rosini E, Pollegioni L, Vignali E, Haidukowski M, Sumarah MW, Logrieco AF, Mulè G. Enzymatic transformation of aflatoxin $B_1$ by Rh_DypB peroxidase and characterization of the reaction products. Chemosphere. 2020;250:126296. DOI: 10.1016/j.chemosphere.2020.126296.

[111] Zhao LH, Guan S, Gao X, Ma QG, Lei YP, Bai XM, Ji C. Preparation, purification and characteristics of an aflatoxin degradation enzyme from *Myxococcus fulvus* ANSM068. Journal of Applied Microbiology. 2011;110:147-155. doi: 10.1111/j.1365-2672.2010.04867.x.

[112] Xu L, Eisa Ahmed MF, Sangare L, Zhao Y, Selvaraj JN, Xing F, Wang Y, Yang H, Liu Y. Novel Aflatoxin-Degrading Enzyme from *Bacillus shackletonii* L7. Toxins (Basel). 2017;9:36. DOI: 10.3390/toxins9010036.

[113] Lapalikar GV, Taylor MC, Warden AC, Scott C, Russell RJ, Oakeshott JG. F420H2-dependent degradation of aflatoxin and other furanocoumarins is widespread throughout the actinomycetales. PLoS One. 2012;7:e30114. DOI: 10.1371/journal.pone.0030114.

[114] Zhang Y, Geary T and Simpson BK. Genetically modified food enzymes: A review. Current Opinion in Food Science. 2019;25:14-18. DOI: 10.1016/j.cofs.2019.01.002.

[115] Wei H, Wang E. Nanomaterials with enzyme-like characteristics (nanozymes): next-generation artificial enzymes. Chemical Society Review. 2013;42:6060-6093. DOI: 10.1039/c3cs35486e.

[116] Liang H, Lin F, Zhang Z, Liu B, Jiang S, Yuan Q, Liu J. Multicopper Laccase Mimicking Nanozymes with Nucleotides as Ligands. ACS Applied Materials and Interfaces. 2017;9:1352-1360. DOI: 10.1021/acsami.6b15124

[117] Chen M, Yang B, Zhu J, Liu H, Zhang X, Zheng X, Liu Q. FePt nanoparticles-decorated graphene oxide nanosheets as enhanced peroxidase mimics for sensitive response to $H_2O_2$. Material Science and Engineering C Materials for Biological Applications. 2018;90:610-620. DOI: 10.1016/j.msec.2018.05.004.

[118] Chi MQ, Chen SH, Zhong MX, Wang C and Lu XF. Self-templated fabrication of FeMnO3 nanoparticle-filled polypyrrole nanotubes for peroxidase mimicking with a synergistic effect and their sensitive colorimetric detection of glutathione. Chemical Communications. 2018;54:5827-5830. DOI:10.1039/C8CC01574K.

[119] Chen M, Yang B, Zhu J, Liu H, Zhang X, Zheng X, Liu Q. FePt nanoparticles-decorated graphene oxide nanosheets as enhanced peroxidase mimics for sensitive response to $H_2O_2$. Materials Science & Engineering C-Materials for Biological Applications. 2018;90:610-620. DOI: 10.1016/j.msec.2018.05.004

[120] Cai S, Han Q, Qi C, Lian Z, Jia X, Yang R, Wang C. Pt74Ag26 nanoparticle-decorated ultrathin MoS2 nanosheets as novel peroxidase mimics for highly selective colorimetric detection of H2O2 and glucose. Nanoscale. 2016;8:3685-3693. DOI: 10.1039/c5nr08038j.

Chapter 7

# Occurrence of Mycotoxins in Certain Freshwater Fish Species and the Impact on Human Health: A General Review

*Muralidharan Velappan and Deecaraman Munusamy*

## Abstract

Mycotoxins are toxic secondary metabolites produced by organisms of the fungus kingdom, which are capable of causing disease and death in humans and animals when present in food. Recent studies evinces fish consumption might become another way for mycotoxins to enter the human food chain. Although the increasing research publications related to the occurrence and prevention of mycotoxin contamination in fish feeds, there was limited studies on bioaccumulation of mycotoxins research in common freshwater fish species. Further this was assumed fish species of salmonid and cyprinids are very sensitive to feed-borne mycotoxins so far. Studies have demonstrated, fish may also carry mycotoxins residue along the food chain, thus compromising human health. This review describes mainly mycotoxin contaminations in certain freshwater fish species and the impact on human health due to their potential proven toxicity. This review also provided comprehensive information on mycotoxins contamination levels in muscle and liver tissue of some freshwater fish species such as *Nile tilapia*, *Labeo rohita*, and *Catla catla* during capturing in fresh water lakes and also fish sold at wet market and hypermarket in Chennai, Tamilnadu.

**Keywords:** Mycotoxins, bioaccumulation, freshwater fish, wet market, hypermarket, Chennai

## 1. Introduction

In many developing countries, fish grew in economic importance during the second half of the twentieth century and by the end of the 1990s, the fisheries sector had become an important source of food, employment and foreign exchange. Worldwide since 1960 consumption of fish has been increasing, on an average fish consumption has varied among continents and countries within each continent, and it always been higher in richer than in poorer countries. Several studies evinces that per capita fish intake will continue to increases worldwide to the next three decades, and the increasing consumption will result as a typical indicator used to measure the country's economic health. In contrast the existing studies of positive income in fish trade, which generally ranges between normal and inferior, however the manner in which consumption responds to increase in wealth seems not only to the level of accomplishment of wealth, but also the quantities of fish that are eaten by the consumers. During the end of the twentieth century, in the developing countries, fishing pressure on inshore underwent increases steadily. This is mainly due to growing populations, changes in the technology, modernization of fishing methods, and access to an increasing number of buyers. According to the Food and Agriculture Organization of the United Nations, overfishing was bringing more inshore fish stocks into a state of overexploitation and the situation was becoming more serious threat for many communities.

Mycotoxins are toxic secondary metabolites produced by organisms of the fungus kingdom and is capable of causing disease and death in humans and animals including aquatic species. Several study reports evinces symptoms like vomiting, abdominal pain, jaundice, pulmonary edema, coma, convulsions, and death are considered as acute aflatoxicosis in humans, chronic symptoms of Long-standing exposure to aflatoxins has been associated with liver diseases, including cancer, cirrhosis, hepatitis [1]. Since 1956, the scientific expert committee jointly convened by FAO/WHO Expert Committee on Food Additives (*JECFA*) is the international body responsible for evaluating the health risk from naturally occurring toxicants and residues of veterinary drugs in food. Goswami et al. [2], Murphy et al. [3] and Marin et al. [4] reported toxigenic fungi can grow on a wide variety of crops, including wheat, maize, and soy bean. Grenier and Oswald [5] and Pal et al. [6] have reported presently more than around 300–400 mycotoxins which are produced by 350 filamentous fungi were identified till date. The most common mycotoxins which are produced by moulds are *Aspergillus, Penicillium, fusarium*, and *Alternaria,* the occurrence of mycotoxicosis only after the consumption of mycotoxin-contaminated by humans and animals [7].

Bennett and Klich [8] and Bryden [9] noted that the fungal genera of *Aspergillus, Fusarium*, and *Penicillium* are most frequent sources of harmful mycotoxins. A number of studies from different regions of Europe evinces *Aspergillus* prefers warmer tropical areas, whereas *Fusarium* and *Penicillium* grow in European temperate areas [10]. However, *Aspergillus flavus* causes a broad spectrum of disease in human beings, ranging from hypersensitivity reactions to invasive infection, *Aspergillus flavus* and *Aspergillus parasiticus* are the major producers of mycotoxins that contaminates foodstuffs such as groundnut, maize, etc., [11]. The toxic symptoms of mycotoxins intake are collectively known as mycotoxicosis are the consequence of ingestion of grains or forage containing toxic metabolites produced by filamentous fungi. Fungi that produce toxins often do so only under specific conditions of warmth, moisture and humidity. Mycotoxins produce their toxic effects in several ways, including impairment of metabolic, nutritional or endocrine functions. According to [12, 13] study reports some mycotoxins are produce teratogenic or carcinogenic. Apart from plant feed stuffs such as soybean meal and cereal grains as a great source of mycotoxins in fishes [14, 15], an aquatic weed, *Eichhornia crassipes*, commonly known as water hyacinth, is one of the most troublesome aquatic weed and also an alternative to fish diets as partial or total fish meal replacement, a fungal phytopathogen *Alternaria alternata* (AL-14) a new strain on water hyacinth has been recorded as lower dissolved oxygen level leading to reduction of aquatic fish production [16]. Gunnarsson and Petersen [17] reported that water hyacinths collection from various sources and some important components namely hemicellulose 22–43.4 percent; cellulose 17.8–31 percent; lignin 7–26.36 percent; and magnesium 0.17 percent. Matai and Bagchi [18] also reported the component levels of fresh water hyacinths ash which contains 28.7 percent K2O, 1.8 percent Na2O and 21 percent Cl. Tacon [19], Santacroce et al. [20] and Anater et al. [21] reported that increased risk of contamination on plant-based diets to the fishes, more specifically increased mycotoxins-contamination tropical regions and developing countries where fish feeds are often made by the farmers themselves under inappropriate conditions with improper milling and storage condition. Gareis and Wolff [22] and Iqbal et al. [23] were observed some mycotoxins contaminating edible tissues in fishes mainly

Aflatoxins (AFs), zearalenone (ZEN), and ochre toxin A (OTA), which represents food safety risk. Persi et al. [24] and Nomura et al. [25] found the residues of aflatoxin B1 (AFB1) in fish muscle under experimental conditions, while [26] hypothesized the presence of mycotoxins in fish tissues could be the result from previous contamination of water ponds or from an accumulation of mycotoxins in mud ponds. Abdel-Wahaab et al. [27] observed, residues of sterigmatocystin (a mycotoxins closely related to AFs) in edible tissue of Nile tilapia, *Oreochromis niloticus*, after the intragastric dosing. Earlier study reports of [28] shows ZEN (a resorcylic acid lactone) and its derivatives are the only known mycotoxins with estrogenic potential and are classified as endocrine-disrupting substance. While analyzing the occurrence of emerging Fusarium mycotoxins in aquacultural fish, [29] reported *Fusarium verticillioides* and *Fusarium proliferatum* are the common ingredient in fish feeds, further he concluded that the risk of contamination with *Fusarium* toxins is higher in maize and wheat than for soybean, however they were isolated in a very small percentage they may cause adverse effects to fish.

Since most studies have concentrated the effects of aflatoxins at high levels in fish feeds, and the establishment of aflatoxins on higher verteberates not on the effects on lower vertebrates. This study mainly discusses the various mycotoxins contamination levels in edible portion of muscle and liver tissues of freshwater fishes of *Nile tilapia*, *Labeo rohita*, and *Catla catla*.

## 2. Mycotoxins

The occurrence of mycotoxins in aquatic feeds and their effects on target species are topics that continue to gain attention due to the general trend of replacing expensive animal protein sources such as fishmeal with cheaper plant-derived proteins. Mycotoxins intoxication occurs when fish and shrimp consume mycotoxins-contaminated feedstuffs [30]. Moreover, the impact of mycotoxins changes depending on the kind of fish that consumes them, especially Aflatoxin B1, was widely investigated mycotoxins as a source of contamination of foods and aquaculture feed worldwide. However great scientific discoveries were made in aflatoxin $B_1$ ($AFB_1$) in the aquaculture feedstuffs, and epizootic of hepatomas in rainbow trout by a number of researchers under the direction of scientists J. Halver, R. 0. Sinnhuber, G. S. Bailey, J. D. Hendricks and colleagues, and very restricted study to a limited number of fish species till date [31].

Mycotoxins primarily found in areas with hot and humid climate, favourable for the growth of molds, they can also be found in temperate zones. In addition, mycotoxins exposure is mostly by ingestion [32]. Several studies performed by [33] shows *A. flavus* and *A. parasiticus* are the major dominant species isolated from fish feed from tropical countries. Fallah [34] and Hussain and Anwar [35] were found fish feed from Egypt and Iran were contaminated with *A. flavus.* Similarly [36, 37] reported fish feeds were contaminated with *A. flavus* at 35% and 55%, whereas *Aspergillus tamarii* were isolated at a frequency of 9.1% and 8% in fish feeds from Brazil, East Africa East Africa and Iran. *Aspergillus niger* (6%, 13.9%, 36%, and 39.1%) and *A. ochraceus* (10.2%) are the potential ochratoxigenic fungi were isolated from fish feed from East Africa, Iran, Portugal, and Brazil [38].

Rodríguez-Cervantes et al. [39] and Alinezhad et al. [40] reported that AFB1, the most dangerous aflatoxin, displays hepatotoxic, carcinogenic, mutagenic, eratogenic, and immunosuppressive effects on a range of animal species, including aquatic vertebrates. Ashley and Halver [41] reported first, aflatoxicosis outbreak in rainbow trout hatcheries in the USA, was related to hepatoma, where trout was fed with AF-contaminated feed. Ashley [42] reported the lethal poisoning by AFs in many other fishes. Most importantly AFB1 mechanism of action is the formation of AFB1–8, 9-epoxide during metabolization by cytochrome P450. Farabi et al. [43] reported that AFB1–8, 9-epoxide forms an adduct with macromolecules in cells, with an affinity in decreasing order of macromolecules of DNA > RNA > protein. Coppock et al. [44] observed, some fish species are extremely sensitive to AFB1 mainly because of differences in the patterns of enzymes involved in AFB1 metabolism. Bailey et al. [45] reported the carcinogenic effect of AFB1 in channel catfish, *Ictalurus punctatus*; Nile tilapia, *Oreochromis niloticus* and the ornamental guppy, *Poecilia reticulata.* Chàvez-Sànchez et al. [46] has been observed marked differences in the susceptibility of different fish species and fish classes with fish fry, for instance, aflatoxicosis being more sensitive and succumbing quicker than adult fish. Dissimilarities in Aflatoxin sensitivity in salmonids with rainbow trout displaying extremely sensitive, while coho salmon, *Oncorhynchus kisutch*, were more resistant. Hendricks [47] reported the occurrence of three forms of Aflatoxicosis: acute, subacute, and chronic. Acute aflatoxicosis in fish appears after ingestion of moderate to high doses of AFs.

Bauer et al. [48] observed, in a experimental study on rainbow trout evinces sublethal doses of AFB1 produces anemia, pale gills, reduced packed cell volume values, edema, haemorrhaging, liver damage, and alterations to nutrient metabolism in rainbow trout. Similarly [49] also reported, acute toxicity was noticed in rohu, *Labeo rohita* following intraperitoneal (i.p.) application of AFB1, with doses of 7.5, 11.25, and 13.75 mg/kg AFB1 caused anorexia, sluggish movement, rapid opercular movement, and also found dose-dependent mortality by the end of the 10-day of the experiment. Histopathological alterations in liver with subcapsular focal congestion, necrotic and vascular changes and gill lamellae, meningitis, brain congestion, degeneration and inflammatory injury of the heart, degenerative and necrotic changes to the kidney tubules, and sloughing of the intestinal mucosa [50, 51]. Sahoo et al. [52] observed AFB1 at concentrations of 1.25 and 2.5 mg/kg (i.p.) in rohu caused cachexia, and preneoplastic liver lesions, along with changes to the spleen, intestine, gill, and pancreas over the 90-d trial. Sahoo et al. [53] were analyzed in rohu, doses of 1.25 and 5.0 mg/kg (i.p.) AFB1 caused disruption of the immune system over 90 days, evinces as a reduction in total protein, globulin levels. Pier et al. [54] also noticed chronic aflatoxicosis after long-term intake of low to moderate doses of AFs. Furthermore, this chronic form of the disease is reported as carcinogenic and genotoxic effects, followed by teratogenic, hormonal, neurotoxic, and hematological changes. Pier et al. [55] demonstrated in sea bass *Dicentrarchus labrax*, AFB1 at concentration of 0.018 mg/kg in feed evinces induced liver damage, increased in serum transaminases and alkaline phosphatase activity with significant decrease in plasma proteins after 42-day of exposure. El-Sayed et al. [56] observed circulation disturbances and reaction induced infiltration around the bile duct, degeneration of liver tissues, nerve cells and renal damages, with the changes of polymorphonuclear in the renal tubules after 120- day of exposure AFB1 at concentrations of 0.2 mg/kg in common carp, *Cyprinus carpio.* Similarly [57] reported that negatively affected growth performance, bactericidal activity, lysozyme activity, and concentration of total serum proteins in yellow catfish, *Pelteobagrus fulvidraco*, after a 12-week trial with the presence of AFB1 in the diet at a level of 0.2 mg/kg. Manning et al. [58] reported AFs in naturally contaminated feed in a concentration of 0.16 mg/kg had no adverse effects on the Production variables of weight gain, feed intake, and feed efficiency ratio (FER) in channel catfish, *I. punctatus.* Similar results were shown by [59] a 12-week study on juvenile channel catfish fed diets containing up to 0.22 mg AFs/kg. No significant reduction in body weight gain, FER, survival, or haematocrit values was noticed. Tuan et al. [60] reported, the species of the genus *Oreochromis* tends to evinces low susceptibility to AFB1 exposure. The effect of diets with 0.25, 2.5, 10, and 100 mg/kg AFB1 on Nile tilapia for 8 weeks. Diets containing 100 mg/kg AFB1 caused weight loss, severe hepatic necrosis, and mortality, while 10.0 mg/kg evoked hepatic injury characterized by an excess of lipofuscin and irregular sized hepatocellular nuclei. Diets containing more than 2.5 mg/kg AFB1 evinces negative values of haematocrit and growth patterns. No significant effects were observed diet containing 0.25 mg/kg AFB1. Deng et al. [61] monitored the toxigenic effects of AFB1 in blue tilapia *Oreochromis aureus* over 20 week by using food containing 0.019, 0.085, 0.245, 0.638, 0.793, and 1.641 mg/kg AFB1. Subsequently reduced cases of mortality rate was noticed in Nile tilapia throughout the experiment and toxic impacts were the only observed in the diet with 0.245 mg/kg or higher between 10 and 20 weeks. At levels of 0.245 mg/kg AFB1, and reduction in the growth rate was noticed along with hepatic damage, and accumulations of inflammatory cells and eosinophilic materials were found in the liver at 0.638 mg/kg of AFB1. [62, 63]. Therefore, based on the several study results, weight gain does not appear to be a sensitive parameter to detect mycotoxins contamination. According to [64] serum Alanine Aminotransferase (ALT) and Lactic Acid Dehydrogenase (LDH) along with lactate concentrations seems to be the delicate to fish with the responses to Deoxynivalenol (DON). Little is known about the impact of ecotoxicology and the consequence of exposure to aquatic organisms [65]. Careful monitoring of the AFs content in fish is essential, particularly in south and Southeast Asia. Thus it can be observed the various effects of mycotoxins reported in fish, as well as the related doses and time that fishes were exposed.

### 2.1 Ochratoxins

Ochratoxins are a group of mycotoxins produced by some *Aspergillus* species (mainly *A. ochraceus* and *A. carbonarius*, but also by 33% of *A. niger* industrial strains) and some *Penicillium* species, especially *P. verrucosum* [66]. Persi et al. [67] reported that *Ochratoxins A* (OTA) is the most prevalent and relevant fungal toxin of this group. According to reports of the International Agency for Research on Cancer (IARC) categorized OTA as possibly carcinogenic to humans under Group 2B carcinogen. As per the reports of [68] Ochratoxins A (OTA) evinces an immunosuppressive, teratogenic, and nephrotoxic compound. However, prevalence of OTA is the highest in South Asian and Eastern European food samples, the average contamination is much higher in South Asia [69]. Human studies are showed that OTA is associated with kidney diseases, such as Balkan endemic nephropathy (BEN). BEN is a chronic tubulointerstitial disease which slowly progressed into terminal renal failure. Doster [70] described the main target organs of OTA toxic impact are the liver and kidney in fishes, and also he recorded an acute toxicity and metabolization of OTA in rainbow trout were developed with 10-days mortalities after single i.p. doses of OTA at 4.0, 6.0, and 8.0 mg/kg body weight. Histopathological study evinces normal architecture of liver specimen in trout dosed with OTA 4.0 mg/kg with many necrotic parenchymal cells. But the apparent effect of OTA on the affected liver was an increased the number of cytoplasmic and nuclear vacuoles at the highest doses of OTA with 8.0 mg/kg evinces necrosis in all parts of the kidney tissues.

Fuchs and Hult [71] and Hagelberg et al. [72] observed an experimental study on rainbow trout with one single intravenous injection of 14C-labeled OTA, further they also noticed this mycotoxins was excreted through the urine and bile in 35.8 and 57.1%, over 24 h, which indicates that the hepatobiliary mode of excretion is more important than urinary excretion in fish. Similarly [73, 74] noticed highest concentrations of OTA in tissue 24 h after exposure were in the pyloric ceca, intestine, and liver and the elimination half-life of OTA in fish is 0.68 h. which evinces much shorter than mammals and birds. El-Sayed et al. [75] observed the acute toxicity of OTA and behavioural changes in marine-reared adult sea bass. They also recorded an acute oral 96-h lethal concentration 50 value of 0.277 mg/kg body weight. Histopathological investigation revealed marked changes in fin and general congestion of the kidneys, gills, and on the periphery of the liver. Diab et al. [76] investigated in an experimental approach on ochratoxicosis in Nile tilapia and its amelioration by some feed additives. He also observed OTA intoxicated positive control group were sluggish swimming, poor growth and off feed before death with reduction in survival was 53% and growth performance. Gross pathological lesions were also observed in liver, kidneys and spleen. Biochemistry results evinces ALT, AST, creatinine and urea were significantly raised with reduced total protein TP, albumin and globulin also compared in ochratoxicated fish group with negative control group.

Bernhoft et al. [77] demonstrated dietary exposure of channel catfish (*Ictalurus punctatus*) and sea bass (*Dicentrarchus labrax*) to OTA led to reduced weight gains, poorer feed conversion rates, lower survival and changes of haematocrit values. Moreover, histopathological changes were observed in liver and posterior kidney tissues and changes of immune parameters were observed in channel catfish, similarly Nile tilapia (*Oreochromis niloticus*) showed increasing dietary OTA levels resulted in decreased growth, and poor feed utilization. In contrast, there have been no studies examining the effect of OTA on contamination levels in muscle and liver tissue of freshwater fish species viz., *Nile tilapia*, *Labeo rohita*, and *Catla catla* during capturing in fresh water lakes and also fish sold at wet market and hypermarket in Chennai, Tamilnadu.

### 2.2 Fusarium mycotoxins

*Fusarium* mycotoxins are a broad class of compounds with different chemical structures, physical and toxicological proprieties. Due to this great diversity, different detoxification strategies are required to deal with this complex group of compounds, Ismaiel et al. [78] and Crisan [79] has proved several studies, adsorption is not a feasible strategy to tackle fusarium mycotoxins, as it is only effective towards aflatoxins and, to a lesser extent, ochratoxins. Fusarium mycotoxins cause acute and chronic toxic effects and have been shown to cause a broad variety of toxic effects in animals [80].

### 2.3 Trichothecenes

Trichothecenes are a very large family of chemically related mycotoxins produced by various species of F*usarium,* Myrothecium, Trichoderma, Trichothecium, Cephalosporium, Verticimonosporium, and Stachybotrys [81]. Hazardous concentrations of trichothecenes have been detected in maize, wheat, oats, and other commodities used as ingredients in aquaculture feeds [82]. The toxicity of trichothecenes is primarily in protein biosynthesis inhibitors, neurotoxins, Immunosuppressive factors, or nephrotoxins and evoke acute and chronic symptoms after uptake [83]. In general, trichothecenes have the ability to affect general cell metabolism due to the tendency of active site thiol groups to attack the 12, 13 carbon epoxide ring, these inhibitory effects mostly seen in actively proliferating cells in the gastrointestinal tract or bone marrow [84]. Trichothecenes represents large group of over 150 chemically related mycotoxins known to date. Structurally each trichothecene consisting of a single six-membered ring containing a single oxygen atom, bounded by two carbon rings, the core ring structure contains an epoxide or tricyclic ether, at the 12, 13 carbon positions, as well as a double bond at the 9, 10 carbon positions, these two functional groups are primarily responsible for trichothecene ability to inhibit protein synthesis and incur cytotoxic effects. Removal of these groups results in a complete loss of toxicity [85]. Further the classification system breaks up the trichothecene family into four groups namely type A, B, C, and D, based on chemical structure, with type A including T-2 toxin, HT-2 toxin, a deacetylated metabolite of T-2 toxin, neosolaniol, and diacetoxyscirpenol and type B, represented by deoxynivalenol (DON), nivalenol, and its 3-acetyl and 15-acetyl derivates [86]. Despite the distinct functional groups of trichothecene classification types give each and unique chemical properties, their classification type does not specifically indicate their relative toxicity, While Type D trichothecenes are pondering to be the most toxic, comparatively, A and B types have mixed toxicity [87]. Trichothecenes toxic effects in animals include decreased plasma glucose, reduced blood cell and leukocyte count, weight loss, alimentary toxic aleukia, as well as pathological changes in the liver and stomach. The mechanism involved in T-2 and DON toxicity is generally via oxidative stress-mediated deoxyribonucleic acid (DNA) damage and apoptosis [88, 89]. Furthermore, T-2 and DON are well-known inhibitors of protein synthesis resulting from the binding of peptidyl-transferase, which is located in the 60s ribosomal subunit. The most important trichothecene mycotoxicosis in animals, including fish are the T-2 toxin and DON [90].

### *2.3.1 T-2 toxin*

T2 Toxin, are trichothecene mycotoxins produced by fungal metabolites of the genus *Fusarium*. They are commonly present in foods and feed of cereal origin, and it was reported T-2 toxin was first isolated from the mould *F. tricinctum (F. sporotrichoides)*. The main toxic effects of T-2 toxin induces DNA damage and cell death on prolonged administration, while these effects can be partially blocked by antioxidants, such as glutathione, coenzyme Q10, or α-tocopherol. In contrast toxic effects have been shown both in experimental animals and in livestock (unpublished data from Sigma Aldrich). Till date, very few investigation have been done on biological effects of T-2 toxin in fish diets. Earlier study reports of [91]. Reported that feeding of T-2 toxin around 16 week >2.5 mg/kg resulted in stunted growth in rainbow trout with reduced feed intake and hematocrit and hemoglobin concentrations evinces dose- dependent depression, while in Adult trout fed 15.0 mg/kg T-2 toxin had focal intestinal hemorrhaging and enlarged spleens and gall bladders. Manning et al. [92] also reported the T-2 toxin, is responsible for significant reduction in growth, significantly poor feed conversion, adversely affected hematocrit value, low survivability and histopathological anomalies of stomach and kidneys in juvenile channel catfish. In addition, LD of T-2 in trout evinces, severe oedema and fluid accumulation in the body cavity and behind the eyes are produced in addition to the loss of the intestinal mucosa. Consumption of T-2 toxin contaminated feed at concentrations of 1.0 and 1.8 mg/kg in the rainbow trout immune system by studying non-specific cellular and humoral immune responses and its effect on red and white blood cells. Both the concentrations evinces significantly increased erythrocyte counts and a decrease in mean corpuscular volume, while haemogram analysis evinces decreased mean corpuscular haemoglobin to both experimental concentrations. In contrast, decreases in plasma haemoglobin was the only significant at the higher T-2 toxin concentration level. However, higher concentration of T-2 toxin resulted in a significant increase of leukocyte and lymphocyte count, while absolute phagocyte count and less mature neutrophil granulocyte forms remained unchanged at both the concentrations. Immunological assay evinces, non-specific humoral immunity was decreased significantly in both experimental groups when compared with the control study. Paradoxically, T-2 toxin in feed at a concentration range of 1.0–1.8 mg/kg influences the immunological defence mechanisms of rainbow trout [93].

### *2.3.2 Deoxynivalenol*

Deoxynivalenol (DON), also known as vomitoxin, is a type B trichothecene, an epoxy- sesquiterpenoid. This mycotoxin occurs predominantly in grains such as wheat, barley, oats, rye, and corn, and less often in rice, sorghum, and triticale, further it is the most economically important mycotoxin [94, 95]. The effects of deoxynivalenol (DON) on fish are still not clear. In vitro study evinces fishes are sensitive animals to (DON) toxin. However this toxin does not seem to be a threat to the health of the fish, and not the case for deoxynivalenol (also called vomitoxin) which is the least toxic trichothecene, and some study reports evinces this can even cause harm to fish and humans [96]. The impact of experimental animals rats after oral exposure of (DON) exhibits both developmental and reproductive toxicity including reduced fertility, embryo toxicity, and skeletal abnormalities, effects on body weight and relative epididymal weight and postnatal mortality [97]. In general, exposure of (DON) among fishes does not cause higher mortality. However, doses of up to 2.6 mg/kg of this (DON) toxin were fed to rainbow trout, symptoms develops poor feeding and reduced feed conversion efficiency, which further leads to poor weight gain and growth rate. Although, feeding a rainbow trout diet with 6.4 mg/kg of deoxynivalenol causes reduced in mortality after *Flavobacterium psychrophilum* infection. Similarly, exposure in channel catfish to deoxynivalenol (2.5 to 10.0 mg/kg) increased their survival rate after *Edwardsiella ictalurid* infection, but no significant negative effects on weight gain and feed conversion efficiency. Therefore, (DON) seems to have some protective effect against Gram positive or Gram negative bacterial infections in some species of fishes [98]. Histopathological examination recorded by [99] morphological changes in the liver, including subcapsular edema, hemorrhages, and fatty infiltration of hepatocytes, while hemorrhages were found in the intestinal tract. According to [100] study reports evinces there was no significant changes in biometric parameters were recorded so far, significant changes were observed in hematological parameters, such as low mean corpuscular hemoglobin values and biochemical parameters, such as a decrease in glucose level, serum cholesterol, and ammonia [101].

## 2.4 Fumonisins

Fumonisins (FUMs) are mycotoxins produced by *F. verticilloides*. Worldwide, the occurrence these mycotoxins a common contaminants of maize and maize by-products. Further several reports evinces these (FUMs) mycotoxins mainly consist of fumonisin $B_1$ ($FB_1$), $FB_2$ and $FB_3$, with $FB_1$ being the most toxic. Clinical signs associated with fumonisin toxicity varies significantly between the species and the primary target organ, further, safe levels of fumonisin in the feed are quite variable between species [102, 103]. Experimental study evinces FB1 is also a cancer promoter and initiator in rat liver cells, hepatotoxicity in higher verteberates such as horses, pigs and vervet monkeys. In vitro cell culture evinces cytotoxicity in mammalian cells and phytotoxicity among various plants. Earlier study reports evinces (FUMs) in home-grown corn have been associated with an elevated risk for human oesophageal cancer in Transkei and China [104]. Voss et al. [105] observed, consumption of feed containing FBs leads to disruption of sphingolipid metabolism and accumulation of sphinganine (SA) in the liver, kidney, and serum in animals. Comparative study was carried out by [106] where the toxic dose for FB1 in fish has a broad range, with pigs and horses [107]. Fumonisin $B_1$ ($FB_1$) have been shown to reduce the productivity of fish. Nile tilapia fingerlings were fed $FB_1$ at 0, 10, 40, 70 and 150 ppm for 8 weeks. The $FB_1$ was extracted from cultures of *Fusarium moniliforme.* Mortalities in all treatment groups were low and were not dose related. Feeding diets containing 150 ppm $FB_1$ shows decreased hematocrit. There was evidence that sphingolipid metabolism was disrupted in fish fed $FB_1$. Observed decreased weight gains among fishes fed with $FB_1$ at 40, 70 and 150 ppm levels. However, fishes are fed 10 ppm of FB1 evinces decreased weight gains for the first 2 weeks, but body weights at 4 weeks not significantly different from controls. Some study evinces Channel catfish are more sensitive and toxic to FB1 [108]. Spring and Burel [109] reported that Channel catfish are more tolerant with FB1 than carp. Exposure of 1-year-old common carp to be feed contaminated with FB1 0.5 and 5.0 mg/kg body weight resulted loss of body weight and alterations of physiological parameters in target organs, including increased activities of liver enzymes. In another study with carp of a similar age, signs of toxicity were observed at dietary levels as low as 10 ppm FB1. Tuan et al. [110] reported in farm animals feed contaminated with FB1, histological sections revealed scattered lesions in the exocrine, endocrine pancreas and interrenal tissues, and this mostly due to ischemia or increased endothelial permeability. FB1 contamination was also found to impair the immune response of fishes were inoculated with killed *Edwardsiella ictaluri* cells. Microscopic hepatic lesions was observed in fish fed diets contaminated with more than 20 ppm. In contrast to these findings, a similar study was reported, there is no histological evidence of toxicity in adult channel catfish fed a diet containing more than 300 ppm FB1 for periods of up to five weeks. David et al. [111] described on Nile tilapia fingerlings, feeding FB1 at 10, 40, 70 or 150 mg/kg feed for eight weeks, affected the growth performance was evident. Similarly, experimental study in fish fed diets containing FB1 at levels of 40,000 μg/kg evinces decreased average weight gains, further, haemogram analysis revealed hematocrit was only decreased in tilapia fed diets containing 150,000 μg FB1/kg. On the other hand, few data's were available that shrimp are sensitive to FB1. So far FB1 has not been extensively studied in shrimp feed contaminants. Wo'zny et al. [112] reported FB1 was not a complete carcinogen in trout, when compared with fumonisin B1 (FB1) in rodents and epidemiological evidence association between FB1 and cancer in humans, for that he designed an experimental approach in rainbow trout with very low spontaneous tumor incidence, firstly, if FB1 was a complete carcinogen, in the absence of an initiator, secondly, promoter of liver tumors in fish initiated as fry with aflatoxin B1 (AFB1) and finally a promoter of liver, kidney, stomach, or swim bladder tumors in fish initiated as the fry with N-methyl-N′-nitro-nitrosoguanidine (MNNG). Despite FBs being the most prevalent mycotoxin in grains (the most common ingredient in commercial aqua feed), and epidemiological evidence suggests the overall concentration is low and does not represent a threat to fish. A slight tendency toward prolonged clotting time and lowered iron concentrations in the liver and ovary after exposing juvenile rainbow trout to 10 mg/kg ZEN i.p. for 24, 72, and 168 h was observed by [113]. ZEN concentrations in commercial fish feed for cyprinids in Central Europe was assessed by [114], while Zhang et al. [115] examined some samples of rainbow trout feed in Argentina, he observed concentrations did not exceed an average level of 0.068 mg/kg (Central Europe) and 0.088 mg/kg (Argentina), suggesting that ZEN poses no threat to fish under aquaculture.

### 2.5 Zearalenone

*Zearalenone* (ZEA), one of the common estrogenic mycotoxins and is mainly produced by Fusarium fungi. Primarily this (ZEA) mycotoxin attacks young crops, also can develop when cereals were stored even dried fully. *In vitro* and *in vivo* study evinces that (ZEA) possess estrogenic activity in mice, swine, donkeys and cattle. According to Southern Regional Aquaculture Centre (SARC) reports, (ZEA) toxin has potent estrogenic effects among farm animals. According to [116] reports, numerous studies have described the (ZEA) toxin worldwide, no data existed in India till date. Greco and Pose [117] reported, the exact mechanism of the reproductive physiology in farm animals with (ZEA) toxin has not been clearly documented. Feed concentrations of zearalenone as low as 1 to 4 ppm can cause transient to permanent reproductive damage in breeding swine, depending on the age of the animals. Susceptibility to (ZEA) toxin older animals are sensitive than younger animals. The effect of ZEA toxin on fish has not been evaluated, but it interferes the reproduction in many animals. Manning et al. [118] examined few samples of rainbow trout feed in Argentina, concluded that the concentrations did not exceed an average level of 0.068 mg/kg (Central Europe) and 0.088 mg/kg (Argentina), and also suggested ZEN poses no threat to fish under aquaculture.

### 2.6 Moniliformin

MON is an uncommon fungal toxin a feed contaminant that is lethal to mainly ducklings [119]. Experimental study were carried out at Auburn University evinces that juvenile channel catfish diets containing moniliformin toxin at 20, 40, 60 and 120 ppm of diet significantly lowered weight gains compared to the control catfish. Moniliformin disrupts the intermediary metabolism of the tricarboxylic acid (TCA) cycle at the conversion of pyruvate to acetyl-CoA, the starting intermediate for the TCA cycle [120]. Yildirim et al. [121] and Thiel [122] described, the MON toxicity, based on the disruption of pyruvate metabolism, since the inhibition of pyruvate dehydrogenase and subsequent pyruvate accumulation in the tissues of the affected animal. Gonçalves et al. [123] performed a comparative study on FB1 and MON toxicity in channel catfish, which evinces fish diets containing 20 mg/kg MON or FB1 led to differences in weight gain and FCR. Catfish fed with an FB1 diet had significantly lowered weight gain and poorer FCR than catfish fed a MON diet, which indicates that FB1 is more toxic than MON to channel catfish. Levels of 60 and 120 mg/kg MON (and the combination of MON and FB1) reduced hematocrit and caused smaller hepatocellular nuclei, whereas 60 mg/kg MON significantly increased serum pyruvate levels. Starostina [124] reported the toxicity of MON over the mineralization, development of bone structures and its influence on survival, growth and gene expression by using zebrafish (*Danio rerio*) as a model species for *in vivo* experiments, while gilthead seabream (*Sparus aurata*) mineralogenic cell line VSa13 as *in vitro* model. *In vivo* and *in vitro* analysis evinces MON did not decrease bone mineralization. This study also reported minimal *in vitro* cytotoxicity concentration at 1000 μg $L^{-1}$ MON, further the occurrence of deformities was also not altered by MON toxicity at the concentration tested (450 μg $L^{-1}$) inspite of larval growth was affected as shown by the decrease in standard length of exposed specimens after 20 dpf. Moniliformin concentrations higher than 900 μg $L^{-1}$ significantly decreased larvae survival when compared to control.

### 2.7 Emerging mycotoxins

According to Fish Site 2016, reports, emerging mycotoxins are a class of compounds that are attracting increasing interest among the scientific community, primarily their high occurrence in feed and food commodities, sometimes at relatively high concentrations, and potential toxicity towards animals and humans. Studies focusing on this class of mycotoxins are still quite low in number, an extensive review published in 2015 showed that among all mycotoxin-related studies, only 7% were directed towards emerging mycotoxins.

Over all, existing literature study evinces the naturally occurring fumonisin toxins produced by various fungal species of fusarium fungi reported to have toxic effects on vital organs, immunological disturbances loss of weight, including metabolic alterations, eventually results in cancer and increased mortality. Further, fusarium have been addressed as the most prevalent fungi that infect agricultural commodities, so far there were no study reports of bioaccumulation of fumonisin toxin in the musculature of fishes. They can also produce a broad array of mycotoxins and secondary metabolites, however, consumption of fish does not seem to be any serious impact reported by food security risk regarding this toxin, more studies are imperative to understand the impacts of these toxins on fish population [125].

#### *2.7.1 Enniatins*

Enniatins (ENNs) are known for their antimicrobial, insecticide and antifungal proprieties. These toxins might have herbicide effects as well. ENNs are commonly found on small cereal grains and derived products in Europe, Africa, Asia, America and Australia, with concentrations ranging from <1 μg/ to 100 mg. Other products can also be contaminated, such as dried fruits, nuts, eggs and fish. The mechanism of action of enniatins is directed towards cellular membrane transport proteins that are inhibited by the toxin. Toxicity of enniatins is particularly severe towards mitochondria [126].

#### *2.7.2 Beauvericin*

Beauvericin (BEA) shows strong antimicrobial activity towards various bacterial species, based on sources of the existing literature review, (BEA) has no distinction between Gram-positive and Gram-negative. This toxin also evinces cytotoxic, apoptotic and immunosuppressive activity. Beauvericin acts on the cellular membranes by increasing the permeability and disrupting the cellular homeostasis. In addition, (BEA) has been reported the toxicity to lymphocytes, skeletomyocytes and cardiomyocytes, with birds and minks being the most sensitive species. However, the mechanism of action has not been fully understood yet, but toxicity study evinces towards mitochondria, there is an assumption with the same mechanism of (ENNs) toxins.

#### *2.7.3 Fusaproliferin*

Studies focused on Fusaproliferin (FUS) evinces is a fungal toxicity towards human B - lymphocytes and some insect cell lines. (FUS) considered as the most emerging mycotoxin, earlier study also reports evinces teratogenic and pathogenic effects on chicken embryos. More recently, some studies were conducted using brine shrimp (*Artemia salina*) as a model organism. The toxin often co-occurs with deacetyl-fusaproliferin, although the toxicity of the latter is much lower compared to fusaproliferin. Studies on the synergistic effects between the two fungal toxins have not been elucidated yet.

### 2.8 Conclusions and future recommendations

The incidence is rapidly increasing mycotoxins, namely toxic fungi are currently of constant interest and concern, and aquatic species have different levels of sensitivity to mycotoxins depending on type and quantity of mycotoxins, duration of exposure, age, species and sex including diet. Outcomes of *mycotoxin* contamination in fish has been increasing during the last few years including rainbow trout, Atlantic salmon, common carp, gibel carp, zebrafish, beluga, sturgeon hybrids, channel catfish and Nile tilapia. However, the effects of the same mycotoxin on two different fish species under the same experimental conditions have not yet been investigated, which makes it difficult to judge species differences in sensitivity to mycotoxins. Most commonly, it was often assumed that salmonids are very sensitive to mycotoxins, but recent investigation evinces that depending on the biological response, similarly, cyprinids are also reported very sensitive to feed-borne mycotoxins. There were no mycotoxin contamination research conducted on *Labeo rohita*, and *Catla catla* during capturing in fresh water lakes and also fish sold at wet market and hypermarket so far, further research is needed to clarify the issue of species-specific sensitivity to certain mycotoxins. Further, the use of appropriate drying methods and improved storage conditions can certainly minimise the formation of mycotoxins in grains independent of the location where they take place, i.e. on a farm, in a warehouse or during transport. Increasing the knowledge on mycotoxins in fish will influence our future strategies for fish nutrition. We suggest that further research should be conducted on the effects of co-occurring mycotoxins and also recommend not only stricter regulations on fish feed, also fish handling (landing centre to retail market) further to reduce the impacts of mycotoxins on fish health and productivity.

## Declaration

No original data is utilized in this review, all information is accessed from published work.

## Author details

Muralidharan Velappan[1*] and Deecaraman Munusamy[2]

1 Department of Marine Biotechnology, AMET University, Chennai, India

2 Department of Biotechnology, Dr. M.G.R Educational and Research Institute, Chennai, India

*Address all correspondence to: muralidharanmicro@gmail.com

## References

[1] World Health Organization, Mycotoxin, 9 May, 2018.

[2] Goswami, R. S. and H. C. Kistler. Heading for disaster: *Fusarium graminearum* on cereal crops. Molecular Plant Pathology. 2004. 5:515-525.

[3] Murphy, P. A., S. Hendrich, C. Landgren, and C. M. Bryant. Food mycotoxins: an update. Journal of Food Science. 2006. 71:51-65.

[4] Marin, S., A. J. Ramos, G. Cano-Sancho, and V. Sanchis. Mycotoxins: occurrence, toxicology, and exposure assessment. Food and Chemical Toxicology. 2013. 60:218-237.

[5] Grenier, B., Oswald, I.P. (2011). Mycotoxin co-contamination of food and feed: Meta-analysis of publications describing toxicological interactions. World Mycotoxin Journal, 4(3), 285-313.

[6] Mahendra Pal, Fikru Gizaw, Firehiwot Abera, Pankaj Kumar Shukla, Hazarika, R.A. (2015). Mycotoxins: A Growing Concern to Human and Animal Health, Beverage & Food World, 42(5)

[7] Grenier, B. and Oswald, I. Mycotoxin co-contamination of food and feed: meta-analysis of publications describing toxicological interactions. World Mycotoxin Journal. 2011. 4 (3): 285-313. DOI: 10.3920/WMJ2011.1281.

[8] Bennett, J. W. and Klich. M. Mycotoxins. Clinical Microbiology Reviews. 2003. 16:497-516.

[9] Bryden, W. L. Mycotoxin contamination of the feed supply chain: implications for animal productivity and feed security. Animal Feed Science and Technology. 2012. 173:134-158.

[10] Iveta Matejova, Zdenka Svobodova,Jan Mares, Helena Modra. Impact of Mycotoxins on Aquaculture Fish Species: A Review. World Aquaculture Society. 2016. DOI: 10.1111/jwas.12371.

[11] Shankar, J. Madan, T. Basir, S. F and Sarma P. U. Identification and characterization of polyubiquitin gene from cDNA library of Aspergillus fumigatus. Indian Journal of Clinical Biochemistry. 2005. vol. 20, pp. 208-212.

[12] Marika Jestoi. Emerging fusarium-mycotoxins fusaproliferin, beauvericin, enniatins, and moniliformin: a review. Critical Review of Food Science Nutrition. 2008. 48(1):21-49. DOI: 1080/10408390601062021.

[13] Iveta Matejova, Zdenka Svobodova, Jan Mares, Helena Modra. Impact of Mycotoxins on Aquaculture Fish Species: A Review. World Aquaculture Society. 2016. DOI: 10.1111/jwas.12371.

[14] Yiannikouris, A. and Jouany, J. P. Mycotoxins in feeds and their fate in animals: a review. Animal Research. 2002. 51:81-99.

[15] Binder, E. M. Managing the risk of mycotoxins in modern feed production. Animal Feed Science and Technology. 2006. 133:149-166.

[16] Kamal Rai Aneja, Romika Dhiman, Neeraj Kumar Aggarwal, and Ashish Aneja, International Journal of Microbiology. 2014. Article ID 758942, 14 pages DOI:10.1155/2014/758942

[17] Carina C Gunnarsson, Cecilia Mattsson Petersen. Water hyacinths as a resource in agriculture and energy production: a literature review. 2005. Waste Management. 27(1):117-29. DOI: 0.1016/j.wasman.

[18] Matai, S. Bagchi, D.K. 1980. Water hyacinth: a plant with prolific bio-productivity and photosynthesis. p. 144-148. In: Gnanam, A,

Krishnaswamy, S., and Kahn, J.S. (eds.), Proc. International. Symposium on Biology. 1980. Applications of Solar Energy. MacMillan Co. of India, Madras.

[19] Tacon, A. G. J. Nutritional fish pathology: morphological signs of nutrient deficiency and toxicity in farmed fish. FAO Fish Technical Paper. 1992. No. 330. Food and Agriculture Organization of the United Nations, Rome, pp. 75.

[20] Santacroce, M. P. M. C. Conversano, E. Casalino, O. Lai, C. Zizzadoro, G. Centoducati, and G. Crescenzo. Aflatoxins in aquatic species: metabolism, toxicity and perspectives. Reviews in Fish Biology and Fisheries. 2008. 18:99-130.

[21] Anater, A. L. Manyes, G. Meca, E. Ferrer, F. B. Luciano, C. T. Pimpão, and G. Font. Mycotoxins and their consequences in aquaculture: a review. 2016. Aquaculture 451:1-10.

[22] Gareis, M. and J. Wolff. Relevance of mycotoxin contaminated feed for farming animals and carryover of mycotoxins in food of animal origin. 2000. Mycoses 43:79-83.

[23] Iqbal, S. Z. S. Nisar, M. R. Asi, and Jinaq, S. Natural incidence of aflatoxins, ochratoxin A and zearalenone in chicken meat and eggs. Food Control. 2014. 43:98-103.

[24] Persi, N. J. Pleadin, D. Kovacevi´ Scortichini, G and S. Milone. Ochratoxin A in raw materials and cooked meat products made from OTA-treated pigs. Meat Science. 2014. 96:203-210.

[25] Nomura, H. M. Ogiso, M. Yamashita, H. Takaku, A. Kimura, M. Chikasou, Y. Nakamura, S. Fujii, M. Watai, and H. Yamada. Uptake by dietary exposure and elimination of aflatoxins in muscle and liver of rainbow trout (*Oncorhynchus mykiss*). Journal of Agricultural and Food Chemistry. 2011. 59:5150-5158.

[26] Julie J Tsafack Takadong, Hippolyte T Mouafo , Linda Manet , Annick M B Baomog , Jorelle, J.B. Adjele, Evrard K Medjo, Gabriel N Medoua. Assessment of the Presence of Total Aflatoxins and Aflatoxin $B_1$ in Fish Farmed in Two Cameroonian Localities. Int J Food Sci. DOI: 10.1155/2020/2506812.

[27] Abdel-Wahaab, M. A. A. M. Hasan, S. E. Aly, and K. F. Mahrous. Adsorption of sterigmatocystin by montmorillonite and inhibition of its genotoxicity in the Nile tilapia fish (*Oreachromis nilaticus*). Mutation Research, Genetic Toxicology and Environmental Mutagenesis. 2005. 582:20-27.

[28] Zinedine, A. J. M. Soriano, J. C. Moltó, and J. Mañes. Review on the toxicity, occurrence, metabolism, detoxification, regulations and intake of zearalenone: an oestrogenic mycotoxin. Food and Chemical Toxicology. 2007. 45:1-18.

[29] Bullerman, LB. Ryu, D. Jackson, LS. Stability of fumonisins in food processing. Advances in Experimental and Medical Biology. 2002. 504:195-204.

[30] Global results of 22318 analyses on the occurrence of mycotoxins – including aflatoxin, zearalenone, deoxynivalenol (vomitoxin), T-2 toxin, fumonisins and Ochratoxin A— in crops such as corn (maize), wheat, soybean, related by-products and finished livestock feeds. Biomin Mycotoxin Survey Q1 2019 Results.

[31] Maria Pia Santacroce, M. C. Conversano, E. Casalino, O. Lai, C. Zizzadoro, G. Centoducati & G. Crescenzo, Springer Link. 2007. 18: pp 99-130.

[32] Bankole, S. M. Schollenberger, S and Drochner, W. "Mycotoxins in food systems in sub-Saharan Africa: a

review," *Mycotoxin Research*, 2006. vol. 22, no. 3, pp. 163-169.

[33] Berthiller, F. Sulyok, M. Krska, R and Schuhmacher, R "Chromatographic methods for the simultaneous determination of mycotoxins and their conjugates in cereals," *International Journal of Food Microbiology*, 2007. vol. 119, no. 1-2, pp. 33-37.

[34] Fallah, A. A. Aflatoxin M1 contamination in dairy products marketed in Iran during winter and summer. Food Control. 2010. 21:1478-1481.

[35] Hussain, I. Anwar, J. A study on contamination of aflatoxin M1 in raw milk in the Punjab province of Pakistan. Food Control.2008. 19:393-395.

[36] El-baradei G, Delacroix-buchet A, Ogier JC Bacterial biodiversity of traditional Zabady fermented milk. Int J Food Microbiol. 2008. 121:295-301.

[37] D'Mello, J. P. F. and A. M. C. Macdonald. Mycotoxins. Animal Feed Science and Technology. 1997. 69:155-166.

[38] Asghar Sepahvand, Masoomeh Shams-Ghahfarokhi, Abdolamir Allameh, Zahra Jahanshiri, Mojdeh Jamali & Mehdi Razzaghi-Abyaneh A survey on distribution and toxigenicity of *Aspergillus flavus* from indoor and outdoor hospital environments. Folia Microbiologica. 2011. **56**, 527-534.

[39] Rodríguez-Cervantes, C.H. A.J. Ramos, A.J. Robledo-Marenco, M.L Sanchis,V. Marín, S & M.I. Girón-Pérez. Determination of aflatoxin and fumonisin levels through ELISA and HPLC, on tilapia feed in Nayarit, Mexico. Food and Agricultural Immunology. 2013. 24:3. DOI:10.1080/09540105.2012.684202.

[40] Alinezhad, S., M. Tolouee, A. Kamalzadeh, A. A. Motalebi, M. Nazeri, M. Yasemi, M. Shams-Ghahfarokhi, R. Tolouei, and M. Razzaghi-Abyaneh. Mycobiota and aflatoxin B1 contamination of rainbow trout (*Oncorhynchus mykiss*) feed with emphasis to *Aspergillus* section *Flavi*. Iranian Journal of Fisheries. 2011. 10:363-374.

[41] Ashley, L.M. and Halver, J.E. Multiple metastasis of rainbow trout hepatoma. Transactions of the American Fisheries Society. 1963. 92:365-371.

[42] Ashley, L. M. Pathology of fish fed aflatoxins and other antimetabolites. A Symposium on Diseases of Fishes and Shellfishes.1970. American Fisheries Society Special Publication No. 5, 366-379.

[43] Farabi, S. M. V. M. Yousefian, M. and Hajimoradloo. A. Aflatoxicosis in juvenile *Huso huso* fed a contaminated diet. Journal of Applied Ichthyology. 2006. 22:234-237.

[44] Coppock, R. W., R. R. G. Christian, and B. J. Jacobsen. Aflatoxins. Pages 1181-1199 *in* R. Gupta, editor. Veterinary Toxicology: Basic & Clinical Principles, 2$^{nd}$ edition. Elsevier, Inc.2012. San Diego, California, USA.

[45] Bailey, G. S. D. Williams, E. Wilcox, E. Loveland, Coulombe, P.M and Hendricks, J.D. Aflatoxin B1 carcinogenesis and its relation to DNA adduct formation and adduct persistence in sensitive and resistant salmonid fish. Carcinogenesis. 1988. 9:1919-1926.

[46] Chàvez-Sànchez, M. C. C. A. Martinez-Palacios, C. A. and Osorio-Moreno, I. Pathological effects of feeding young *Oreochromis niloticus* diets supplemented with different levels of aflatoxin B1. Aquaculture. 1994. 127:49-60.

[47] Hendricks, J. D. Carcinogenicity of aflatoxins in non-mammalian organisms. Pages 103-136 *in* D. L. Eaton

and J. D. Groopman, editors. The toxicology of aflatoxins: human health, veterinary, and agricultural significance.1994. Academic Press, New York, New York, USA.

[48] Bauer, D. H. Lee,D.J and Sinnhuber.R.O Acute toxicity of aflatoxins B1 and G1 in the rainbow trout (*Salmo gairdneri*). Toxicology and Applied Pharmacology. 1969. 15:415-419.

[49] Sahoo, P. K. Mukherjee, S.C Nayak, S. K. and Dey. S. Acute and sub chronic toxicity of aflatoxin B1 to rohu, *Labeo rohita* (Hamilton). Indian Journal of Experimental Biology.2001. 39:453-458.

[50] Hamilton, P. Problems with mycotoxins persist, but can be lived with. Feedstuffs.1990. 62:22-23.

[51] Santacroce, M. P. M. C. Conversano, E. Casalino, O. Lai, C. Zizzadoro, G. Centoducati, and G. Crescenzo. Aflatoxins in aquatic species: metabolism, toxicity and perspectives. Reviews in Fish Biology and Fisheries. 2008. 18:99-130.

[52] Sahoo, P. K. Mukherjee, S.C Nayak, S. K. and Dey. S. Acute and sub chronic toxicity of aflatoxin B1 to rohu, *Labeo rohita* (Hamilton). Indian Journal of Experimental Biology.2001. 39:453-458.

[53] Sahoo, P. K. S. C. Mukherjee, S.CS. Nayak, S.K. and S. Dey. Acute and sub chronic toxicity of aflatoxin B1 to rohu, *Labeo rohita* (Hamilton). Indian Journal of Experimental Biology.2001. 39:453-458.

[54] Pier, A. C. Richard, J.L and Cysewski. S.J. Implications of mycotoxins in animal disease. Journal of the American Veterinary Medical Association. 1980. 176:719-724.

[55] Pier, A. C. Richard, J.L and Cysewski. S.J. Implications of mycotoxins in animal disease. Journal of the American Veterinary Medical Association. 1980. 176:719-724.

[56] El-Sayed, Y. S. and Khalil. R.H. Toxicity, biochemical effects and residue of aflatoxin B1 in marine water-reared sea bass (*Dicentrarchus labrax* L.). Food and Chemical Toxicology. 2009. 47:1606-1609.

[57] Wang, X. Y. Wang, Y. Li, M. Huang, Y. Gao, X. Xue, H. Zhang, P. Encarnação, G. A. Santos, and R. A. Gonçalves. Response of yellow catfish (*Pelteobagrus fulvidraco*) to different dietary concentrations of aflatoxin B1 and evaluation of an aflatoxin binder in offsetting its negative effects. Ciencias Marinas. 2016. 42: 15-29.

[58] Manning, B. B. Wise, D. J. Abbas, H. K. and Peterson, B. C. Channel catfish, *Ictalurus punctatus*, fed diet containing aflatoxin from moldy corn do not experience increased mortality after challenge with *Edwardsiella ictaluri*. Journal of the World Aquaculture Society. 2011. 42:598-602.

[59] Manning, B. B. Wise, D. J. Abbas, H. K. and Peterson, B. C. Channel catfish, *Ictalurus punctatus*, fed diet containing aflatoxin from moldy corn do not experience increased mortality after challenge with *Edwardsiella ictaluri*. Journal of the World Aquaculture Society. 2011. 42:598-602.

[60] Tuan, N. A. Grizzle, J.M. Lovell, R.T. Manning, B.B and Rottinghaus, G.E. Growth and hepatic lesions of Nile tilapia (*Oreochromis niloticus*) fed diets containing aflatoxin B1. Aquaculture. 2002. 212:311-319.

[61] Deng, S. X. Tian, L. X. F. J. Liu, S. J. Jin, G. Y. Liang, H. J. Yang, Z. Y. Du, and Liu, Y. J. Toxic effects and residue of aflatoxin B1 in tilapia (*Oreochromis niloticus* × *O. aureus*) during long-term dietary exposure. Aquaculture. 2010. 307:233-240.

[62] Ashley, L.M. and Halver, J.E. Multiple metastasis of rainbow trout hepatoma. Transactions of the American Fisheries Society. 1963. 92:365-371.

[63] Bailey, G. S. Williams, D. E. Wilcox, J. Loveland, P.M. Coulombe, R.A and Hendricks, J.D. Aflatoxin B1 carcinogenesis and its relation to DNA adduct formation and adduct persistence in sensitive and resistant salmonid fish. Carcinogenesis. 1988. 9:1919-1926.

[64] Pietsch, C. Kersten, S. Burkhardt-Holm, P. Valenta, H and Dänicke, S. Occurrence of deoxynivalenol and zearalenone in commercial fish feed: an initial study. Toxins. 2013. 5:184-192.

[65] Shams, M. Mitterbauer, R. Corradini, R. Wiesenberger, G. Dall'Asta, C. Schuhmacher, R.Berthiller, F. Isolation and characterization of a new less-toxic derivative of the fusarium mycotoxin diacetoxyscirpenol after thermal treatment. Journal of Agricultural and Food Chemistry.2011. 59(17), 9709-9714.

[66] Forgacs, J. Mycotoxicoses-the neglected diseases. Feedstuffs. 1962. 34: 124-134.

[67] Persi, N. J. Pleadin, D. Kovacevi´ Scortichini, G and S. Milone. Ochratoxin A in raw materials and cooked meat products made from OTA-treated pigs. Meat Science. 2014. 96:203-210.

[68] Ladeira, C. Frazzoli, C. and Orisakwe, O. E. Engaging one health for non-communicable diseases in Africa: perspective for mycotoxins. Front. Public Health.2017. 5:266. DOI: 10.3389/fpubh.2017.00266.

[69] Schatzmayr, G. and Streit, E. Global occurrence of mycotoxins in the food and feed chain: facts and figures. World Mycotoxin Journal.2013. 6:213-222.

[70] Doster, R. C. Toxicity and metabolism of ochratoxins in rainbow trout (*Salmo gairdneri*). PhD dissertation. Oregon State University, Corvallis, Oregon. 1973. USA.

[71] Fuchs, R. and Hult, K. Ochratoxin A in blood and its pharmacokinetic properties. Food and Chemical Toxicology.1992. 30:201-204.

[72] Hagelberg, S. K. Hult, K and Fuchs, R. Toxicokinetics of ochratoxin A in several species and its Plasma-binding properties. Journal of Applied Toxicology. 1989. 9:91-96.

[73] Doster, R. C. Toxicity and metabolism of ochratoxins in rainbow trout (*Salmo gairdneri*). PhD dissertation. Oregon State University, Corvallis, Oregon. 1973. USA.

[74] Fuchs, R. and Hult, K. Ochratoxin A in blood and its pharmacokinetic properties. Food and Chemical Toxicology. 1992. 30:201-204.

[75] El-Sayed, Y. S. Khalil, R.H and Saad, T.T Acute toxicity of ochratoxin-A in marine water-reared sea bass (*Dicentrarchus labrax* L.). Chemosphere. 2009. 75:878-882.

[76] Amany M. Diaba, Salem, R.M.b El-Keredy M.S. Abeerc Gehan I.E. Alic Nagwan El-Habashi. Experimental ochratoxicosis A in Nile tilapia and its amelioration by some feed additives. International Journal of Veterinary Science and Medicine. 2018. 149-158. DOI:org/10.1016/j.ijvsm.2018.09.004.

[77] Bernhoft, A. Høgåsen, H.R. Rosenlund, G. Moldal, T. Grove, S. Berntssen, M.H.G. Thoresen, S.I. Alexander, J. Effects of dietary deoxynivalenol or ochratoxin A on performance and selected health indices in Atlantic salmon (*Salmo salar*). *Food Chem. Toxicol.* 2018, *121*, 374-386.

[78] Ismaiel, A.A. Ghaly, M.F. El-Naggar, A.K. Milk kefir: Ultrastructure,

antimicrobial activity, and efficacy on aflatoxin B1 production by Aspergillus flavus. Curr. Microbiol. 2011. 62, 1602-1609.

[79] Crisan, E.V. Effects of aflatoxin on seedling growth and ultrastructure in plants. Appl. Microbiol. 1973, 12, 991-1000.

[80] Placinta, C.M. Mello, J. P. F. D and Macdonald, A. M. C. A review of worldwide contamination of cereal grains and animal feed with *Fusarium mycotoxins*. Animal Feed Science and Technology.1999 78:21-37.

[81] Arukwe, A. T. Grotmol, T. Haugen, T.B. Knudsen, F.R and Goksøyr. A. Fish model for assessing the in vivo estrogenic potency of the mycotoxin zearalenone and its metabolites. Science of the Total Environment. 1999. 236:153-161.

[82] Meronuck, R. and Xie. W.1999. Mycotoxins in feed. Feedstuffs 71:123-130.

[83] Pestka, J. J. Zhou, H.R. Moon, Y and Chung, Y.J. Cellular and molecular mechanisms for immune modulation by deoxynivalenol and other trichothecenes: unraveling a paradox. Toxicology Letters. 2004. 153:61-73.

[84] Ueno, Y. Trichothecene mycotoxins: mycology, chemistry, and toxicology. Advances in Nutritional Research.1989. 3:301-353.

[85] Escrivá, L., G. Font, and L. Manyes. In vivo toxicity studies of fusarium mycotoxins in the last decade: a review. Food and Chemical Toxicology. 2015. 78:185-206.

[86] Escrivá, L., G. Font, and L. Manyes. In vivo toxicity studies of fusarium mycotoxins in the last decade: a review. Food and Chemical Toxicology. 2015. 78:185-206.

[87] Meronuck, R. and W. Xie. Mycotoxins in feed. Feedstuffs. 1999 71:123-130.

[88] Wu, F. and G. P. Munkvold. Mycotoxin in ethanol co-products: modelling economic impacts on the livestock industry and management strategies. Journal of Agricultural and Food Chemistry. 2008. 56:3900-3911.

[89] Winnie-Pui-Pui Liew and Sabran Mohd-Redzwan. Mycotoxin: It's Impact on Gut Health and Microbiota. Frontiers in Cellular and Infection Biology. 2018. DOI:.org/10.3389/fcimb.2018.00060.

[90] Yuan, G. Y.Wang, X. Yuan, T. Zhang, Zhao, J. Huang, L and S. Peng. T-2 toxin induces developmental toxicity and apoptosis in zebrafish embryos. Journal of Environmental Sciences. 2014. 26:917-925.

[91] Poston, H. A. Coffin, J.L and Combs.G.F. Biological effects of dietary T-2 toxin on rainbow trout, *Salmo gairdneri*. Aquatic Toxicology. 1982. 2:79-88.

[92] Manning, B. B., M. H. Li, and E. H. Robinson. Aflatoxin from moldy corn cause no reductions in channel catfish *Ictalurus punctatus* performance. Journal of the World Aquaculture Society. 2005. 36:59-67.

[93] Helena Modra, Miroslava Palikova, Pavel Hyrsl, Jana Bartonkova, Ivana papezikova, Zdenka Svobodova, Jana Blahova & Jan Mares. Effects of trichothecene mycotoxin T-2 toxin on haematological and immunological parameters of rainbow trout (*Oncorhynchus mykiss*). Mycotoxin Research. 2020. 36, 319-326.

[94] Marin, S. Ramos, A.J. Cano-Sancho, G and Sanchis, V. Mycotoxins: occurrence, toxicology, and exposure assessment. Food and Chemical Toxicology. 2013. 60:218-237.

[95] Mariana Oliveira and Vitor Vasconcelos. Occurrence of Mycotoxins in Fish Feed and Its Effects: A Review. Toxins. 2020. 12, 160: DOI: 10.3390/toxins12030160.

[96] Mariana Oliveira and Vitor Vasconcelos. Occurrence of Mycotoxins in Fish Feed and Its Effects: A Review. Toxins. 2020. 12, 160: DOI: 10.3390/toxins12030160.

[97] Hussein, H. S. and Brasel.J.M. Toxicity, metabolism, and impact of mycotoxins on humans and animals. Toxicology. 2001 167:101-134.

[98] Mariana Oliveira and Vitor Vasconcelos. Occurrence of Mycotoxins in Fish Feed and Its Effects: A Review. Toxins. 2020. 12, 160: DOI: 10.3390/toxins12030160.

[99] Hooft, J. Elmor, A. E. H. I. Encarnação, P and Bureau. D.P. Rainbow trout (*Oncorhynchus mykiss*) is extremely sensitive to the feed-borne Fusarium mycotoxin deoxynivalenol (DON). Aquaculture. 2011. 311:224-232.

[100] Matejova, I. H. Modra, H. Blahova, J. Franc, A. Fictum, P. Sevcikova, M and Svobodova. Z. The effect of mycotoxin deoxynivalenol on haematological and biochemical indicators and histopathological changes in rainbow trout (*Oncorhynchus mykiss*). BioMed Research International 2014:5. DOI: 10.1155/2014/310680.

[101] Matejova, I. H. Modra, H. Blahova, J. Franc, A. Fictum, P. Sevcikova, M and Svobodova. Z. The effect of mycotoxin deoxynivalenol on haematological and biochemical indicators and histopathological changes in rainbow trout (*Oncorhynchus mykiss*). BioMed Research International 2014: 5. DOI: 10.1155/2014/310680.

[102] Scott, P. M. Recent research on fumonisins: a review. Food Additives and Contaminants: Part A, Chemistry, Analysis, Control, Exposure and Risk Assessment.2012. 29:242-248.

[103] Ahangarkani, F. S. Rouhi, and Azizi.I.G. A review on incidence and toxicity of fumonisins. Toxin Reviews. 2014. 33:95-100.

[104] Riley, R. T. and K. A. Voss. Differential sensitivity of rat kidney and liver to fumonisin toxicity: organ-specific differences in toxin accumulation and sphingoid base metabolism. Toxicological Sciences. 2006. 92:335-345.

[105] Voss, K. A. Smith, G.W and Haschek, W.M. Fumonisins: toxicokinetics, mechanism of action and toxicity. Animal Feed Science and Technology.2007. 137:299-325.

[106] Voss, K. A. Smith, G.W and Haschek, W.M. Fumonisins: toxicokinetics, mechanism of action and toxicity. Animal Feed Science and Technology.2007. 137:299-325.

[107] Robert W Coppock , Barry J Jacobsen. Mycotoxins in animal and human patients. Toxicology and Industrial Health. 2009. DOI: org/10.1177/0748233709348263.

[108] Peter Spring and Christine Burel. Effect of mycotoxins in aqua culture. Mycotoxins in farm animals. Transworld Research Network, Kerala, India.2008. pp.71-90.

[109] Peter Spring and Christine Burel. Effect of mycotoxins in aqua culture. Mycotoxins in farm animals. Transworld Research Network, Kerala, India.2008. pp.71-90.

[110] Tuan, N. A. Grizzle, J.M. Lovell, R. T. Manning, B.B and Rottinghaus. G.E. Growth and hepatic lesions of Nile tilapia (*Oreochromis niloticus*) fed diets containing aflatoxin B1. Aquaculture.2002. 212:311-319.

[111] David, B. Carlson David, E. Williams Jan, M. Spitsbergen, P. Frank Ross Charles, W. Bacon Filmore, I. Meredith Ronald, T. Riley. Fumonisin $B_1$ Promotes Aflatoxin $B_1$ and *N*-Methyl-*N′*-nitro-nitrosoguanidine-Initiated Liver Tumors in Rainbow Trout. ScienceDirect. 2001. Volume 172, Issue 1, pp 29-36. DOI:org/10.1006/taap.2001.9129.

[112] Wo'zny, M. P. Brzuzan, M. Gusiatin, E. Jakimiuk, S. Dobosz, and Ku'zmi´ nski, H. Influence of zearalenone on selected biochemical parametres in juvenile rainbow troat. Polish Journal of Veterinary Sciences. 2012. 15:221-225.

[113] Pietsch, C. S. Kersten, P. Burkhardt-Holm, H. Valenta, and Dänicke, S. Occurrence of deoxynivalenol and zearalenone in commercial fish feed: an initial study. Toxins. 2013. 5:184-192.

[114] Greco, M. A. Pardo, and Pose, G. Mycotoxigenic fungi and natural co-occurrence of mycotoxins in rainbow trout (*Oncorhynchus mykiss*) feeds. Toxins. 2015. 7:4595-4609.

[115] Guo-Liang Zhang, Yu-Long Feng, Jun-Lin Song and Xiang-Shan Zhou, Zearalenone: A Mycotoxin with Different Toxic Effect in Domestic and Laboratory Animals' Granulosa Cells. Frontiers in Genetics. 2018. Front. Genet. 18: DOI:org/10.3389/fgene.2018.00667.

[116] Constanze Pietsch. Risk assessment for mycotoxin contamination in fish feeds in Europe. Springer. 2019. DOI:org/10.1007/s12550-019-00368-6.

[117] Greco, M. A. Pardo, and Pose, G. Mycotoxigenic fungi and natural co-occurrence of mycotoxins in rainbow trout (*Oncorhynchus mykiss*) feeds. Toxins. 2015. 7:4595-4609.

[118] Manning, B. B. Wise, D.J. Abbas, H.K and Peterson, B.C. Channel catfish, *Ictalurus punctatus*, fed diet containing aflatoxin from moldy corn do not experience increased mortality after challenge with *Edwardsiella ictaluri*. Journal of the World Aquaculture Society. 2011. 42:598-602.

[119] The factsheet by the Southern Regional Aquaculture Center (SRAC) gives information on managing high pH in freshwater ponds. 2013.

[120] Thiel, P. G. A molecular mechanism for the toxic action of moniliformin, a mycotoxin produced by *Fusarium moniliforme*. Biochemical Pharmacology. 1978. 27:483-486.

[121] Yildirim, M. B. B. Manning, B.B. Lovell, R.T. Grizzle, J.M and Rottinghaus, G.E Toxicity of moniliformin and fumonisin B1 fed singly and in combination in diets for young channel catfish *Ictalurus punctatus*. Journal of the World Aquaculture Society. 2000. 31:599-608.

[122] Thiel, P. G. A molecular mechanism for the toxic action of moniliformin, a mycotoxin produced by *Fusarium moniliforme*. Biochemical Pharmacology. 1978. 27:483-486.

[123] Rui A. Gonçalves, Marco Tarasco, Dian Schatzmayr and Paulo Gavaia. Preliminary Evaluation of Moniliformin as a Potential Threat for Teleosts. Fishes. 2018. DOI: 10.3390/fishes3010004.

[124] Emerging Mycotoxins: Overview and Occurrence. Biomin, 2016.

[125] Constanze Pietsch. Risk assessment for mycotoxin contamination in fish feeds in Europe. Springer Link. 2019. 36, pages41-62.

[126] Nazia Hoque, Choudhury Mahmood Hasan, Md. Sohel Rana, Amrit Varsha, Mohamed Hossain Sohrab, and Khondaker Miraz Rahman. Fusaproliferin, a Fungal Mycotoxin, Shows Cytotoxicity against Pancreatic Cancer Cell Lines. 2018. 23(12): pp. 3288.

Chapter 8

# Aflatoxins Occurrence in Spices

*Farman Ahmed and Muhammad Asif Asghar*

## Abstract

A wide range of spices are used in most dishes as seasoning, colouring, texture developer, palatability or preserving food and beverages worldwide. However, the spices are produced mainly in developing countries where tropical and/or subtropical climate such as high temperature, heavy rainfall and humidity encourage fungal growth leading to increased occurrence of aflatoxins (AFs) in spices. Moreover, the inadequate implementation of good agricultural practice, good manufacturing practice and good hygienic practice in these countries are great alarming situation. AFs are considered as a carcinogenic, mutagenic, teratogenic and immunosuppressive to humans and are classified as hazardous food toxins. This chapter provides the worldwide production and regulations of spices, suitable conditions for the AFs production, worldwide occurrence of AFs, detection techniques and some aspect for the reduction of AFs in spices.

**Keywords:** detoxification techniques, climatic variation, potential exposure in human

## 1. Introduction

Nowadays, scientists are focusing on efficient control of the occurrence of xenogenous constituents in foodstuffs which might be risk for the public health. Spices native to India were grown as early as the 8th century BC in the gardens of Babylon. Spices are considered one of the valuable crops in the world due their important characteristic such as flavoring, colouring and aromatizing as well as antimicrobial and antioxidant effect [1]. Spices are extensively used as a staple crop and cultivated in tropical and sub-tropical regions.

Spices are considered as the non-leafy fragments of plant such as seed, bud, bark, fruit, rhizome or bulp. However, the leaf and flower are designated as different group known as herbs. However, all parts of a plant should be considered to be spices if they possess the aforementioned properties for meal enhancement such as its color, flavor or even texture [2]. Unfortunately, many spices are very susceptible to toxigenic fungal strains and are likely to produce aflatoxins (AFs) contamination [3–5]. Fungal growth is also exaggerated by the landform, soil natures and properties along with interactions between the micro-fungus and micro- or macro-organisms in soil. In addition, harvesting, drying, handling, packing, carrying, due to probable physical rupturing, insect damage, growth and metabolic action of fungal are also responsible to propagate the fungal proliferation. Moreover, spices purchased in loose or open packing are proved to be considerably more contaminated than spices purchased in sealed or close packing [6].

AFs are naturally occurring metabolites mostly created by *Aspergillus flavus* and *A. parasiticus*. *A. bombysis, A. ochraceoroseus, A. nomius*, and *A. pseudotamari* are rarely AFs-producing species. From the mycological viewpoint, each strain shows different qualitative and quantitative abilities to produce AFs. For instance, only about half of *A. flavus* strains produced AFs-producing species more than $10^6$ μg/kg [7]. Aflatoxins B and G are produced by the *A. parasiticus* and more improved to a soil environment with limited spreading. Presently, 18 different types of AFs have been recognized, aflatoxin $B_1$, $B_2$, $G_1$ and $G_2$ ($AFB_1$, $AFB_2$, $AFG_1$ and $AFG_2$) is considered more toxic but $AFB_1$ is the most recurrently arising amongst all of them [8]. The order of chronic and acute poisonousness is $AFB_1 > AFG_1 > AFB_2 > AFG_2$. AFs are among the most studied mycotoxins globally. AFs are linked with several diseases such as aflatoxicosis in humans, birds, fishes and livestock domestic animals [9]. AFs are the most harmful and tremendously mutagenic mycotoxins [10]. Moreover, AFs have been designated as the first class carcinogens by the International Agency for Research on Cancer (IARC) [11]. $AFB_1$ is deliberated as most toxic due to its extreme hepatotoxigenic and hepatocarcinogenic ability. The liver is recognized as the prime target organ [12]. Furthermore, the cyclic nucleotide phosphodiesterase action in the heart, kidney, liver and brain tissues could be inhibited by $AFB_1$. This results in the malfunctioning of these body parts.

Due to above declared facts; many countries have enforced strict guidelines concerning AFs occurrence in food and their products [4]. In addition, spices are frequently vulnerable to AFs contamination, as reported in assessments from various states [13–15]. Spices are mainly produced in tropical climatic regions with higher range of humidity, temperature and rainfall [16]. Moreover, inadequate storage, prolonged drying periods and higher moisture contents may cause improvement of AFs in spices. The lacking of infrastructure against fungal attack on food commodities in developing countries (e.g. India, Sri Lanka and Pakistan) causes AFs problems. Limited execution of Good Hygienic Practice (GHP), Good Agricultural Practice (GAP), Good Manufacturing Practice (GMP), Good Storage Practice (GSP), improper storing and inadequate shipping could also liable to *Aspergillus* growth and proliferation the hazard of AFs contamination. The condition regarding AFs contamination in spices is well accepted [3]. Still there is a need to collect information regarding AFs in different states around the world. Consequently, this chapter provides the comprehensive facts regarding occurrence of AFs in spices.

## 2. Worldwide spices cultivation

During the last 5 years (2015–2019), the average production of spices was c. 602126902 tonnes and 127787137 tonnes in 2019. These spices includes anise, badian, fennel, coriander, chilies and peppers, cinnamon, cloves, garlic, ginger, nutmeg, mace, cardamoms, mustard seed, pepper (piper spp.), peppermint and vanilla". Asia is considered the largest producer of spices in the world with the production share of 76.2% (197818212 tonnes in 2019). Whereas, India provides most to this segment (9508837 tonnes in 2019), followed by China (5307696 tonnes in 2019) [17]. Currently, the global spices and seasonings market is undergoing a healthy growth. Looking forward, the market is predicted to reveal a CAGR of around 4.7% during 2020–2025 [18].

## 3. Suitable climatic conditions for AFs production

The climate is considerably influence on the accessibility and quality of the spices. The change in climate simultaneously impacts the complex of AF-producers to change its fungal community's structure. The temperature and water activity (aw) in the atmosphere alters by the climate which further impacts the gene appearance to produce AFs [19]. The AF-producing genes are clustered on the genome and express the main regulatory genes as transcription activator aflatoxin (*aflR*), pathway regulator aflatoxin (*aflS*) as well as structural genes such as reductase aflatoxin (*aflD*) which are subjective by the contact of temperature and aw conditions [20]. As revealed by the [21], the expression fraction of *aflR*/*aflS* significantly connects with the amount of $AFB_1$ produced. Most examinations in regions with warm climates have emphasized the occurrence of fungal species of the genus Aspergillus in spices. Generally, the greater contamination is found in warm, humid and even hot deserts and drought environments [22]. However, ideal situations for the AFs formation is considered as moisture content between 18 to 20%, water activity >0.82, pH 3.0 to 8.5 and ambient temperature between 12 to 40 °C (54 to 104 °F) with an optimal at 25 to 30 °C (77 to 86 °F). Nutrition aspects such as carbohydrate, nitrogen sources, zinc, phosphates and other trace metals also influence the development of AFs [23].

| Country | Commodities | Maximum acceptable limits (μg/kg) | |
|---|---|---|---|
| | | $AFB_1$ | $AFB_1$, $AFB_2$ + $AFG_1$ + $AFG_2$ |
| United States (FDA & FAO) | All foods | — | 20 |
| EU | Spices | 5 | 10 |
| Bulgaria | Spices | 2 | 5 |
| Croatia | Spices | 30 | 15 |
| Brazil | Spices | — | 20 |
| China | Spices | 5 | — |
| Czech Republic | Spices | 20 | — |
| Finland | All Spices | — | 20 |
| Indonesia | Spices powder | 15 | 5 |
| Brazil | Spices | 20 | 30 |
| India | All foods | 30 | — |
| Turkey | Spices | 10 | — |
| Iceland | All Spices | 30 | — |
| Iran | Spices | 5 | 10 |
| Republic of South Africa | All foods | 5 | 10 |
| Australia | All foods | — | 5 |
| Uruguay | All Spices | 5 | 20 |
| Hong Kong | All foods | — | 15 |
| Malaysia | All foods | — | 35 |
| Japan | All foods | 10 | — |
| Singapore | All foods | — | 0 |
| New Zealand | All foods | — | 5 |
| Sri Lanka | All foods | — | 30 |
| Pakistan | Selected Spices | — | 30 |

**Table 1.**
*MTL as established by various countries for $AFB_1$ and AFs ($B_l$, $B_2$, $G_1$ and $G_2$) in spices and foods.*

## 4. Regulations of aflatoxins in spices

Though large number of mycotoxins occur in nature however only few toxins (e.g. Aflatoxins) creates food safety and security problems. Therefore, it is necessary, to prevent dangerous outbreaks of these toxins in humans and animals, also to control them within tolerance limits assigned by international agencies. The international regulatory agencies & authorities establish maximum tolerated limit (MTL) for AFs in spices because of severe toxicity of these toxins. The MTL relating to AFs differ from country to country, as developed nations have set lower tolerance limits as compare to developing countries where these susceptible commodities are produced [24]. In addition, the MTL differ from one country to another because of different agricultural practices and climatic conditions. The Food and Agriculture Organization (FAO) has stated that nearly 100 countries have been established MTL for mycotoxins or minimum only for AFs. While 13 countries are uncertain to provide specific regulations and almost 50 countries have no regulations or no data exist [25].

As it is evident from these data, at present, a fair number of the Codex member states have fixed the maximum limits on AFs in spices. These limits range from 1 μg/kg (Honduras) to 30 μg/kg (India) [4]. The first tolerance level of 30 μg/kg for total AFs in all foods was legislated in 1965 by the USFDA. Later, it was reduced to 20 μg/kg due to the potent toxicity of AFs [26]. The European Union' Scientific Committee on Food (SCF) established the MTL in spices i.e. 5 μg/kg for $AFB_1$ and 10 μg/kg for total AFs [27]. In 2017, the National Standard of China has been updated by the National Food Safety Standard for Maximum Levels of Mycotoxins in Foods (GB 2761–2017) and in January 2020, the public consultation on its revision was launched. While under the National Standard, the maximum level is set at 5 μg/kg for $AFB_1$ in spices [4]. In India, the MTL prescribed for AFs in spices by the Food Safety and Standards Authority is 30 μg/kg. Also, MTL have also been established for AFs in different spices in many countries as listed in **Table 1**.

## 5. Aflatoxins detection techniques in spices

To develop effective and valid analytical methods extensive researches have been carried out for qualitative and quantitative detection or determination of AFs in spices. Generally, the determination of AFs is performed in two steps, (i) extraction or clean-up of samples and (ii) detection or quantification of AFs. The purpose for the use of different extraction and clean-up methods is to separate AFs from other matrix components and to minimize the impact of heterogeneous distribution of AFs [28]. As a result, reduce the background signal during the instrumental analysis. Conventional extraction approaches are unable to precisely & accurately analyse AFs in spices. It is because of the presence of natural colour/pigment producing background interference in HPLC Analysis results masking of toxin [29]. In addition, the complexity of natural constituents in spices matrix frequently makes it challenging to efficiently extract the AFs. Various extraction solvents are currently is in use such as Methanol: Water (80:20), Acetonitrile: Water (60:40), Acetone: Water (75:25) and Methanol: Water (60:40). The reported maximum recovery was achieved by Methanol: Water (80:20) [30, 31]. However, various clean-up methods have been proposed as mentioned below:

- Liquid–Liquid Extraction (LLE)

- Solid Phase Extraction (SPE)

- Immunoaffinity Column Clean-up (IAC)
- Supercritical Fluid Extraction (SFE)
- Energy-Assisted Extraction (EAE)

To clean up AFs in foodstuffs, SPE using a silica gel column, a florisil column, or multifunctional columns has been used. Recently, immunoaffinity (IA) chromatography utilizing immunological interaction which has a high clean-up effect has been employed as well [32]. In addition, the Quick, Easy, Cheap, Effective, Rugged and Safe (QuEChERS) method is a simple and straightforward technique has also been utilized for AFs extraction [33, 34]. Furthermore, the detection methods are based on the emission and absorption characteristics such as thin layer chromatography (TLC), 2D-TLC (Two Dimensional), Enzyme linked immunosorbent assay (ELISA), Fluorometric determination, High performance liquid chromatography (HPLC), Gas chromatography (GC) and Liquid chromatography linked with tandem mass spectrometry (LC–MS–MS). Still, there are certain advantages and disadvantages linked with these developed techniques e.g. reduced sensitivity, unsatisfied accuracy, scope restriction, cost, laborious and sometimes extended analysis time [35, 36].

Thin layer chromatographic technique is considered as preliminary analytical testing method for mycotoxins. From time to time, TLC is performed for the confirmation of other methods or techniques outcomes & effectively being practiced in developing countries because of low cost. The difficulties of TLC method of analyses are low sensitivity, sometimes poor separation and unsatisfactory accuracy. Special skills are also required to observe the separated spots of compounds (toxin) on TLC cards in presence of ultraviolet or fluorescent lamps. The analyte is difficult to separate from sample matrix in this technique. Also, the poor reproducibility or repeatability in TLC because of factors e.g. sample extraction in solvents, application of extracted sample as spots on TLC card or plate and observer visualization [37]. The fluorometric system is relatively sensitive and accurate as compare to conventional spectrophotometric systems. More consideration and sensitive equipment technique is also prerequisite regarding environmental factors [38].

ELISA technique is widely applied since few years, because of its simplicity, sensitivity and fast quantification of AFs. More benefits of ELISA include simplicity of sample preparation and probably low analysis cost. However, ELISA is established on the immunological mechanism & it needed very specific monoclonal & polyclonal sera for sensitive and specific quantification of antigen. Also, it consume long incubation time, mixing & washing steps and it is unable to analyse AFs individually [39].

On the contrary to ELISA & TLC, the HPLC method has taken more attention because of its accuracy, sensitivity, specificity and reproducibility, also, the HPLC instrumental analysis is capable to measure single toxin exclusively. In other food matrices, HPLC has increased attraction where determination of $AFB_1$ is necessary requirement solely. HPLC determination is remarkably sensitive as compare to the TLC system and it can measure $AFB_1$ toxin even if less than 0.1 μg/kg [40]. Conversely, the disadvantage of HPLC is the toxins need derivatization to improve their fluorescence properties. AFs have natural fluorescence characteristics due to the rigid and conjugated molecular structure. In these circumstances, small alterations in the molecular structure may increase fluorescence characteristic significantly. Hence, prerequisite derivatization with aid of chemicals boosts their fluorescence property. For instance, $AFG_2$ and $AFB_2$ are more fluorescent in comparison with $AFB_1$ and $AFG_1$.

Several derivatization methods of $AFB_1$ and $AFG_1$ are presently in practice. The frequent techniques include (i) pre-column treatment with trifluoroacetic acid (TFA) [41], (ii) post-column derivatization with iodine [42], (iii) cyclodextrins [43] and (iv) pyridinium hydrobromide perbromide [44]. The drawbacks related to the TFA based treatment method are the longer reaction time with elevated temperature, TFA toxicity and its corrosiveness [45]. Similarly, iodine based method also does have prolonged reaction time (up to 2 min) at elevated temperatures along with chromatogram peak broadening and need of supplementary HPLC pump. Also, daily preparation of the iodine solution is not recommended because of its corrosiveness to avoid capillary blockage and draining of the reagent pump seals [46]. All of the above four methods are prolonged and linked with the some weaknesses. In these circumstances, an exciting methodology of photochemical derivatization is known as Kobra Cell™ (R-Biopharm, Rhone Ltd., UK). This derivatization does not need everyday preparation of any reagent. There is no instability or corrosiveness issues and photochemical derivatization time is 4 seconds only at ambient temperature [40]. Likewise the method with a low maintenance cost no supplementary pump is needed.

The Gas Chromatography methodology is also operated for the determination of particular AFs which are challengingly measured by HPLC. Unfortunately, this technique is time-consuming and expensive. Sometimes it is required to transform analyte into the volatile compound compared to other methods [47]. Sometimes, pre-derivatization is prerequisite for the AFs before GC injection. Thermal stability of the AFs extract is also an issue because AFs decomposes at high temperature. In addition, the GC is not widespread using for the commercial testing of AFs because of greater running cost than HPLC analysis.

Nowadays, the advanced version of Liquid Chromatography Mass Spectrometry i.e. LC/MS/MS system has achieved more attention for AFs determination. The LC/MS/MS benefits over other techniques are of extra ordinary sensitivity (lower level detection), greatly specific and the confirmation support of mass spectral fragments and identification of interfering impurities [48]. A single run of LC/MS/MS can support the quantification and determination of multiple mycotoxins [49]. Conversely, to get desire selectivity and sensitivity, there is need of additional accuracy in the sample preparation steps. The LC/MS/MS is an expensive equipment unit and it requires more skill for analytics hence it is more recommended for R & D. The extraction specific solvents for LC/MS/MS sample preparation is an additional requirement.

The variation in these approaches could be established because of the effect of matrix and matrix parameters, the intensity of AFs contamination in product. A validated method is desirable in these situations, a method which avoid maximum matrix effect and close by the tolerable limits as obligatory by the international legislative authorities.

## 6. Worldwide contamination of aflatoxins in spices

This section of the chapter describes the studies regarding AFs in spices over the last few years. A total of 27 studies altogether covering 19 spices were included. AFs incidence in spices differs place to place due to temperature & moisture differences, microflora and agronomics variations [31]. The worldwide occurrence of $AFB_1$ and total AFs with respect to each unique spice are shown in **Table 2**. In terms of AFs, studies are most often concerned with red chilli, black pepper, caraway, cinnamon, aniseed, cumin, ginger, red pepper, clove, fenugreek, coriander, cardamom, turmeric, paprika, curry, garlic and mix spices. The occurrence of total AFs in the above-mentioned spices is usually high to very high.

| Country | Category of spices | n | Positive samples (%) | $AFB_1$ | | Total AFs | | Study Year | References |
|---|---|---|---|---|---|---|---|---|---|
| | | | | Range | Mean | Range | Mean | | |
| Pakistan | 1 | 331 | 97 | — | — | 1.3–93.7 | 17.2 | 2006–2011 | [31] |
| Turkey | 2,3,5,6,8,9,19 | 93 | 58 | 0.5–52.5 | 20.7 | — | — | 2010–2011 | [50] |
| Pakistan | 1 | 69 | 67 | — | — | 1.2–600.0 | 57.5 | 2012 | [51] |
| Turkey | 9 | 42 | 90 | — | — | 0.4–86.0 | 17.1 | 2013 | [52] |
| Turkey | 1 | 182 | 82 | 0.2–165.0 | — | — | — | 2013 | [53] |
| India | 1,3 | 18 | 18 | 31.1–174.7 | — | — | — | 2013 | [54] |
| Iran | 3,9 | 76 | 54 | 0.88–28.6 | 15.5 | 1.4–30.2 | 15.5 | 2014 | [55] |
| Algeria | 2,3,4,5,6,7,8,9,11 | 36 | 63.9 | 0.1–26.5 | — | — | — | 2015 | [5] |
| Iran | 3,5,9,13 | 80 | 40 | 0.8–17.9 | — | 0.8–24.1 | | 2015 | [56] |
| South Africa | 1,8,15,19 | 70 | 40 | 3.0–19.0 | — | — | — | 2015 | [57] |
| Iran | 3,7, 8,9,13 | 120 | 31 | 0.2–57.5 | — | 0.7–57.5 | | 2015 | [58] |
| Malaysia | 1,3,5,6,7,13 | 25 | 88 | 0.3–28.4 | 7.3 | 0.32–31.17 | 8.4 | 2015 | [59] |
| Pakistan | 19 | 75 | 77 | — | — | 0.7–25.7 | 4.6 | 2015 | [6] |
| Saudi Arabia | 1 | 60 | 57 | — | — | 0–200 | 16.0 | 2015 | [60] |
| USA | 1 | 169 | 64 | ND–94.9 | 4.8 | — | — | 2015–2016 | [14] |
| Nigeria | 1 | 55 | 93 | ND–156.0 | 13.5 | — | — | | |
| Italy | 12 | 45 | 31 | LOQ–155.7 | 12.8 | LOQ–529.1 | 13.9 | 2017 | [61] |
| Tanzania | 5,8,10,16 | 120 | 57 | 0.15–11.2 | 0.8 | 0.1–11.9 | 1.4 | 2017–2018 | [62] |
| Pakistan | 1,3 | 50 | 30 | 23.9–75.8 | — | — | — | 2018 | [63] |
| Lebanon | 1,2,5,6,7, 8,10,11,13,15,16,17,18,19 | 94 | 19 | 2.2–1118.2 | 193.4 | 2.2–1118.2 | 168.1 | 2018 | [64] |
| Pakistan | 1,3,13,19 | 120 | 100 | 1.0–30.4 | 6.54 | 1.5–44.3 | 9.7 | 2018 | [13] |

| Country | Category of spices | n | Positive samples (%) | $AFB_1$ | | Total AFs | | Study Year | References |
|---|---|---|---|---|---|---|---|---|---|
| | | | | Range | Mean | Range | Mean | | |
| Bangladesh | 1 | 50 | 75 | — | — | 12.0–68.7 | | 2018 | [65] |
| Iran | 3,5,9,13 | 80 | 50 | — | — | 1.2–77.3 | 8.6 | 2019 | [66] |
| Malaysia | 1,20 | 20 | 40 | 4.7–16.9 | — | — | — | 2019 | [67] |
| Nigeria | 1 | 70 | 69 | — | — | 0–97.0 | 8.9 | 2019 | [68] |
| Greece | 2,5,6,7,8,9,13,14,15,16,18,19 | 29 | 69 | LOD–132.7 | 9.9 | — | — | 2020 | [69] |
| Indonesia | 1 | 6 | 50 | 39.3–139.5 | — | — | — | 2020 | [70] |

*$AFB_1$ = Aflatoxin B1, Total AFs = Total Aflatoxins, n = number of tested samples.*
*Number of spice category: [1] Red chilli; [2] Aniseed; [3] Black pepper; [4] Caraway; [5] Cinnamon; [6] Coriander; [7] Cumin; [8] Ginger; [9] Red pepper; [10] Clove; [11] Sweet cumin; [12] Sweet pepper; [13] Turmeric; [14] Curry; [15] Paprika; [16] Cardamom; [17] Garlic; [18] Fenugreek; [19] Mix spices.*

**Table 2.**
*The worldwide occurrence of $AFB_1$ and total AFs with respect to each unique spice.*

Composite spices are common in South Asian countries (Bangladesh, India, Pakistan and Sri Lanka) due to enrich aroma, color and flavor in variety of cooked meals. Yet no survey is accessible on AFs incidence in composite spices. Some studies have informed that spices are considerably more contaminated with AFs than other foods [71]. Furthermore, chilli, red and black peppers were found to be more contaminated as compare to other spices as reported from India, Pakistan, Turkey, Iran, Bangladesh, Indonesia and Nigeria [4, 72]. The samples of ground chilli were found more exposed to AFs occurrence than whole or uncut red chilli. It is because of the possibility of inferior raw material usage for powder chilli production. Also, the tendency of powder to be hygroscopic makes it susceptible for high AFs contamination [73]. The inappropriate handling, processing and high amount of fat content in black pepper and the solubility of AFs in fat is most likely the reason of high level of AFs contamination. In addition, the presence of essential oils may prevent the occurrence of AFs in crude spices [74].

The antifungal and anti-toxicogenic properties of ginger, turmeric, clove, cinnamon, garlic and cumin can maintain the AFs occurrence at lower level [75, 76]. Some spices show antifungal activity and disrupt the integrity of fungi cell wall which creates AFs [77]. Also, some stated that the extract of turmeric can downregulate the gene expression in the biosynthesis of AFs in *A. flavus* [78]. The lack of AFs in cinnamon and cumin is due to the inhibition of the aflatoxigenic fungi by essential oils and aromatic constituents in these plants. The cinnamon is likely not to be a good substrate for aflatoxigenic fungi development and accumulation. Additionally, the effect of 09 oils studied against the growth and the toxicity of *A. parasiticus* [79]. The clove oil was found capable to inhibit the development of fungi to limit the formation of discontinue the AFs biosynthesis [80].

Considering highly reported contamination with AFs in spices particular chillis and peppers regular monitoring of the imported spices are highly recommended to maintain the food quality. Advance studies are still needed to address the source of occurrence and to control the AFs level in the spice from pre-harvesting to post-harvesting and from packaging, storage and shipment stages. A worldwide potential risk for AFs contamination may occur during prolonged storing of spices in poor temperature and moisture control. The factor of storage environmental conditions plays a major role in the occurrence of secondary metabolites such as AFs.

## 7. Mitigation of aflatoxins in spices

The widespread elimination or inhibition of AFs contamination during pre- and post-harvest steps is not an easy work however strategies to control fungal growth are essential to minimize the exposure to humans. Numerous methods for the detoxification or elimination of AFs by means of physical, chemical and biological approaches have been proposed [81]. The product safety outcomes of these methods and reducing agents are not clear.

Approaches to address AFs fall under two main areas. The first includes reducing AFs occurrence in the growing cycle by applying good agricultural practices and the other is mitigating the accelerated toxin growth in the post-harvest supply chain both approaches reduce AFs levels in food commodities. Farmers need to use those crop varieties robust to native growing environment, mainly drought, insects and pests, also show resistance to fungal contamination. Postharvest control of humidity is a key to reducing chances of AFs contamination. Irrigation and fungicides can develop plant health to resist the AFs-producing fungus. Solar dryer is also a solution to control moistness in spices earlier to storage.

AFs occurrence could be reduced by different inhibition methods. The toxins toxins levels could be minimized when the defected chilies like midget, dwarf, damaged and broken are physically sorted from achieving an average of 78% reduction in toxin content [82]. The use of gamma radiation can be helpful for the protection of chilies with respect to the production of AFs during storage [83]. In addition, some novel detoxification technologies including a microwave, ultraviolet, electrolyzed water, ozone, pulsed light, cold plasma and gamma irradiation in a support with biological, physical, chemical or genetic engineering methods have the potential to detoxify [84–87]. The application of each technique has its benefits and drawbacks. Consequently, biocontrol processes in synchrony with other physical and chemical methods with improved packaging materials should be implemented to attain spices safety and security.

By the execution of advanced agricultural technologies, good agricultural practices, good manufacturing practices and good storage practices can mitigate the AFs occurrence or contamination [88]. AFs contamination occurs in pockets of high concentration which are not randomly dispersed throughout the commodity [89]. Thus, sampling is of key importance before sample preparation in laboratory. The sampling, sample handling and analyses are not yet standardized at growers and farmers eventually the users are at risk. Therefore, attention must be taken in the determination of laboratory results and quality testing should be performed from ISO-17025 accredited or similar laboratories.

Furthermore, the unpacked composite spices are susceptible to the AFs occurrence because of direct exposure to climate. The higher levels of AFs presence could be credited to tropical condition which may favor the spread of toxigenic fungi [90]. Organization of American States and Mayan Reserve Foundation jointly reported the corrective measures to reduce AFs contamination in chilies such as storage at low relative humidity and temperature, shorten the drying time and quick supplying to the user. And last but not least, the skilled personnel to involve in these processes [91]. Hence, consumers are guided to take measures such as procure from reliable retailers, store food in cool conditions and avoid unpacked products.

## 8. Conclusion

Aflatoxins contaminated spices are associated with severe risks to the consumers as these spices are part of food particularly in the Asian cooking. It is essential for legislative bodies to monitor AFs occurrence and harmful effects in spices to endorse that toxins are not prevailing at levels that may harmful to consumer health. Also, harvesting, drying, storage and transportation should be cautiously organized to control fungus growth. AFs occurrence can be controlled at pre- and post-harvest positions by applying good agricultural, good manufacturing and good storage practices. Further, the unique innovative processing technologies in combination either with genetic engineering or with physical, chemical or biological approaches have the potential to improve the capability of AFs decontamination as well as to overcome the limitations of any specific technology.

## Acknowledgements

The authors are enthusiastically thanks to the Pakistan Council of Scientific & Industrial Research (PCSIR), Karachi Laboratories Complex, Pakistan for the support of Food & Feed Safety research.

## Conflict of interest

The authors declare no conflict of interest.

## Author details

Farman Ahmed* and Muhammad Asif Asghar
Food and Feed Safety Laboratory, Food and Marine Resources Research Centre, Pakistan Council of Scientific and Industrial Research (PCSIR), Karachi Laboratories Complex, Karachi, Pakistan

*Address all correspondence to: ahmed.farman@gmail.com

## References


[1] Alirezalu K, Pateiro M, Yaghoubi M, Alirezalu A, Peighambardoust SH, Lorenzo JM. Phytochemical constituents, advanced extraction technologies and techno-functional properties of selected Mediterranean plants for use in meat products. A comprehensive review. Trends in Food Science & Technology. 2020.

[2] Pitt JI, Miller JD. A concise history of mycotoxin research. Journal of agricultural and food chemistry. 2017;65(33):7021-33.

[3] Kabak B, Dobson AD. Mycotoxins in spices and herbs–An update. Critical reviews in food science and nutrition. 2017;57(1):18-34.

[4] Pickova D, Ostry V, Malir J, Toman J, Malir F. A Review on Mycotoxins and Microfungi in Spices in the Light of the Last Five Years. Toxins. 2020;12(12):789.

[5] Azzoune N, Mokrane S, Riba A, Bouras N, Verheecke C, Sabaou N, et al. Contamination of common spices by aflatoxigenic fungi and aflatoxin B1 in Algeria. Quality Assurance and Safety of Crops & Foods. 2015;8(1):137-144.

[6] Asghar MA, Zahir E, Rantilal S, Ahmed A, Iqbal J. Aflatoxins in composite spices collected from local markets of Karachi, Pakistan. Food Additives & Contaminants: Part B. 2016;9(2):113-119.

[7] Bennett JW. An overview of the genus Aspergillus. Aspergillus: molecular biology and genomics. 2010:1-17.

[8] Arce-López B, Lizarraga E, Vettorazzi A, González-Peñas E. Human biomonitoring of mycotoxins in blood, plasma and serum in recent years: a review. Toxins. 2020;12(3):147.

[9] Asghar MA, Ahmed A, Iqbal J. Aflatoxins and ochratoxin A in export quality raisins collected from different areas of Pakistan. Food Additives & Contaminants: Part B. 2016;9(1):51-58.

[10] Alshannaq A, Yu J-H. Occurrence, toxicity, and analysis of major mycotoxins in food. International journal of environmental research and public health. 2017;14(6):632.

[11] Cancer IAfRo. Monographs on the evaluation of carcinogenic risks to humans. http://monographsiarcfr/ENG/Classification/indexphp. 2006.

[12] Shi D, Liao S, Guo S, Li H, Yang M, Tang Z. Protective effects of selenium on aflatoxin B 1-induced mitochondrial permeability transition, DNA damage, and histological alterations in duckling liver. Biological trace element research. 2015;163(1):162-168.

[13] Akhtar S, Riaz M, Naeem I, Gong YY, Ismail A, Hussain M, et al. Risk assessment of aflatoxins and selected heavy metals through intake of branded and non-branded spices collected from the markets of Multan city of Pakistan. Food Control. 2020;112:107132.

[14] Singh P, Cotty PJ. Aflatoxin contamination of dried red chilies: Contrasts between the United States and Nigeria, two markets differing in regulation enforcement. Food Control. 2017;80:374-379.

[15] Do KH, An TJ, Oh S-K, Moon Y. Nation-based occurrence and endogenous biological reduction of mycotoxins in medicinal herbs and spices. Toxins. 2015;7(10):4111-4130.

[16] Cho S-H, Lee C-H, Jang M-R, Son Y-W, Lee S-M, Choi I-S, et al. Aflatoxins contamination in spices and processed

spice products commercialized in Korea. Food Chemistry. 2008;107(3):1283-1288.

[17] FAOSTAT. Food and Agriculture Organization of the United Nations. Available online: http://wwwfaoorg/faostat/en/#data/QC/visualize. (accessed on 05 February 2021).

[18] Seasoning and Spices Market - Growth T, COVID-19 Imapct, and Forecasts (2021-2026). Available online: https://www.mordorintelligence.com/industry-reports/seasoning-and-spices-market. (accessed on 05 February 2021). 2013.

[19] Dövényi-Nagy T, Rácz C, Molnár K, Bakó K, Szláma Z, Jóźwiak Á, et al. Pre-Harvest Modelling and Mitigation of Aflatoxins in Maize in a Changing Climatic Environment—A Review. Toxins. 2020;12(12):768.

[20] Olarte RA. Population Dynamics of Intra-and Inter-Specific Crosses and the Effect of Biocontrol on Natural Populations of Aspergillus Species: North Carolina State University; 2014.

[21] Schmidt-Heydt M, Rüfer CE, Abdel-Hadi A, Magan N, Geisen R. The production of aflatoxin B 1 or G 1 by Aspergillus parasiticus at various combinations of temperature and water activity is related to the ratio of aflS to afl R expression. Mycotoxin Research. 2010;26(4):241-246.

[22] Cotty PJ, Jaime-Garcia R. Influences of climate on aflatoxin producing fungi and aflatoxin contamination. International journal of food microbiology. 2007;119(1-2):109-115.

[23] Herrera M, Anadón R, Iqbal SZ, Bailly J, Ariño A. Climate change and food safety. Food Safety: Springer; 2016. p. 149-160.

[24] Dohlman E. Mycotoxin hazards and regulations. International Trade and Food Safety. 2003;97.

[25] Food U, Administration D. Guidance for industry: action levels for poisonous or deleterious substances in human food and animal feed. USFDA, Washington, DC. 2000.

[26] Food, Administration D. Guidance for industry: Action levels for poisonous or deleterious substances in human food and animal feed. 2000. 2010.

[27] Commission E. Commission Regulation (EC) No 165/2010 of 26 February 2010 amending Regulation (EC) No 1881/2006 setting maximum levels for certain contaminants in foodstuffs as regards aflatoxins. Off J Eur Union. 2010;50:8-12.

[28] Zhang K, Banerjee K. A Review: Sample Preparation and Chromatographic Technologies for Detection of Aflatoxins in Foods. Toxins. 2020;12(9):539.

[29] Bae SE, Cho SY, Won YD, Lee SH, Park HJ. A comparative study of the different analytical methods for analysis of S-allyl cysteine in black garlic by HPLC. LWT-Food Science and Technology. 2012;46(2):532-535.

[30] O'Riordan MJ, Wilkinson MG. Comparison of analytical methods for aflatoxin determination in commercial chilli spice preparations and subsequent development of an improved method. Food Control. 2009;20(8):700-705.

[31] Khan MA, Asghar MA, Iqbal J, Ahmed A, Shamsuddin ZA. Aflatoxins contamination and prevention in red chillies (Capsicum annuum L.) in Pakistan. Food Additives & Contaminants: Part B. 2014;7(1):1-6.

[32] Delaunay N, Combès A, Pichon V. Immunoaffinity Extraction and Alternative Approaches for the Analysis of Toxins in Environmental, Food or Biological Matrices. Toxins. 2020;12(12):795.

[33] Sirhan A, Tan G, Wong R. Method validation in the determination of aflatoxins in noodle samples using the QuEChERS method and high performance liquid chromatography coupled to a fluorescence detector (HPLC-FLD). Food Control. 2011;22:1839-1843.

[34] Sirhan AY, Tan GH, Al-Shunnaq A, Abdulra'uf L, Wong RC. QuEChERS-HPLC method for aflatoxin detection of domestic and imported food in Jordan. Journal of Liquid Chromatography & Related Technologies. 2014;37(3):321-342.

[35] Sapsford KE, Taitt CR, Fertig S, Moore MH, Lassman ME, Maragos CM, et al. Indirect competitive immunoassay for detection of aflatoxin B1 in corn and nut products using the array biosensor. Biosensors and bioelectronics. 2006;21(12):2298-2305.

[36] Iqbal J, Asghar MA, Ahmed A, Khan MA, Jamil K. Aflatoxins contamination in Pakistani brown rice: a comparison of TLC, HPLC, LC–MS/MS and ELISA techniques. Toxicology mechanisms and methods. 2014;24(8):544-551.

[37] Turner NW, Subrahmanyam S, Piletsky SA. Analytical methods for determination of mycotoxins: a review. Analytica chimica acta. 2009;632(2):168-180.

[38] Bueno D, Istamboulie G, Muñoz R, Marty JL. Determination of mycotoxins in food: a review of bioanalytical to analytical methods. Applied Spectroscopy Reviews. 2015;50(9):728-774.

[39] Hosseini S, Vázquez-Villegas P, Rito-Palomares M, Martinez-Chapa SO. Advantages, disadvantages and modifications of conventional ELISA. Enzyme-linked Immunosorbent Assay (ELISA): Springer; 2018. p. 67-115.

[40] Asghar MA, Iqbal J, Ahmed A, Khan MA, Shamsuddin ZA, Jamil K. Development and validation of a high-performance liquid chromatography method with post-column derivatization for the detection of aflatoxins in cereals and grains. Toxicology and industrial health. 2016;32(6):1122-1134.

[41] Espinosa ET, Askar KA, Naccha Torres LR, Olvera RM, Santa Anna JPC. Quantification of aflatoxins in corn distributed in the city of Monterrey, Mexico. Food Additives & Contaminants. 1995;12(3):383-386.

[42] Jansen H, Jansen R, Brinkman UT, Frei R. Fluorescence enhancement for aflatoxins in HPLC by post-column split-flow iodine addition from a solid-phase iodine reservoir. Chromatographia. 1987;24(1):555-559.

[43] Chiavaro E, Dall'Asta C, Galaverna G, Biancardi A, Gambarelli E, Dossena A, et al. New reversed-phase liquid chromatographic method to detect aflatoxins in food and feed with cyclodextrins as fluorescence enhancers added to the eluent. Journal of Chromatography A. 2001;937(1-2):31-40.

[44] Garner RC, Whattam MM, Taylor PJ, Stow MW. Analysis of United Kingdom purchased spices for aflatoxins using an immunoaffinity column clean-up procedure followed by high-performance liquid chroma. Journal of Chromatography A. 1993;648(2):485-490.

[45] Shepherd MJ, Gilbert J. An investigation of HPLC post-column iodination conditions for the enhancement of aflatoxin B1 fluorescence. Food Additives & Contaminants. 1984;1(4):325-335.

[46] Kok WT. Derivatization reactions for the determination of aflatoxins by liquid chromatography with

fluorescence detection. Journal of Chromatography B: Biomedical Sciences and Applications. 1994;659(1-2):127-137.

[47] Shephard GS. Determination of mycotoxins in human foods. Chemical Society Reviews. 2008;37(11):2468-2477.

[48] Jeswal P, Kumar D. Mycobiota and natural incidence of aflatoxins, ochratoxin A, and citrinin in Indian spices confirmed by LC-MS/MS. International journal of microbiology. 2015;2015.

[49] Herebian D, Zühlke S, Lamshöft M, Spiteller M. Multi-mycotoxin analysis in complex biological matrices using LC-ESI/MS: Experimental study using triple stage quadrupole and LTQ-Orbitrap. Journal of separation science. 2009;32(7):939-948.

[50] Tosun H, Arslan R. Determination of aflatoxin B1 levels in organic spices and herbs. The Scientific World Journal. 2013;2013.

[51] Akhund S, Akram A, Hanif NQ, Qureshi R, Naz F, Nayyar BG. Pre-harvest aflatoxins and Aspergillus flavus contamination in variable germplasms of red chillies from Kunri, Pakistan. Mycotoxin Research. 2017;33(2):147-155.

[52] Karaaslan M, Arslanğray Y. Aflatoxins B 1, B 2, G 1, and G 2 contamination in ground red peppers commercialized in Sanliurfa, Turkey. Environmental monitoring and assessment. 2015;187(4):1-9.

[53] Golge O, Hepsag F, Kabak B. Incidence and level of aflatoxin contamination in chilli commercialised in Turkey. Food Control. 2013;33(2):514-520.

[54] Mozaffari Nejad AS, Sabouri Ghannad M, Kamkar A. Determination of aflatoxin B1 levels in Iranian and Indian spices by ELISA method. Toxin Reviews. 2014;33(4):151-154.

[55] Barani A, Nasiri Z, Jarrah N. Natural occurrence of aflatoxins in commercial pepper in Iran. Food and Agricultural Immunology. 2016;27(4):570-576.

[56] Jalili M. Natural occurrence of aflatoxins contamination in commercial spices in Iran. Iranian Journal of Health, Safety and Environment. 2016;3(2):513-517.

[57] Motloung L, De Saeger S, De Boevre M, Detavernier C, Audenaert K, Adebo O, et al. Study on mycotoxin contamination in South African food spices. World Mycotoxin Journal. 2018;11(3):401-409.

[58] Khazaeli P, Mehrabani M, Heidari MR, Asadikaram G, Najafi ML. Prevalence of aflatoxin contamination in herbs and spices in different regions of Iran. Iranian journal of public health. 2017;46(11):1540.

[59] Ali N, Hashim NH, Shuib NS. Natural occurrence of aflatoxins and ochratoxin A in processed spices marketed in Malaysia. Food Additives & Contaminants: Part A. 2015;32(4):518-532.

[60] Gherbawy YA, Shebany YM, Hussein MA, Maghraby TA. Molecular detection of mycobiota and aflatoxin contamination of chili. Archives of Biological Sciences. 2015;67(1):223-234.

[61] Gambacorta L, Magistà D, Perrone G, Murgolo S, Logrieco A, Solfrizzo M. Co-occurrence of toxigenic moulds, aflatoxins, ochratoxin A, Fusarium and Alternaria mycotoxins in fresh sweet peppers (Capsicum annuum) and their processed products. World Mycotoxin Journal. 2018;11(1):159-174.

[62] Fundikira SS. Aflatoxin contamination of marketed spices in

Tanzania: a case study of Dar es salaam: Sokoine University of Agriculture; 2018.

[63] Zahra N, Khan M, Mehmood Z, Saeed M, Kalim I, Ahmad I, et al. Determination of aflatoxins in spices and dried fruits. Journal of Scientific Research. 2018;10(3):315-321.

[64] El Darra N, Gambacorta L, Solfrizzo M. Multimycotoxins occurrence in spices and herbs commercialized in Lebanon. Food Control. 2019;95:63-70.

[65] Hossain MN, Talukder A, Afroze F, Rahim MM, Begum S, Haque MZ, et al. Identification of aflatoxigenic fungi and detection of their aflatoxin in red chilli (Capsicum annuum) samples using direct cultural method and HPLC. Advances in Microbiology. 2018;8(1):42-53.

[66] Zareshahrabadi Z, Bahmyari R, Nouraei H, Khodadadi H, Mehryar P, Asadian F, et al. Detection of Aflatoxin and Ochratoxin A in Spices by High-Performance Liquid Chromatography. Journal of Food Quality. 2020;2020.

[67] Alsharif AMA, Choo Y-M, Tan G-H. Detection of five mycotoxins in different food matrices in the Malaysian market by using validated liquid chromatography electrospray ionization triple quadrupole mass spectrometry. Toxins. 2019;11(4):196.

[68] Ezekiel CN, Ortega-Beltran A, Oyedeji EO, Atehnkeng J, Kössler P, Tairu F, et al. Aflatoxin in chili peppers in Nigeria: extent of contamination and control using atoxigenic Aspergillus flavus genotypes as biocontrol agents. Toxins. 2019;11(7):429.

[69] Koutsias I, Kollia E, Makri K, Markaki P, Proestos C. Occurrence and Risk Assessment of Aflatoxin B1 in Spices Marketed in Greece. Analytical Letters. 2020:1-14.

[70] Wikandari R, Mayningsih IC, Sari MDP, Purwandari FA, Setyaningsih W, Rahayu ES, et al. Assessment of microbiological quality and mycotoxin in dried chili by morphological identification, molecular detection, and chromatography analysis. International journal of environmental research and public health. 2020;17(6):1847.

[71] El-Dawy EGAE, Yassein AS, El-Said AH. Detection of mycobiota, aflatoxigenic and ochratoxigenic genes, and cytotoxic ability in spices. Food science & nutrition. 2019;7(8):2595-2604.

[72] Jacxsens L, De Meulenaer B. Risk assessment of mycotoxins and predictive mycology in Sri Lankan spices: Chilli and pepper. Procedia food science. 2016;6:326-330.

[73] Iqbal SZ, Paterson RRM, Bhatti IA, Asi MR. Comparing aflatoxin contamination in chilies from Punjab, Pakistan produced in summer and winter. Mycotoxin Research. 2011;27(2):75-80.

[74] Hammami W, Fiori S, Al Thani R, Kali NA, Balmas V, Migheli Q, et al. Fungal and aflatoxin contamination of marketed spices. Food Control. 2014;37:177-181.

[75] Kaefer CM, Milner JA. Herbs and spices in cancer prevention and treatment. Herbal Medicine: Biomolecular and Clinical Aspects 2nd edition. 2011.

[76] Císarová M, Hleba L, Medo J, Tančinová D, Mašková Z, Čuboň J, et al. The in vitro and in situ effect of selected essential oils in vapour phase against bread spoilage toxicogenic aspergilli. Food Control. 2020;110:107007.

[77] Liu Q, Meng X, Li Y, Zhao C-N, Tang G-Y, Li H-B. Antibacterial and antifungal activities of spices.

International journal of molecular sciences. 2017;18(6):1283.

[78] Mohajeri M, Behnam B, Cicero AF, Sahebkar A. Protective effects of curcumin against aflatoxicosis: A comprehensive review. Journal of cellular physiology. 2018;233(4):3552-3577.

[79] Juglal S, Govinden R, Odhav B. Spice oils for the control of co-occurring mycotoxin-producing fungi. Journal of food protection. 2002;65(4):683-687.

[80] Combrinck S, Regnier T, Kamatou GP. In vitro activity of eighteen essential oils and some major components against common postharvest fungal pathogens of fruit. Industrial Crops and Products. 2011;33(2):344-349.

[81] Jalili M. A review on aflatoxins reduction in food. Iranian Journal of Health, Safety and Environment. 2016;3(1):445-459.

[82] Khan M, Asghar M, Ahmed A, Iqbal J, Shamsuddin Z. Reduction of aflatoxins in dundi-cut whole red chillies (Capsicum indicum) by manual sorting technique. Science Technology and Development. 2013;32(1):16-23.

[83] Iqbal SZ, Bhatti IA, Asi MR, Zuber M, Shahid M, Parveen I. Effect of γ irradiation on fungal load and aflatoxins reduction in red chillies. Radiation Physics and Chemistry. 2013;82:80-84.

[84] Pankaj S, Shi H, Keener KM. A review of novel physical and chemical decontamination technologies for aflatoxin in food. Trends in Food Science & Technology. 2018;71:73-83.

[85] Guo Y, Zhao L, Ma Q, Ji C. Novel strategies for degradation of aflatoxins in food and feed: A review. Food Research International. 2020:109878.

[86] Tripathi S, Mishra H. Enzymatic coupled with UV degradation of aflatoxin B1 in red chili powder. Journal of Food Quality. 2010;33:186-203.

[87] Kamber U, Gülbaz G, Aksu P, Doğan A. Detoxification of aflatoxin B1 in red pepper (*Capsicum annuum* L.) by ozone treatment and its effect on microbiological and sensory quality. Journal of Food Processing and Preservation. 2017;41(5):e13102.

[88] Watson I, Kamble P, Shanks C, Khan Z, El Darra N. Decontamination of chilli flakes in a fluidized bed using combined technologies: Infrared, UV and ozone. Innovative Food Science & Emerging Technologies. 2020;59:102248.

[89] George W, Latimer J. Official method of analysis of AOAC. AOAC International. 2019.

[90] Afsah-Hejri L, Jinap S, Hajeb P, Radu S, Shakibazadeh S. A review on mycotoxins in food and feed: Malaysia case study. Comprehensive Reviews in Food Science and Food Safety. 2013;12(6):629-651.

[91] Sinha A, Petersen J. Caribbean hot pepper production and post harvest manual. FAO/Caribbean Agricultural Research and Development Institute, Rome, Italy. 2011.

Chapter 9

# Aflatoxin and Disruption of Energy Metabolism

*Adewale Segun James, Emmanuel Ifeanyichukwu Ugwor, Victoria Ayomide Adebiyi, Emmanuel Obinna Ezenandu and Victory Chukwudalu Ugbaja*

## Abstract

Aflatoxins constitute a cluster of mycotoxins that are derived from fungal metabolites and are produced from diverse fungi species, especially *Aspergillus.* They are a collection of closely linked heterocyclic compounds produced predominantly by two filamentous fungi, *Aspergillus flavus* and *Aspergillus parasiticus.* They are also known to cause severe health threats to humans and animals, thereby resulting to several complications like immunotoxicity, teratogenicity hepatotoxicity. Aflatoxins interfere with normal metabolic processes. This interference encompasses the regulatory processes that occur throughout the progression of energy metabolism. Thus, the effects of aflatoxins are seen in the inhibition of ATP generation, carbohydrate and lipid metabolism, mitochondrial structure and proteins synthesis. This chapter will focus on the mechanisms of aflatoxin-induced disruption of lipids, carbohydrates, and proteins metabolism, and how they affect the bioenergetic systems.

**Keywords:** aflatoxin, mitochondria, lipids, carbohydrates, proteins, energy

## 1. Introduction

Aflatoxins constitute a cluster of mycotoxins that are derived from fungal metabolites and are produced from diverse fungi species, especially *Aspergillus* [1]. They are a collection of closely linked heterocyclic compounds produced predominantly by two filamentous fungi, *Aspergillus flavus* and *Aspergillus parasiticus* [2]. These fungi are generally infectious to cereal produces like wheat, walnut, rice, cotton, peanuts, tree nuts and corn [3]. Aflatoxins are members of the difuranocoumarins with two significant chemical structure series. These series include – (a) difurocoumarocyclopentenone series (b) difurocoumarolactone series [4]. They are also known to cause severe health threats to humans and animals, thereby resulting to several complications like immunotoxicity, teratogenicity hepatotoxicity [5]. The key aflatoxins are B1, B2, G1, and G2. They are noted for their ability to induce huge amplification of inflammatory responses during the body's, cutaneous and mucous respiratory cycles [6].

Food contamination by aflatoxin is a global concern particularly in the tropical and subtropical areas of the biosphere whereby warm temperatures and moisture enhance the growth of the Aspergillus fungi. Aflatoxins are well recognized carcinogens specifically aflatoxin B1 (AFB1) to man and animals [4]. Currently, there are over 18 identified aflatoxins of which have been inadequately researched for their occurrence, health-risk, and mechanisms of toxicity [7]. Owing to their extensive distribution in foods and feeds, Aflatoxins are the mycotoxins of utmost concern to food security. As a result of the public health fears that these toxicants add and their relationship with energy metabolism disruption, intensive findings have been carried out since their discovery to elucidate their interference with energy metabolism and related concerns. The elucidation of these toxic features is a criterion to the design of therapeutic or protective means, and to sufficiently regulate their existence in foods and feeds [8].

Aflatoxins are extremely lipo-soluble compounds; hence they are readily absorbed via the gastrointestinal tract and respiratory tract which is usually their site of exposure into blood stream [9, 10]. Aflatoxins are found in human and animals based on two significant routes. They are either directly ingested as aflatoxin-contaminated foods or inhaled from dust particles containing aflatoxin, usually expelled from industries and factories [9, 11]. In the body, aflatoxins are absorbed across the cell membranes where they enter the blood stream. From the blood stream, they are distributed in blood to various tissues, especially the liver which is the primary organ for metabolism of xenobiotic [11]. Aflatoxins are predominantly metabolized by the liver to yield a reactive epoxide intermediate, to be converted to a less harmful aflatoxin [12, 13]. In humans and predisposed animal species, aflatoxins, particularly Aflatoxin B1 (AFB1) are metabolized by cytochrome P450 (CYP450) microsomal enzymes to yield aflatoxin-8, 9-epoxide. This metabolite is a responsive form that binds to DNA and to albumin usually in the blood serum, giving rise to adducts and thus triggering DNA impairment [12, 13].

## 2. Aflatoxin-induced disruption of energy metabolism

Aflatoxins interfere with normal metabolic processes. This interference encompasses the regulatory processes that occur throughout the progression of energy metabolism. Thus, the effects of aflatoxins are seen in the inhibition of ATP generation, carbohydrate and lipid metabolism, mitochondrial structure and proteins synthesis [14].

### 2.1 Inhibition of ATP generation

Aflatoxin B1 (AFB1), a member of the mycotoxins inhibits the electron transport chain (ETC) in the mitochondria which is a major tissue in energy metabolism. This inhibition occurs at both ADP-coupled and dDNDP-uncoupled stages [15]. At the cytochrome oxidase level and also between cytochrome b and c, AFB1 inhibits the electron transport chain. This however, can be reversed by the electron acceptor N′-tetramethylphenylenediamine (TMPD) [4]. AFB1 gives rise to reduction in cellular ATP synthesis. Consequently, an enlargement of the mitochondria develops and then sodium, potassium gradient is distressed within the cell [16].

### 2.2 Effect of aflatoxins on mitochondrial DNA

In the mitochondria, AFB causes radical structural changes [17–19]. Similarly, it causes mitochondrial directed apoptosis, consequently reducing their function [17, 18, 20]. The presence of aflatoxins may also disturb the telomere length and the different check points in the cell cycle, thereby initiating further harm to the regulatory processes of the cell cycle [20]. Furthermore, the degree of aflatoxin binding to DNA and its injured state, the stages of various protein modifications ranging from cell cycle and apoptotic pathways like protein kinase C (PKC), protein kinase A (PKA), c-Myc, pRb, Ras, Bcl-2, p53, NF-kB, CKI, cyclins and CDK have significant implications to the life processes that may lead to the deregulation of cell proliferation resulting in the development of cancer [17, 18].

During hepatocarcinogenesis, the reactive aflatoxin-8,9-epoxide binds to mitochondrial DNA (mitDNA) when compared to nuclear DNA which prevents the production of ATP and FAD/NAD-linked enzymatic roles [19]. This results in the disturbance of mitochondrial functions in different body parts that require energy production in form of ATP [19]. Mitochondrial damage as a result of aflatoxin influence can give rise to mitochondrial illnesses and may account for aging mechanisms [19]. Reports have stated that specific mitochondrial diseases occur as a result of the nucleus being able to detect energy deficits in its region. The nucleus then tries to recompense the ATP shortages by initiating the replication of any neighboring mitochondria; however, the feedback enhances replication of the original mitochondria that causes the energy deficit, thus, causing further complications [15]. Gene mutations are also seen when AFBI binds to DNA. This is such that structural alterations are formed, which results in length changes of the telomeres and the cell cycle check points [17, 18]. Also, the binding of Aflatoxin B1 to DNA at the guanine base in hepatic cells corrupts the genomic code that controls cell growth, thereby resulting in the formation of tumors [17–19]. The injury to mitochondrial DNA is initiated by mutations of mitochondrial membranes resulting in heightened apoptosis as well as a disruption in the production of energy [18, 21, 22].

### 2.3 Carbohydrate and lipid metabolism

Metabolites of aflatoxin react with various cells, which in turn cause the inhibition of carbohydrate and lipid metabolism, as well as reduced liver function [23, 24]. The gluconeogenesis process is inhibited by AFB1. This is done by a reduction in the activity of glycogen synthase and transglycolase. This accounts for the rearrangement and elongation of glycogen molecules [15]. Furthermore, AFB1 lowers the enzymatic function of phosphorglucomutase, which reversibly converts glucose −6-phosphate to glucose −1-phosphate. It also lowers the amount of glycogen present in the liver via the oxidation of glucose −6- phosphate [4]. A major interference caused by aflatoxins, especially AFB1, is the process of lipid deposition in the hepatic tissue. This can be attributed to impaired lipid transport in contrast with a prediction of increased lipid biosynthesis [15]. This lipid deposition in the hepatic tissue can be ascribed to a decreased oxidation of fat as the mitochondria are being compromised [15]. Also increased fat contents have been reported in plasma, liver, and adipose tissues in several studies [25–27] and linked to reduced oxidation of lipids and increased fatty acid synthesis, owing to altered expression of genes involved in lipid and lipoprotein metabolism, following AFB1 exposure [26].

### 2.4 Inhibition of proteins synthesis

Metabolites of Aflatoxins exhibit negative effects with diverse cells, which inhibit the synthesis of protein [28]. AFB1 directly inhibits the production of protein via the inactivation of enzymes involved in protein synthesis; that is initiation, transcription and translation processes of protein synthesis. Indirectly, AFBI inhibits protein production by changing the activity of DNA template. They obstruct pyrimidine and purines nucleosides subsequently leading to the inhibition of protein synthesis via the development of DNA, RNA and protein adducts [4].

Furthermore, the decrease in protein content of body tissues such as the kidney, heart, skeletal muscle and liver could be due to increased liver and kidney necrosis [29].

AFB1 is known to be mutagenic, immunosuppressive and teratogenic. These features may interfere with regular processes of protein production as well as inhibition of several metabolic systems; consequently, initiating harms to several organs particularly the kidney, heart and liver [15, 30]. The precise reversible non-covalent and nonspecific-irreversible covalent binding with aflatoxins can alter the activities and structure of proteins [21].

## 3. Conclusion

Aflatoxins, a cluster of mycotoxins produced by *Aspergillus* and other fungal species, are known to interfere with normal metabolic processes, thereby posing severe health threats to humans and animals. This chapter focused on mechanisms underlying aflatoxin-induced inhibition of energy metabolism, which involve disruption of lipids, carbohydrates, and proteins metabolism, as well as mitochondrial function, culminating in depletion of ATP pools.

## Author details

Adewale Segun James*, Emmanuel Ifeanyichukwu Ugwor,
Victoria Ayomide Adebiyi, Emmanuel Obinna Ezenandu
and Victory Chukwudalu Ugbaja
Department of Biochemistry, College of Biosciences, Federal University of Agriculture, Abeokuta, Nigeria

*Address all correspondence to: whljaymz@gmail.com

## References

[1] Bennett, J. W., & Klich, M. (2003). Mycotocins. *Clinical Microbiology Reviews*, 497-516. doi:http://dx.doi.org/10.1128/CMR.16.3.497-516.2003

[2] Mishra, H., & Chitrangada, D. (2003). A Review on Biological Control and Metabolism of Aflatoxin. Critical Reviews in Food Science and Nutrition, *43(3)*, 245-264.

[3] Rashid, N., Bajwa, M., Rafeek, M. M., Tariq, F., Abbas, M. A., Awan, M. A., Ahmad, Z. (2013). Prevalence of Aflatoxicosis in broiler chickens in Quetta, Pakistan. Pakistan Journal of Zoology, *45(4)*, 1021-1026.

[4] Bbosa, G. S., Kitya, D., Odda, J., & Okeng, J. O. (2013). Aflatoxins metabolism, effects on epigenetic mechanisms and their role in carcinogenesis. Health, *5(10)*, 14-34.

[5] Rawal, S. J., Kim, E., & Jr, C. E. (2010). Aflatoxin B1 in poultry: Toxicology, metabolism and prevention. Veterinary Science, *89*, 325-331.

[6] Romani, L. (2004). Immunity to fungal infections. Nature Reviews Immunology, *4*(1), 11-24.

[7] Noreddine, B. (2020). Chronic and Acute Toxicities of Aflatoxins: Mechanisms of Action. *International Journal of Environmental Research and Public Health, 17*, 1-28. doi:http://dx.doi.org/10.3390/ijerph17020423

[8] Adebayo-Tayo, B. C., Onilude, A. A., & Patrick, U. G. (2008). Mycofloral of smoke-dried fishes sold in Uyo, Eastern Nigeria. World Journal of Agricultural Sciences, 4(3), 346-350.

[9] Agag, B. I. (2004). Mycotoxins in foods and feeds : Aflatoxins. Association of Universal Bulletin of Environmental Research, *7(1)*, 173-191.

[10] Larsson, P., & Tjalve, H. (2000). Intranasal instillation of Aflatoxin B1 in rats: Bioactivation in the nasal mucosa and neuronal transport to the olfactory bulb. Toxicological Science, 383-391.

[11] Godfrey, S. B., David, K., Lubega, J. O., William, W. A., & David, B. K. (2013). Review of the Biological and Health Effects of Aflatoxins on Body Organs and Body Systems. *Intech*. doi:http://dx.doi.org/10.5772/51201

[12] Wild, C. P., & Montesano, R. (2009). A model of interaction: Aflatoxins and hepatitis viruses in liver cancer aetiology and prevention. Cancer Letters, 22-28.

[13] Wu, F., & Khlangwiset, P. (2010). Health economic impacts and cost-effectiveness of aflatoxin reduction strategies in Africa: Case studies in biocontrol and postharvest interventions. Food Additives & Contaminants, *27*, 496-509.

[14] Lahiani, A., Yavin, E., & Lazarovici, P. (2017). The molecular basis of toxins' interactions with intracellular signaling via discrete portals. Toxins, *9*(3), 107.

[15] Syeda, M. H., Shahzad, S. M., Syed, K. H., Asif, I., & Huma, H. (2020). Cellular Interactions, Metabolism, Assessment and Control of Aflatoxins: An Update. *Computational Biology and Bioinformatics, 8*(2), 62-71. doi: 10.11648/j.cbb.20200802.15

[16] Khatun, S., Chakraborty, M., Islam, A., Cakilcioglu, U., & Chatterjee, N. C. (2012). Mycotoxins as health hazard. Biological Diversity and Conservation, *5(3)*, 123-133.

[17] Jacotot, E., Ferri, K. F., & Kroemer, G. (2000). Apoptosis and cell cycle: distinct check points with overlapping upstream control. Pathological Biology, *48(3)*, 271-279.

[18] Tuppen, H. A., Blakely, E. L., Turnbull, D. M., & Taylor, R. W. (2010). Mitochondrial DNA mutations and human disease. Biochimica et Biophysica Acta (BBA)-Bioenergetics, *1797*(2), 113-128.

[19] WHO. (2008). World Health Statistics. *World Health Organisation, Geneva,*. Retrieved from http://www.who.int/whosis/whostat/EN_WHS08_Full.pdf.

[20] Hornsby, P. J. (2007). Senescence: As an Anticancer Mechanism. Journal of Clinical Oncology, *25(14)*, 1852-1857.

[21] Thrasher, J. D., & Crawley, S. L. (2012). Neurotoxicity of Mycotoxins. Retrieved from http://www.drthrasher.org/page189.html

[22] Thrasher, J. D., & Crawley, S. L. (2012b). Neurotoxicity of Mycotoxins. Retrieved from http://www.drthrasher.org/page189.html

[23] Edrington, T. S., Sarrb, A. B., Kubenaa, L. F., & Harvey, R. B. (1996). Hydrated sodium calcium aluminosilicate (HSCAS), acidic HSCAS, and activated charcoal reduce urinary excretion of aflatoxin M1, in turkey poults. Lack of effect by activated charcoal on aflatoxicosis. Toxicology Letters, *89*, 115-122.

[24] Hussain, I., Anwar, J., Munawar, M. A., & Asi, M. R. (2008). Variation of levels of aflatoxin M1 in raw milk from different localities in the central areas of Punjab, Pakistan. Food Control, *19(12)*, 1126-1129.

[25] El-Nekeety, A. A., Abdel-Azeim, S. H., Hassan, A. M., Hassan, N. S., Aly, S. E., & Abdel-Wahhab, M. A. (2014). Quercetin inhibits the cytotoxicity and oxidative stress in liver of rats fed aflatoxin-contaminated diet. Toxicology Reports, *1*, 319-329.

[26] Rotimi, O. A., Rotimi, S. O., Duru, C. U., Ebebeinwe, O. J., Abiodun, A. O., Oyeniyi, B. O., & Faduyile, F. A. (2017). Acute aflatoxin B1–Induced hepatotoxicity alters gene expression and disrupts lipid and lipoprotein metabolism in rats. Toxicology reports, *4*, 408-414.

[27] Zhang, L., Ye, Y., An, Y., Tian, Y., Wang, Y., & Tang, H. (2011). Systems responses of rats to aflatoxin B1 exposure revealed with metabonomic changes in multiple biological matrices. Journal of proteome research, *10*(2), 614-623.

[28] Hussain, I., & Anwar, J. (2008). A study on contamination of aflatoxin M1 in raw milk in the Punjab province of Pakistan. Food Control, *19*, 393-395.

[29] Sharma, V. E. (2011). Ameliorative Effects of Curcuma Longa and Curcumin on Aflatoxin B1 Induced Serological and Biochemical Changes In Kidney of Male Mice. Asian Journal of Biochemical and Pharmaceutical Research, *1(2)*, 338-351.

[30] Mohammed, A. M., & Metwally, N. S. (2009). Antiaflatoxicogenic activities of some aqeous plant extracts against AFB1 induced Renal and Cardiac damage. Journal of Pharmacology and Toxicology, *4(1)*, 1-16.

Chapter 10

# Chromatographic Techniques for Estimation of Aflatoxins in Food Commodities

*Mateen Abbas*

## Abstract

Aflatoxins, produced mainly by Aspergillus *flavus* Aspergillus *parasiticus*, have been documented as one of the major food contaminants throughout the world. Because of their toxic nature, these food contaminants have acknowledged considerable attention in recent years. Among the different types of Aflatoxins, the most prevalent and predominant Aflatoxins are AFB1, AFB2, AFG1, AFG2, AFM1, AFM2 which are considered the more lethal as compared to others. Several analytical and immunological methods are available for testing and estimating aflatoxins in different food commodities. However, chromatographic techniques have been considered superior regarding the estimation of aflatoxins both qualitatively and quantitatively. Chromatographic techniques have numerous applications for the separation and identification of chemical and biological compounds in food industry. It has grown to be the most popular and versatile of all analytical techniques in laboratories used for the analysis of multiple components in different matrices. For preliminary qualitative detection of Aflatoxins, Thin layer chromatography (TLC) is considered the best analytical technique which is being used broadly in food industry. However, liquid chromatographic techniques including High Performance Liquid Chromatography (HPLC) and Liquid chromatography-mass Spectrometry (LC–MS) are the best analytical techniques developed so far for the quantification of Aflatoxins in food commodities.

**Keywords:** Food, Aflatoxins; TLC, HPLC, LC–MS

## 1. Introduction

Aflatoxins are toxic substances formed by certain kind of fungi (molds) that have the potential to contaminate food, feed, crops and pose a serious health risk to humans and livestock. Aflatoxins are also assumed to be responsible for the annual loss of 25% or more of the world's food crops, which has significant economic implications. Various procedures for the detection and analysis of aflatoxins are available in feed and food, as they are highly specific, practical, and useful [1].

Aflatoxins are cancerous secondary metabolites produced primarily by Aspergillus *flavus* and Aspergillus *parasiticus* in foodstuff. Basically the chemical composition of aflatoxins contain the difurano-coumarin molecules which are synthesized following the polyketide pathway [2]. Eighteen different types of aflatoxins have been identified however six are well-known and recognized as B1, B2,

G1, G2, M1, and M2, respectively, [3]. Aflatoxins B1, B2, G1 & G2 found in different kinds of food & feed which are metabolized in animal body and then excreted mainly via milk as aflatoxins M1 and M2. All these aflatoxins have molecular differences; the aflatoxin B-group (B1 and B2) contains the cyclopentane ring which shows blue fluorescence under ultraviolet (UV) light whereas the aflatoxin G-group (G1 and G2) comprises the lactone ring and shows yellow-green fluorescence under UV light [4]. The different color fluorescence is important for identifying and differentiating between the aflatoxins B & G groups. Aflatoxin B1 is most commonly found in different kind of food matrixes [5] and widespread maximally [6, 7] in the world and accounts for 75% of all aflatoxins contamination in food commodities [8]. Aflatoxins M1 and M2 are hydroxylated products (metabolites) of aflatoxins B1 and B2, respectively, which are concomitant with animal milk upon ingestion of aflatoxins B1 and B2 contaminated feed. Furthermore, once converted from B1 and B2 forms, aflatoxins M1 and M2 remain stable during milk processing [9].

To protect consumer health, maximum levels (MLs) for mycotoxins in foodstuffs have been established worldwide. In particular, the European Union legislation (often considered as the most stringent one) has established MLs for aflatoxins [10].

International organizations for example AOAC (Association of Official Analytical Chemists), CEN (European Committee for Standardization) and ISO (International Organization for Standardization) have continued rendezvous experts over the years to develop internationally recognized analytical standards. The main objective is to evade the discrepancies in outcomes that may arise from the use of different analytical methodologies, with the risk to partial worldwide food trade. Currently, seventy-two official methods are offered from these organizations for scrutinizing the mycotoxins in food commodities.

A variety of methods to detect aflatoxins in food and feed are available for different needs and different techniques for their detection and analysis have been extensively researched to develop those that are highly specific, useful and practical.

Owing to its common incidence and toxic nature, numerous analytical and immunological methods were developed. However, there are minor modifications actually in most of these analytical methods from the officially adopted basic methods for certain food commodities. They differ only in the analytical techniques used for assessing the strength of fluorescence of the analyzed mycotoxins and in the extraction solvents used to extract the mycotoxins from different food matrixes. A plethora of methods are available for different needs, ranging from techniques/methods for regulatory control in Official laboratories starting from simple rapid test kits (AgraStrip®, CHARM EZ-M) to advanced methods [including immunochemical methods comprises radioimmunoassay (RIA), Enzyme-Linked Immunosorbent Assay (ELISA), Immunoaffinity column assay (ICA), Immunodipstick and immunosensors; Spectroscopic methods including Fluorometer, Spectrophotometer, Fourier-transform infrared spectroscopy (FTIR), Quartz Crystal Microbalances (QCMs), Surface Plasmon resonance Spectroscopy (SPRS); and some Chromatographic methods such as Thin Layer Chromatography (TLC) with densitometer, High-performance Thin Layer Chromatography (HPTLC), High-Performance Liquid Chromatography (HPLC), Gas Chromatography (GC), Liquid Chromatography-Mass Spectrometry (LC–MS)] for factories and grain silos (**Table 1**).

Quickness and effortlessness in analysis are the other features that have gain worldwide consideration recently. When a large number of samples have to be analyzed in a short time period then enzyme-linked immunosorbent assay (ELISA), mini-column quick methods, and radio-immunoassay (RIA) techniques may be used.

| Method | Sample preparation | LOD | Field Applicable | Reference |
|---|---|---|---|---|
| AgraStrip® | Simple extraction with Methanol | 4 ppb | Appropriate | [11] |
| Immunodipstick | Extraction only | 5 μg/Kg | Appropriate | [12] |
| CHARM EZ-M | Water based extraction | 1 ppb | Inappropriate | [13] |
| Fluorometer | IAC | 5–5000 μg/Kg | Inappropriate | [14] |
| TLC densitometer | Liquid Extraction, SPE | 1–20 ng/kg | Inappropriate | [15, 16] |
| HPTLC | Liquid Extraction | Pictogram | Inappropriate | [17] |
| RIA | Liquid Extraction | 1 μg/Kg | Inappropriate | [18] |
| FTIR | Liquid Extraction | <10 μg/Kg | Inappropriate | [19] |
| ELISA | Liquid Extraction | 1 μg/Kg | Inappropriate | [20] |
| HPLC | IAC or SPE | 0.5 μg/Kg | Inappropriate | [21] |
| LC-MS | Liquid Extraction | 0.1 μg/Kg | Inappropriate | [22] |
| QCMs | Liquid Extraction | 0.01–10 ng/mL | Inappropriate | [23, 24] |
| SPRS | Liquid Extraction | 3.0–98 ng/mL | Inappropriate | [25] |
| Electrochemical | Liquid Extraction | 0.1–2 μg/Kg | Inappropriate | [26, 27] |

**Table 1.**
*Evaluation of different methods for analysis of aflatoxins in food and feed.*

Potential innovative aflatoxins-detection techniques, based on the emerging techniques, include electronic noses, dip-stick kits, molecularly imprinted polymers, hyper-spectral imaging, and aptamer-based biosensors (small organic molecules that can bind specific target molecules). The latter techniques may have significance in remote areas because of their use, stability and ease of production. However, any method recommended for aflatoxin analysis should be economical and convenient to the handlers, taking into account their available laboratory facilities, as well as providing greater accuracy in the results.

All analytical methods for aflatoxins involve basically the same steps: sampling and sample extraction, clean-up, work-up, detection, and confirmation, as well as estimation of the toxin.

## 2. Sampling procedures are problematic

Adequate sampling techniques as well as appropriate sample preparation procedures are the most significant steps before performing the chemical analysis of aflatoxins. Aflatoxins are present in only a few grains and kernels obviously and have highly crooked distribution in food and feed commodities therefore, some variations in analytical results might be possible if the sample collected for analysis is not representative of the bulk [28–31].

As molds and aflatoxins aren't equally dispersed all through the bulk shipments and batches of stored grain, proper sampling is essential for obtaining a representative result. Proper protocols for sampling have been established, particularly in the perspective of regulatory control. For example, the Codex Alimentarius Commission has set the protocols to be used for various food commodities in setting maximum levels for aflatoxins. The United Nation's Food and Agriculture Organization (FAO) has established a mycotoxins sampling contrivance that is available on-line. The use of recommended sampling methods is a problem, especially for subsistence farmers in rural areas who do not produce enough grain to allow for accurate testing. As a result, to improve surveillance and control in rural areas, low-cost, rapid and low-technology aflatoxins detection techniques are required. Food organizations trying their best to control aflatoxins in Africa and the World Food Programme's are also addressing these issues, for example, the World Food Programme has introduced the appropriate Purchase guidelines to ensure grain quality.

A precise and accurate sample can be selected by collecting a representative sample in large quantity and then dividing it into three equal parts. Differences in weight of selected samples may also be critical which depend on the regulations of a specific country. For example; the United Kingdom (UK) has proposed a sample weight of 10.5 kg, while the United States (US) has recommended the sample weight of 66 kg, greatly a larger amount. However, an average sample weight of 5–10 kg has been adopted by most of the countries. Precise grinding and sub-division of the sample would also be critical for accurate determination of aflatoxins. Spinning riffles, rotary sample divisors, and cascade samplers may also be used to select the representative sub-samples [31–33]. The size of the sub-samples may vary from 20 to 100 g. However, in most of the methods 50 g sample was used for analysis of aflatoxins, which looks to be the best in terms of economy in using costly extraction solvents.

## 3. Aflatoxins extraction and clean-up methods

The frequently used extraction and clean-up techniques for aflatoxins analysis are liquid–liquid extraction (LLE), solid-phase extraction (SPE) and "Quick, Easy, Cheap, Effective, Rugged, and Safe" (QuEChERS) methods. Furthermore, some other extraction methods are also offered in the literatures that are not commonly used in routine analysis at the moment.

### 3.1 Liquid–Liquid extraction (LLE)

Liquid–liquid extraction procedures are the simple, easy and cheap methods for the extraction of aflatoxins. It is based on the partition coefficient and different solubility properties of the mycotoxin in the organic or aqueous phase or in their combination mixtures. However, the shortcomings of these extraction techniques are that it does not provide appropriately clean analyte in all cases.

An efficient extraction method is required for the qualitative detection and quantification of aflatoxins in food and feed samples. Aflatoxins are commonly soluble in the polar-protic solvents like acetone, acetonitrile, chloroform and methanol. Hence, aflatoxins can be extracted by using either any of the mentioned pure solvents or in combination of these solvents as well as with small quantity of water [34, 35]. Several studies have been conducted on different food matrices to determine the extraction efficiency of various aqueous-organic solvents [36–38] and the different extraction recoveries have been reported. Since methanol has a minor negative effect on antibodies than other organic solvents like acetone and acetonitrile therefore aflatoxins extraction using a mixture of methanol with water (e.g.; 8 + 2 v/v) [37, 39] is required for determination of aflatoxins on immunoassay technique.

### 3.2 Liquid–Solid extraction (LSE)

Liquid–solid extraction technique is another simple and easy extraction method for the extraction of aflatoxins using solid matrices of different consistency.

Initially, the selection of an appropriate and the most effective extraction solvents is a crucial step to extract the component of interest. Most frequently used extraction solvents are mixtures of methanol/water or acetonitrile/water in different ratios [40]. For instance, the 80% methanol/water mixture proved to be the most optimal for extraction of aflatoxins in the case of nutmeg samples. The choice of methanol for further use is also preferable, because the antibodies better tolerate higher concentrations of methanol than acetonitrile. Methanol was also suitable for chromatographic separation, as aflatoxins were measurable without interference [41]. The extraction efficiency is significantly influenced by the composition of the extraction agents, the sample/solvent ratio, and the time of extraction. Sometimes, the use of only LSE method is inadequate to extract aflatoxins without interference and additionally some purification step(s) are required for proper extraction. The extraction process comprises the different steps including the weighing of homogenized sample which will be properly grind having appropriate particle size, addition of suitable extraction solvents and then dissolution or disintegrating the mixture applying, e.g., vortex, blender, shaker, or other approaches to extract the required components. After extraction, sample is filtered and cleaned prior to analysis.

### 3.3 Ultrasound extraction

Liquid–solid extraction efficiency can substantially be improved with the use of ultrasound. In the ultrasound extraction process the container (e.g., flask, centrifuge tube or vials) containing the sample to be extracted and the extraction solvent is most often immersed into an ultrasonic bath that contains water. After a few minutes, the acoustic cavitation under the influence of ultrasonic field in liquids significantly increases the transfer of the analytes and matrix components from the sample to the extraction solvent, thereby increasing the recovery and efficiency of extraction [42].

### 3.4 Supercritical fluid extraction (SFE)

Supercritical fluid extraction uses a supercritical fluid for the extraction of the required compound from the matrix. The SFE procedure is mainly used efficiently for the extraction of apolar organic molecules [43]. During the extraction of polar aflatoxins with SFE a number of problems have arisen, e.g., low recoveries and high concentrations of co-extracts. Furthermore, lipids may cause difficulties during further cleanup and chromatographic separation [44].

### 3.5 Solid phase extraction (SPE)

Solid phase extraction techniques are considered the most accurate and reliable approaches to clean-up the mixtures before qualitative and quantitative estimations. With the help of SPE, required analyte can be separated and unwanted components which may interfere during analysis can be removed accurately. Two types of SPE are used.

SPE is a multi-step process, starting from the conditioning then followed by the sample loading, washing and at the end elution of required analyte. In the SPE, the required analyte either bound to the matrix component(s) or removed from the sample [45]. Various extenders are used in the SPE columns. Aflatoxins are often analyzed by using C-18 (octadecylsilane) column. A specific application of SPE is the so-called immunoaffinity clean-up columns (IAC) and Multi-functional clean-up columns (MFC) including MultiSep®, MycoSep®, and Myco6in1 column [46]. The extraction of aflatoxins is usually followed by a cleanup step. The common cleanup technique used is immunoaffinity column (IAC) chromatography and Mycosep multi-functional cleanup (MFC) columns [47]. These purification techniques are considered the best choice for isolation of target analyte (like aflatoxins) and to clean-up or remove the unwanted components before their quantitative estmation using HPLC [48].

Immunoaffinity chromatographic technique proved to be the accurate and highly specific which reversibility of binding between an antigen and antibody to isolate, purify and separate the target molecule from matrices [49]. During the cleanup process, the extracted liquid sample is applied to the IAC which holding the specific antibodies to bind with aflatoxins that immobilized on a solid surface such as silica or agarose. As the extracted sample moves down the IAC column, the aflatoxins bind to the antibodies and are retained onto the column. To remove the unbound proteins and impurities washing step is generally required using appropriate ionic strength buffers or distilled water. Thereafter, the aflatoxins are recovered or removed from the IAC by using pure solvents like acetonitrile or methanol which breaks the bond between the antibody and the aflatoxins.

Mycosep multi-functional cleanup (MFC) columns are also recognized a best approach for purification of aflatoxins. It is simple, easy, handy to use and a rapid one-step purification technique. These columns are designed to retain certain groups of basic compounds that may create interferences in HPLC analysis. On the other hand, MFC purification columns allow the molecules of interest to pass through the columns. During the MFC cleanup procedure, after extraction of aflatoxins using suitable solvents a portion of the extract is passed through an MFC column designed particularly for aflatoxins analysis. Compounds that may create interferences are retained in MFC, whereas aflatoxins pass through the column. Ideal recovery (> 95%), precision and coefficient of variation (< 3%) of aflatoxins were observed by these columns [50].

## 4. Work-up

After the clean-up step, the extract must be worked up to make it suitable for the estimations. The purified pooled extract can be treated with sodium sulphate (anhydrous) to remove the moisture if present in the extract. To concentrate the extracted solvent evaporated it to dryness using nitrogen stream or in a rotary evaporator at 50°C. On the other hand, evaporation of solvents can be achieved with the help of steam bath under the nitrogen stream preferably. Finally, reconstituted the residues using pure organic solvents like acetonitrile or methanol and used for estimations.

## 5. Methods for detection and quantification of aflatoxins

The most commonly used chromatography techniques for analysis of aflatoxins are Thin-Layer Chromatography (TLC), High-Performance Liquid Chromatography (HPLC), Gas chromatography (GC) and Liquid Chromatography-Mass Spectrometry (LC–MS). Although many of the chromatographic techniques are very sensitive, they require trained skilled technician, cumbersome pretreatment of sample, and expensive apparatus/equipment [51].

### 5.1 Thin-layer chromatography (TLC)

Thin-layer chromatography is one of the most widely used separation techniques for detection of aflatoxins. TLC has been regarded by the Association of Official

Analytical Chemist (AOAC) as the method of choice since 1990. It consists of a solid immobilized stationary phase may contain either alumina or cellulose or silica on an inert material such as plastic or glass, called the matrix. The mobile phase is contained of acetonitrile: methanol: water mixture [52], which brings the sample along as it moves through the stationary phase. In TLC, aflatoxins are distributed between the mobile phase and stationary phases on the basis of partition coefficient or differences in solubility of the analytes in the two phases. Different types of aflatoxins (B1, B2, G1 & G2), according to their interaction with the stationary and mobile phases as well as due to the different molecular structures, either adhere to the solid surface of stationary phase more or remain in the mobile phase, thus allowing for effective and quick separation. TLC technique has been commonly used in food industry for the determination of aflatoxins [53–55] and detection limit of 1–20 ppb of different types of aflatoxins has been reported. The major advantage the TLC is that it can detect different types of mycotoxins with good resolution and excellent sensitivities [56]. It also requires pre-treatment of sample, skilled and trained technician, and expensive equipment as well [57]. In addition, there are also some drawbacks of TLC which may probably be occurring during spotting, TLC plate development, and interpretation.

Quantification of aflatoxins on TLC plates using fluoro-densitometer is considered to be a more precise and accurate method than visual estimates [58] with the minimum limit of detection (LOD) is 1 μg/kg. Although fluoro-densitometers are commercially available, but not commonly used due to its high cost and visual fluorescence identification method is still to be continue for identification of aflatoxins [59].

Attempts to improve TLC have led to the development of automated form of TLC, called the high-performance thin-layer chromatography (HPTLC).

### 5.2 High performance thin layer chromatography (HPTLC)

The conventional TLC method has improved through the automation of sample spotting, plate development and interpretation in HPTLC. Currently, HPTLC is one of the best analytical methods for estimation of aflatoxins [60, 61].

Automated sample applicator, digital scanner, and a computing integrator, lead to improve the sensitivity and precision in the quantification of aflatoxins. The other benefit of HPTLC method is the use of minimum amount (only 1 μl) for sample spotting, instead of 10-20 μl used for the conventional TLC method. With the use of HPTLC minimum concentrations of aflatoxins (5 pg) can be possibly detected [59].

However, the costly equipment, extensive sample treatment procedure and the requirement for skilled researcher, limit the HPTLC technique to the laboratory and thus it is inapplicable in field situations.

### 5.3 High-performance liquid chromatography (HPLC)

The most commonly used chromatographic technique for separation and determination of organic compounds is High Performance Liquid Chromatography (HPLC). Worldwide, approximately 80% of all organic compounds are estimated using HPLC [62].

The HPLC technique for estimation of aflatoxins has high automation, high sensitivity and high precision. There are two types of phase systems comprising normal phase (wherein mobile phase: non-polar & stationary phase: polar) and reverse phase (wherein mobile phase: polar & stationary phase: non-polar)) in combination with UV/VIS absorption and fluorescence detection. Reverse phase HPLC is broadly used for estimation of aflatoxins [59].

In HPLC, the stationary phase is confined to either a plastic or glass tube and the mobile phase containing the organic/aqueous solvents that pass through the solid adsorbent. The sample to be examined is introduced on top of the column which passes through and distributes between both the stationary and mobile and phases.

The components present in the sample move through the column with the mobile phase at different speeds because of their different relative affinities and interactions. Separate fractions containing individual components in the sample elute from the HPLC column at different rates. The HPLC technique involves the use of a stationary phase (polar or non-polar columns), a pump that moves the mobile phase(s) through the column or other parts of HPLC at constant flow rate, a degasser to remove the trapped gases or air bubbles in the mobile phase, a detector to quantify the analytes and read out device to display the retention times of individual components.

Reversed phase chromatographic mode is most commonly used in HPLC for the identification and quantification of aflatoxins. Chemical derivatization of aflatoxins B1 and G1 typically required to improve the sensitivity because the natural fluorescence of aflatoxins B1 and G1 may be inadequate to meet the necessary detection limit [63]. **Figure 1** depicts derivatization reactions of aflatoxin B1 with the acid and halogens. In the first reaction, Trifluoro Acetic Acid (TFA) hydrolyzes the second furan ring of aflatoxin B1 to produce highly fluorescent aflatoxin B2a, while bromine and iodine are used as chemical reagents in the second and third derivatization reactions, respectively. When these halogens react with aflatoxin B1, they produced highly fluorescent aflatoxin B1 derivatives.

HPLC provides quick, accurate and reliable aflatoxins results within a short time. FLD has been presented an excellent sensitivity of 0.1 ng/kg [65]. However, the shortcoming of using HPLC to analyze the aflatoxins is the requirement of laborious purification columns to clean-up the sample. Furthermore, HPLC involves the tedious pre-column or post-column derivatization processes to improve the sensitivity of aflatoxins [62]. To overcome the challenges of derivatization processes

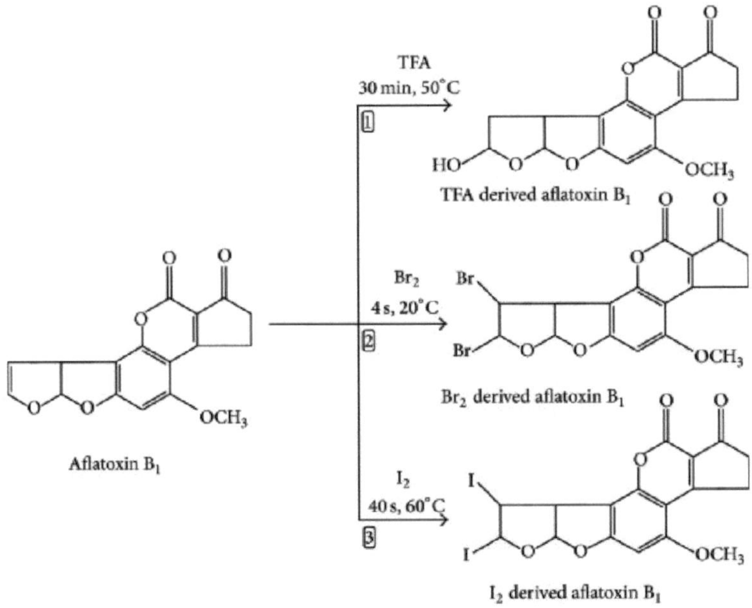


**Figure 1.**
*Derivatization of aflatoxin B1 with trifluoroacetic acid, bromine ($Br_2$) and iodine ($I_2$) [64].*

in aflatoxins testing, a modification of the HPLC protocol in which the HPLC is coupled to mass spectrometry has been developed and is currently used in aflatoxin determination [66].

Since the mass spectrometry does not requires the use of UV/VIS fluorescence or absorbance of analyte, thus chemical derivatization of compounds is no longer required. HPLC–MS/MS produces structural information using small amount of sample and has low detection limits developed up to now [21]. On the other hand, HPLC–MS/MS is costly equipment that can only be handled by trained, qualified and professional person. Furthermore, this also restricts its use to only well-equipped laboratory environment and not field conditions.

### 5.4 Liquid chromatography-mass spectrometry (LC: MS)

Although different HPLC methods are available for quantitative determination of aflatoxins with selective sample clean-up techniques, still the methods are required to confirm the identity of the substances. A method other than the commonly used UV/VIS and fluorescent methods, for the confirmation is mass spectrometry method that coupled with HPLC.

LC–MS technique has become the fastest growing technique available for analysis of mycotoxins. The potential benefits of LC–MS technique for mycotoxin analysis have long been recognized and exploited. Simultaneous determination of multi-mycotoxins can be possible with LC–MS according to the mass to charge ratio (m/z) of analytes, an intrinsic property that provides more specific identification based on molecular weight of the target analyte. The impact of modern LC–MS technique has been signified by the unmatchable sensitivity in quantitation, specificity in identification and number of mycotoxins that could be analyzed in one analysis [67].

A modern LC–MS instrument, particularly LC–MS-triple quadrupole (LC–MS-QQQ), has been developed and introduced with increasing sensitivity for quantitative analysis of mycotoxins. Despite high capital costs of LC–MS instruments, many efforts have been exerted to quantitate aflatoxins using this technique [68].

### 5.5 Gas chromatography (GC)

In gas chromatography, an inert gas is used as the mobile phase instead of liquid and the stationary phase may be a liquid coated onto inert solid particles or solid. GC analysis, like other chromatographic approaches, is based on the differential partitioning of analytes between the two phases. The stationary process is made up of inert particles covered with a liquid layer that confined in a long stainless steel or glass tube known as a column fixed in oven to maintain the specific temperature. The sample to be tested is vaporized into a gaseous form and transported by a carrier gas into the stationary phase.

The different chemical components within the sample will distribute themselves between the stationary phase and mobile phase. Components of the sample mixture with a higher affinity for the stationary phase travel through the column more slowly, while those with a lower affinity move through the column faster. Each portion of the analyte should, in reality, have its own partition coefficient, which will dictate how quickly it passes through the column [69]. After the separation of volatile compounds, these are detected using a universal GC detector known as Flame Ionization Detector (FID) or an Electron Capture Detector (ECD) and the most recent and advanced mass spectrometer (MS) detector [70].

Since aflatoxins are non-volatile, thus derivatization will be required to be detected [71]. However, GC is not commonly used in commercial analysis of aflatoxins because some other cheaper and simple chromatographic techniques are existed [72]. Furthermore, gas chromatography is limited to the analysis of a few mycotoxins, such as A-trichothecenes and B-trichothecenes, due to the requirement of preliminary cleanup step prior to analysis. GC technique has some other disadvantages including drifting responses, non-linearity of calibration curves, memory effects from previous samples, and high variation in repeatability and reproducibility [73].

Earlier, gas chromatography mass spectrometry with negative ion chemical ionization has been used for confirmation of aflatoxin B1 [74], injection was applied using an on-column injector, which is necessary because of the thermos-lability of the aflatoxins. Gas chromatography mass spectrometry have also been used with electron impact for aflatoxins B1, B2, G1 and G2 [75].

## 6. Conclusions

Several qualitative as well as quantitative methods have been explored for analysis of aflatoxins in food commodities, crops and feeds. Among all the different developed methods, chromatographic techniques are considered the most appropriate methods in aflatoxins analysis. Analytical methods based on immunochemistry and spectroscopy have also been added to the chromatographic methods, some of which emerged as better alternatives for routine and on-site estimation of aflatoxins. Although a large number of analytical techniques are constantly being optimized, the LC/MS/MS technique is considered the most valuable confirmation technique for analyzing multiple mycotoxins as it is high specific, sensitive, accurate and reliable.

## Acknowledgements

I would like to thanks the Director, Quality Operations Laboratory (QOL), Institute of Microbiology, University of Veterinary and Animal Sciences (UVAS) and all colleagues for helpful suggestions and support for the preparation of manuscript.

## Conflict of interest

The authors declare that there is no conflict of interests regarding the publication.

## Author details

Mateen Abbas
Quality Operations Laboratory (QOL), Institute of Microbiology, University of Veterinary and Animal Sciences, Lahore, Pakistan

*Address all correspondence to: mateen.abbas@uvas.edu.pk

## References

[1] Evaluation of certain contaminants in food (Eighty-third report of the Joint FAO/WHO Expert Committee on Food Additives). WHO Technical Report Series WHO Technical Report Series, No.1002, 2017.

[2] Bennett JW, Klich M. "Mycotoxins," Clinical Microbiology Reviews. 2003; 16(3): 497-516.

[3] Dors GC, Caldas S, Feddern V. "Aflatoxins: contamination, analysis and control," in Aflatoxins-Biochemistry and Molecular Biology. InTech, Shanghai, China, 2011. 415-438 p.

[4] Gourama H, Bullerman LB. "Detection of molds in foods and feeds: potential rapid and selective methods," Journal of Food Protection. 1995; 58(12): 1389-1394.

[5] Hussein HS, Brasel JM. "Toxicity, metabolism, and impact of mycotoxins on humans and animals," Toxicology. 2001; 167(2): 101-134.

[6] Cullen JM, Newberne PM, Eaton D, Groopman J. "Acute hepatotoxicity of aflatoxins," in The Toxicology of Aflatoxins: Human Health, Veterinary and Agricultural Significance. 1993; 3-26.

[7] Kok WT. "Derivatization reactions for the determination of aflatoxins by liquid chromatography with fluorescence detection," Journal of Chromatography B: Biomedical Sciences and Applications. 1994; 659(1-2): 127-137.

[8] Ayub M, Sachan D. "Dietary factors affecting aflatoxin bi carcinogenicity," Malaysian Journal of Nutrition. 1997; 3: 161-197.

[9] Stroka J, Anklam E. "New strategies for the screening and determination of aflatoxins and the detection of aflatoxin producing moulds in food and feed," TrAC—Trends in Analytical Chemistry. 2002; 21(2): 90-95.

[10] European Union. Commission Regulation (EC) No 1881/2006 of 19 December 2006 setting maximum levels for certain contaminants in foodstuffs. Off. J. Eur. Union 2006, L 364, 5-24.

[11] Romer Labs Division Holding GmbH Erber Campus 13131 Getzersdorf, Austria, https://www.romerlabs.com/en/analytes/mycotoxins/aflatoxin-testing/

[12] Luppa PB, Sokoll LJ, Chan DW. "Immunosensor-principles and applications to clinical chemistry," Clinica Chimica Acta. 2001; 314 (1-2): 1-26.

[13] Charm Sciences, Inc. (Headquarters) 659 Andover Street Lawrence, MA 01843-1032 USA, https://www.charm.com/products/test-and-kits/mycotoxin-tests/

[14] Malone BR, Humphrey CW, Romer TR, Richard JL. "Determination of aflatoxins in grains and raw peanuts by a rapid procedure with fluorometric analysis," Journal of AOAC International. 2000; 83(1): 95-98.

[15] Balzer I, Bogdani´c C, Pepeljnjak S. "Rapid thin layer chromatographic method for determining aflatoxin B1, ochratoxin A, and zearalenone in corn," Journal of the Association of Official Analytical Chemists. 1978; 61(3): 584-585.

[16] Park DL, Trucksess MW, Nesheim S, Stack M, Newell RF. "Solvent-efficient thin-layer chromatographic method for the determination of aflatoxins B1, B2, G1, and G2 in corn and peanut products: collaborative study," Journal of AOAC International. 1994; 77(3): 637-646.

[17] Liang Y, Baker ME, Yeager BT, Denton MB. "Quantitative analysis of aflatoxins by high-performance thin layer chromatography utilizing a scientifically operated charge coupled device detector," Analytical Chemistry. 1996; 68(22): 3885-3891.

[18] Sun P, Chu Y. "A simple solid-phase radioimmunoassay for aflatoxin b1," Journal of Food Safety. 1979; 1: 67-75.

[19] Pearson T, Wicklow D, Maghirang E, Xie F, Dowell F. "Detecting aflatoxin in single corn kernels by transmittance and reflectance spectroscopy," Transactions of the American Society of Agricultural Engineers. 2001; 44(5): 1247-1254.

[20] Omar SS, Moawiya AH, Salvatore P. "Validation of HPLC and Enzyme-Linked Immunosorbent Assay (ELISA) Techniques for Detection and Quantification of Aflatoxins in Different Food Samples", Foods. 2020; 9(661). doi:10.3390/foods9050661

[21] Rahmani A, Jinap S, Soleimany F. "Qualitative and quantitative analysis of mycotoxins," Comprehensive Reviews in Food Science and Food Safety. 2009; 8(3): 202-251.

[22] Kokkonen M, Jestoi M, Rizzo A. "Determination of selected mycotoxins in mould cheeses with liquid chromatography coupled tandem with mass spectrometry," Food Additives and Contaminants. 2005; 22(5): 449-456.

[23] Gaag BV, Spath S, Dietrich H. "Biosensors and multiple mycotoxin analysis," Food Control. 2003; 14(4): 251-254.

[24] Liron Z, Tender LM, Golden JP, Ligler FS. "Voltage induced inhibition of antigen-antibody binding at conducting optical waveguides," Biosensors and Bioelectronics. 2002; 17(6-7): 489-494.

[25] Yu H, Eggleston CM, Chen J, Wang W, Dai Q, Tang J. "Optical waveguide lightmode spectroscopy (OWLS) as a sensor for thin film and quantum dot corrosion," Sensors. 2012; 12(12): 17330-17342.

[26] Masoomi L, Sadeghi O, Banitaba MH, Shahrjerdi A, Davarani SSH. "A non-enzymatic nanomagnetic electroimmunosensor for determination of Aflatoxin B1 as a model antigen," Sensors and Actuators B: Chemical. 2013; 177: 1122-1127.

[27] Linting Z, Ruiyi L, Zaijun L, Qianfang X, Yinjun F, Junkang L. "An immunosensor for ultrasensitive detection of aflatoxin B1 with an enhanced electrochemical performance based on graphene/conducting polymer/gold nanoparticles/the ionic liquid composite film on modified gold electrode with electrodeposition," Sensors and Actuators B: Chemical. 2012; 174: 359-365.

[28] Whitaker TB, Dickens JW, Monroe RJ. Variability of aflatoxin test results. J Am Oil Chem Soc. 1974; 51: 214-218.

[29] Horwitz W, Albert R. The reliability of aflatoxin assay. Assoc Food Drug Officials Q Bull. 1982; 46: 14-24.

[30] Coker RD. Control of aflatoxin in groundnut products with emphasis on sampling, analysis and detoxification. In: McDonald D, Mehan VK, eds. Aflatoxin contamination of groundnut: Proceedings of the International Workshop. Patancheru, India: International Crops Research Institute for the Semi-Arid Tropics, 1989:124-132.

[31] Coker RD. Design of sampling plans for determination of mycotoxins in foods and feeds. In: Sinha KK, Bhatnagar D, eds. Mycotoxins in agricultural and food safety. New York: Marcel Dekker, 1998:109-133.

[32] Coker RD, Jones BD, Nagler MJ, Gilman GA, Wallbridge AJ, Panigrahi S. Mycotoxin training manual. London: Tropical Development and Research Institute, 1984.

[33] Coker RD. High performance liquid chromatography and other chemical quantification methods used in analysis of mycotoxins in foods. In: Gilbert J, ed. Analysis of food contaminants. London: Elsevier, 1984: 207-263 p.

[34] Bertuzzi T, Rastelli S, Mulazzi A, Pietri A. "Evaluation and improvement of extraction methods for the analysis of aflatoxins B1, B2, G1 and G2 from naturally contaminated maize," Food Analytical Methods. 2012; 5(3): 512-519.

[35] Taylor SL, King JW, Richard JL, Greer JI. "Analyticalscale supercritical fluid extraction of aflatoxin b1 from fieldinoculated corn," Journal of Agricultural and Food Chemistry. 1993; 41(6): 910-913.

[36] Stroka J, Petz M, Joerissen U, Anklam E. "Investigation of various extractants for the analysis of aflatoxin B1 in different food and feed matrices," Food Additives and Contaminants.1999; 16(8): 331-338.

[37] Arranz I, Sizoo E, Van Egmond H. "Determination of aflatoxin B1 in medical herbs: interlaboratory study," Journal of AOAC International. 2006; 89(3): 595-605.

[38] Gallo A, Masoero F, Bertuzzi T, Piva G, Pietri A. "Effect of the inclusion of adsorbents on aflatoxin B-1 quantification in animal feedstuffs," Food Additives and Contaminants—Part A Chemistry, Analysis, Control, Exposure and Risk Assessment. 2010; 27(1): 54-63.

[39] Lee NA, Wang S, Allan RD, Kennedy IR. "A rapid aflatoxin B1 Elisa: development and validation with reduced matrix effects for peanuts, corn, pistachio, and soybeans," Journal of Agricultural and Food Chemistry. 2004; 52(10): 2746-2755.

[40] Sheibani A, Ghaziaskar HS. Pressurized fluid extraction for quantitative recovery of aflatoxins B1 and B2 from pistachio. Food Contr. 2009; 20: 124-128. doi: 10.1016/j.foodcont.2008.03.001

[41] Kong WJ, Liu SY, Qiu F, Xiao XH, Yang MH. Simultaneous multi-mycotoxin determination in nutmeg by ultrasound-assisted solid liquid extraction and immunoaffinity column clean-up coupled with liquid chromatography and on-line post-column photochemical derivatization fluorescence detection. Analyst. 2013; 7: 2729-2739. doi: 10.1039/c3an00059a

[42] Xie L, Chen M, Ying Y. Development of methods for determination of aflatoxins. Food Sci. Nutr. 2016; 56: 2642-2664. doi: 10.1080/10408398.2014. 907234

[43] Anklam E, Berg H, Matthiasson L, Sharman M, Ulberth F. Supercritical fluid extraction (SFE) in food analysis: a review. Food Addit. Contam. 1998; 15: 729-750. doi: 10.1080/02652039809374703

[44] Shephard GS. Aflatoxin analysis at the beginning of the twenty-first century. Anal. Bioanal. Chem. 2009; 395: 1215-1224. doi: 10.1007/s00216-009-2857-y

[45] Yao H, Hruska Z, Diana D, Mavungu J. Developments in detection and determination of aflatoxins. World Mycotoxin J. 2015; 8: 181-191.

[46] Tang YY, Lin YH, Chen CY, Su TW, Wang CS, Chiueh CL. Development of a quantitative multi-mycotoxin method in rice, maize, wheat and peanut using UPLC-MS/MS. Food Anal. Meth. 2013; 6: 727-736. doi: 10.1007/s12161-012-9473-8

[47] Ma F, Chen R, Li P, Zhang Q, Zhang W, Hu W. "Preparation of an immunoaffinity column with amino-silica gel microparticles and its application in sample cleanup for aflatoxin detection in agri-products," Molecules. 2013; 18(2): 2222-2235.

[48] Scott PM, Trucksess MW. "Application of immunoaffinity columns tomycotoxin analysis," Journal of AOAC International. 1997; 80(5): 941-949.

[49] Shelver WL, Larsen GL, Huwe JK. "Use of an immunoaffinity column for tetrachlorodibenzo-p-dioxin serum sample cleanup," Journal of Chromatography B: Biomedical Applications. 1998; 705(2): 261-268.

[50] Wilson TJ, Romer TR. Use of the Mycosep multifunctional cleanup column for liquid chromatographic determination of aflatoxins in agricultural products. J Assoc Off Anal Chem. 1991; 74(6): 951-956.

[51] Sapsford KE, Taitt CR, Fertig S. "Indirect competitive immunoassay for detection of aflatoxin B1 in corn and nut products using the array biosensor," Biosensors and Bioelectronics. 200; 21(12): 2298-2305.

[52] Betina V, "Thin-layer chromatography of mycotoxins," Journal of Chromatography. 1985; 334(3); 211-276.

[53] Gulyas H. "Determination of aflatoxins b1, b2, g1, g2 and m1 by high pressure thin layer chromatography," Journal of Chromatography A. 1985; 319: 105-111.

[54] Abdel-Gawad KM, Zohri AA. "Fungal flora and mycotoxins of six kinds of nut seeds for human consumption in Saudi Arabia," Mycopathologia,. 1993; 124(1): 55-64.

[55] Younis YMH, Malik KM. "Tlc and hplc analysis of aflatoxin contamination in sudanese peanut and peanut products," Kuwait Journal of Science and Engineering. 2003;30(1): 2003.

[56] Trucksess M, Brumley W, Nesheim S. "Rapid quantitation and confirmation of aflatoxins in corn and peanut butter, using a disposable silica gel column, thin layer chromatography, and gas chromatography/mass spectromety," Journal of the Association of Official Analytical Chemists. 1984; 67(5): 973-975.

[57] Papp E, H-Otta K, Z´aray G, Mincsovics E. "Liquid chromatographic determination of aflatoxins," Microchemical Journal. 2002; 73 (1-2): 39-46.

[58] Pons WA Jr, Goldblatt LA. Instrumental evaluation of aflatoxin resolution on TLC plates. J Assoc Off Anal Chem. 1968; 51: 1194-1197.

[59] Mehan VK. Analytical and immuno-chemical methods for the analysis of aflatoxins in groundnuts and groundnut products. In: Mehan VK, Gowda CLL, eds. Aflatoxin contamination problems in groundnut in Asia. Proceedings of the First Asia Working Group Meeting. Patancheru, India: International Crops Research Institute for the Semi-Arid Tropics. 1997; 49-65.

[60] Ramesh J, Sarathchandra G, Sureshkumar V. "Analysis of feed samples for aflatoxin b1 contamination by hptlc-a validated method," International Journal of Current Microbiology and Applied Sciences. 2013; 2: 373-377.

[61] Nawaz S, Coker RD, Haswell SJ. "Development and evaluation of analytical methodology for the determination of aflatoxins in palm kernels," Analyst. 1992; 117(1): 67-74.

[62] Li P, Zhang Q, Zhang D. "Aflatoxin measurement and analysis," in Aflatoxins—Detection, Measurement

and Control, I. Torres-Pacheco, Ed., Intech, Shanghai, China. 2011. 183-208 p.

[63] Kok WT, Van Neer TCH, Traag WA, Tuinstra LGT. "Determination of aflatoxins in cattle feed by liquid chromatography and post-column derivatization with electrochemically generated bromine," Journal of Chromatography A. 1986; 367: 231-236.

[64] Kok WT. "Derivatization reactions for the determination of aflatoxins by liquid chromatography with fluorescence detection," Journal of Chromatography B: Biomedical Sciences and Applications. 194; 659(1-2): 127-137.

[65] Herzallah SM. "Determination of aflatoxins in eggs, milk, meat and meat products using HPLC fluorescent and UV detectors," Food Chemistry. 2009; 114(3): 1141-1146.

[66] Takino M and Tanaka T. Determination of Aflatoxins in Food by LC-MS/MS, Agilent Technologies, 2008.

[67] Di Stefano V, Avellone G, Bongiorno D, Cunsolo V, Muccilli V, Sforza S, Dossena A, Drahos L, Vékey K. Applications of liquid chromatography—Mass spectrometry for food analysis. J. Chromatogr. A 2012; 1259: 74-85.

[68] Sforza, S, Dall'Asta C, Marchelli R. Recent advances in mycotoxin determination in food and feed by hyphenated chromatographic techniques/mass spectrometry. Mass Spectrom. Rev. 2005; 25: 54-76.

[69] Boyer RF. Modern Experimental Biochemistry, Benjamin/Cummings Publishing Company, 1993.

[70] Pascale MN. "Detection methods for mycotoxins in cereal grains and cereal products," Matica Srpska Proceedings for Natural Sciences, 2009. vol. 117, 15-25 p.

[71] Scott P. "Mycotoxin methodology," Food Additives & Contaminants, 1995. vol. 12, no. 3, 395-403 p.

[72] Liang Y, Zhang C, and Liu L. "Chromatographic analysis of mycotoxins," ZhongguoWeisheng Jianyan Zazhi; 2005. vol. 15, 1273 p.

[73] Petterson H and Langseth W. "Intercomparison of trichothecenes analysis and feasibility to produce certified calibrants," EU Reports EUR 20285, European Commission BCR Information Project, 2002.

[74] Trucksess MW, Brumley WC and Nesheim S. Rapid quantitation and confirmation of aflatoxins in com and peanut butter, using a disposable silica gel column, thin layer chromatography, and gas chromatography/mass spectrometry. J. Assoc. Off Anal. Chem., 1984; 67: 973-975.

[75] Goto T, Matsui M and Kitsuwa T. Analysis of Aspergillus mycotoxins by gas chromatography using fused silica capillary column. Maikotokishin. 1990; 31: 43-47.

Chapter 11

# Determination of Aflatoxins by Liquid Chromatography Coupled to High-Resolution Mass Spectrometry

*Natalia Arroyo-Manzanares, Natalia Campillo, Ignacio López-García and Pilar Viñas*

## Abstract

The most common mycotoxins are aflatoxins (AFs), which are produced by strains of various species of molds in the genus Aspergillus (*A. flavus, A. parasiticus, A. nomius and A. tamarii*) and can grow on many foods, mainly peanuts, maize and cottonseed. AFs are currently considered to be the most hazardous mycotoxins to health, in particular because of their hepatocellular carcinogenic potential. The main aflatoxins are B1 (AFB1), B2 (AFB2), G1 (AFG1) and G2 (AFG2) although many other derivatives have been described. In addition, animals consuming contaminated feeds are able to metabolize them by hydroxylation in a certain position, yield for example aflatoxin M1 (AFM1) and aflatoxin M2 (AFM2) from AFB1 and AFB2, respectively. Nowadays, only the four main AFs and one hydroxylated metabolite (AFM1) are routinely analyzed. High resolution mass spectrometry (HRMS) using Orbitrap or time-of-flight (TOF) mass analysers is a trend for AFs determination, allowing to determine AFs and their derivatives for which there are no commercial standards available, in order to carry out metabolization studies, exposure assessment or monitoring modified AFs in food. The aim of this study is to show the recent trends in analytical methods based on LC-HRMS for determination of AFs.

**Keywords:** aflatoxins, high resolution mass spectrometry, liquid chromatography, biological samples, foods

## 1. Introduction

Aflatoxins (AFs) are highly toxic secondary metabolites produced by fungi belonging to several *Aspergillus* species, mainly found in hot and humid climates [1]. Currently, more than 15 different types of AFs have been identified; the naturally occurring are aflatoxin B1 (AFB1), B2 (AFB2), G1 (AFG1) and G2 (AFG2). *Aspergillus flavus* colonizes mostly the aerial parts of plants (leaves, flowers) producing B AFs, while *Aspergillus parasiticus* produces B and G AFs, being more adapted to soil environments [2]. The structures of the main AFs and their derivatives are shown in **Figure 1**.

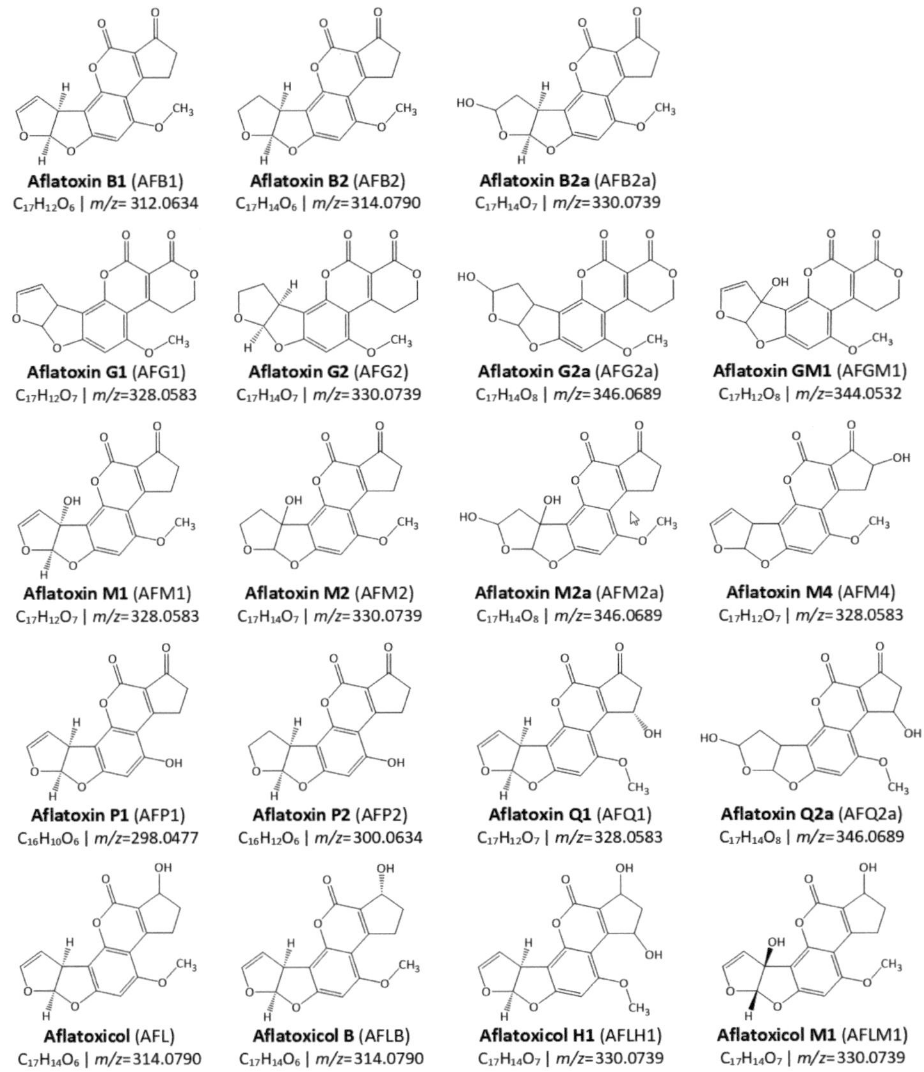


**Figure 1.**
*Chemical structure of the most important AFs and their derivatives.*

Raw materials usually used for human food and animal feed are contaminated by this type of fungi and their metabolites. Cereals (maize, wheat, rice, barley, soy, etc.), dried fruits, nuts, coffee and other foods could be contaminated during plant growth or postharvest, depending on different factors such as temperature, humidity, water activity, concurrent mycobiota, physical damage, and other storage conditions [2]. AFs are very stable and may resist cooking processes, resulting a problem in processed foods. Human exposure to AFs can result directly from ingestion of contaminated foods, or indirectly from consumption of animal foods previously exposed to contaminated feeds. AFs have a great risk for human health, especially by their carcinogenic potential [3]. Degradation or enzymatic transformation of mycotoxins led to the appearance of modified mycotoxins, usually lesser toxic than the parent compounds. Thus, aflatoxin M1 (AFM1) is formed from the hydroxylation of AFB1 and eliminated in the milk of animals that consumed feed contaminated with this mycotoxin [4].

Therefore, it is important to develop reliable methods for the determination of AFs and their derivatives in foods and feeds, as well as toxicokinetic and toxicodynamic studies for assessment of human or animal exposure. The target and non-target qualitative and quantitative analysis using high resolution mass spectrometry (HRMS) instruments, such as time-of-flight (TOF) and Orbitrap, brings great challenges for screening of AFs [5]. Main advantages include high sensitivity, accurate mass measurement, and retrospective data analysis, allowing both the target determination of AFs and the non-targeted screening of modified AFs or unknown metabolites.

## 2. Toxicity of aflatoxins

AFs are potent carcinogenic, mutagenic, teratogenic, and immunosuppressive agents. Their carcinogenicity has mainly been associated with liver and kidney, although the effect of AFs has also been reported in pancreas, bladder, bone, viscera or central nervous by some epidemiological and animal studies [6]. Their inhalation and direct contact could also cause lung and skin [7, 8] occupational cancers, respectively. In addition, feeds contaminated by AFs can involve high susceptibility to diseases, low productivity and low reproductive performance in animals [9].

Among AFs, AFB1 is considered the highest risk. The Scientific Committee on Food has established that AFs are genotoxic carcinogens [10, 11], being the order of toxicity as follows: AFB1 > AFG1 > AFB2 > AFG2. Indeed, AFB1 has been shown to be carcinogenic in all experimental animals and has been classified since 1988 by the World Health Organization (WHO) as a human carcinogen. Consequently, the International Agency for Research on Cancer (IARC) [12] has classified AFB1 within the category of Group 1 substances based on the existence of sufficient evidence about its carcinogenicity to humans, both alone and in natural mixtures with the other AFs [13, 14].

The most common route of entry of AFs into the human body is the ingestion. In the case of AFB1, the best studied aflatoxin, is absorbed in the gastrointestinal tract, due to its liposolubility, and transported by red blood cells and plasma proteins to the liver. In the liver, it is metabolized producing intermediate metabolites that have been related with the toxic and carcinogenic effects of AFs [15]. Specifically, AFB1 is biotransformed in the liver by microsomal enzymes of the cytochrome superfamily P450. Microsomal biotransformation can result in the hydrolyzation of aflatoxin B1, producing less toxic metabolites such as AFM1, aflatoxin Q1 (AFQ1), aflatoxin P1 (AFP1) and aflatoxin B2a (AFB2a). In addition, AFB1 can produce aflatoxicol (AFL) via NADPH reductase. The formation of these compounds is considered a detoxification process although the protein binding of some of them can lead to additional toxicities [16]. They are excreted in urine and feces, although AFM1 is also commonly detected in breast milk.

The action of CYP450 enzymes can also metabolize AFB1 resulting in the appearance of a reactive intermediate metabolite, AFB1–8,9-epoxide (AFBO), which has two isomers (*endo*-8,9-epoxide and *exo*-8,9-epoxide). AFBO can be detoxified by glutathione S-transferase (GST) action, yield the adduct AFB1-glutathione (AFB1-GSH), that is eventually excreted as AFB1-mercapturic acid in the urine [17]. The formation of AFB-mercapturic acid is catalyzed by γ-glutamyltransferase (GGT), dipeptidase (DPEP), and N-acetyltransferase (NAT) [16]. However, due to its high electrophilic nature, AFBO can form covalent bonds with diverse macromolecules, such as nucleic acids and proteins. The protein binding is responsible for AFB1 toxicity, giving rise to adduct AFB1-lysine (AFB1-lys) with serum albumin. AFBO can also undergo rapid non-enzymatic hydrolysis to AFB1–8,9-dihydrodiol, which is in equilibrium with AFB1-dialdehyde. AFB1-dialdehyde can protein bind or be detoxified by the action of AF aldehyde reductase (AFAR) via conversion to the dialcohol [18].

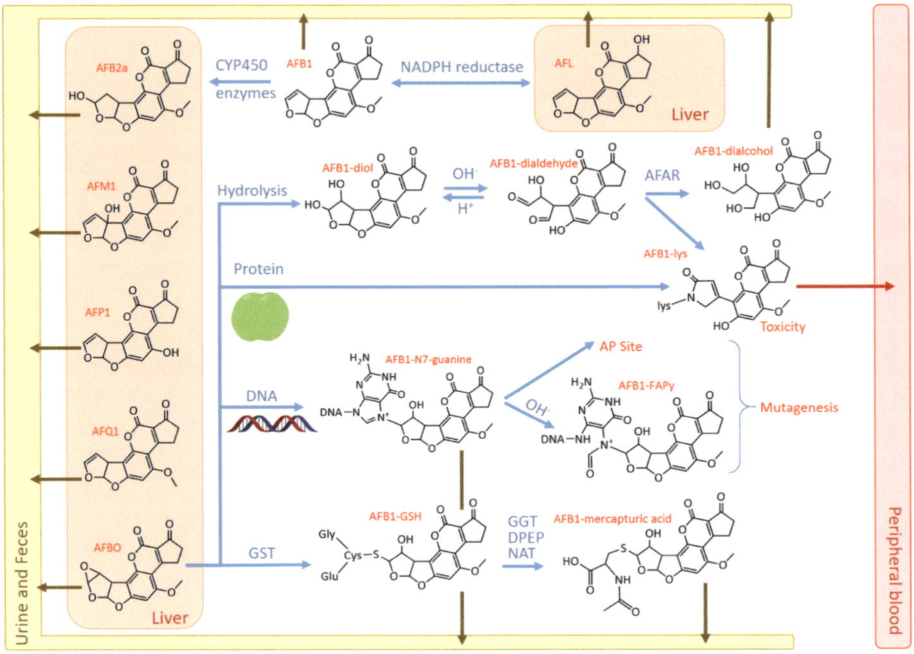


**Figure 2.**
*Metabolic pathway of AFB1.*

The interaction AFB1-DNA causes AFB1-N7-guanine adduct, which is chemically unstable and undergoes rapid urinary excretion resulting in an aputinic (AP) site on the DNA backbone [16]. Alternatively, the adduct AFB-N7-guanine may be stabilized by rearranging to a ring-opened formamidopyramidine structure (AFB1-FAPy) [17]. Both AP and AFB1-FAPy can produce mutagenesis. **Figure 2** summarizes the action mechanism of AFB1.

From the action mechanism of AFB1 it can be deduced that AFB1-lys, AFB1-N7-guanine, AFB1-mercapturic acid or the hydroxylated forms (AFM1, AFQ1, AFP1, AFL and AFB2a) could be effective biomarkers for assessing AF exposure.

Due to the high lesions produced by AFs, especially cancer, the European Union has established maximum permitted levels of these contaminants in various foods through Regulation No. 1881/2006 [19]. Specifically, the maximum contents for AFB1, AFB2, AFG1, AFG2 and AFM1 in nuts, cereals, milk and baby foods are included in this regulation the maximum contents are between 4 and 15 μg $kg^{-1}$.

In the field of animal nutrition, the specifications regarding the presence of mycotoxins in feed are reflected in Directive 2002/32/EC [20]. Only AFB1 has been legislated. The maximum levels ranged between 5 and 50 μg $kg^{-1}$. The lower limit was set for feed intended for milk-producing animals (5 μg $kg^{-1}$).

## 3. Applications of HRMS for determination of aflatoxins

### 3.1 HRMS: a useful tool for aflatoxins determination

Liquid chromatography (LC)-HRMS is a powerful tool for metabolomic approaches, allowing simultaneous quantitative and qualitative analysis of a wide variety of mycotoxins, as well as the search of related metabolites derived from mycotoxin biotransformation or degradation, enabling the detection and identification of unknown compounds. In addition, HRMS offers the ability to work in various modes, such as target analysis and non-target screening, or retrospective analysis. The relative incompatibility of HRMS ion sources with the continuous liquid flow of LC limited the progress of LC-HRMS coupling for years, but the development of interfaces such as electrospray ionization (ESI) and atmospheric pressure chemical ionization (APCI), where LC effluent is de-solvated, has allowed the proposal of a high number of LC-HRMS methods. Thus, complex mixtures can be separated in the chromatographic system and their components are unequivocally detected by HRMS with high sensitivity.

For AFs determination, quadrupole (Q)-TOF, Orbitrap and its hybrid Q-Orbitrap are the mass analysers most widely used. Comparing both instruments, Orbitrap shows better resolution and accuracy (Q-TOF: 60,000 full width at half maximum (FWHM) and between 1 and 10 ppm; Orbitrap: 240,000 FWHM and less than 1 ppm), and a greater range of *m/z* (Q-TOF: <4000 and Orbitrap: <6000), although this is not important for the aflatoxin determination, since the expected masses are around 300–350 Da and both mass spectrometers cover this range. However, Q-TOF instruments have shown to have a greater linear dynamic range (Q-TOF: $>10^5$ and Orbitrap: $>10^4$) [21]. Multiclass mycotoxin (including the main AFs) methods based on the hybrid ion trap (IT)-Orbitrap have also been developed and validated [22, 23]. In addition, AFB1 has also been monitored by TOF [24, 25].

ESI or its variant heated ESI (HESI) working in positive mode are the best options for AF determination. Although it should be noted that many of the methods described in this chapter are multiclass methods, i.e., they determine a greater number of mycotoxins, not just AFs, and in this case, authors usually prefer two independent runs using both positive and negative polarities.

Regarding LC instruments, ultra-high-performance LC (UHPLC) is normally coupled to HRMS. Although NanoLC coupled to Q-Orbitrap for the determination of AFB1-lys in human plasma [26] and high performance LC (HPLC)-TOF for the determination of AFB1 in beer [24] have also been proposed. In addition, Qi et al. used a multiple heart-cutting two-dimensional liquid chromatography (Heart-cutting 2D-LC) coupled to Q-Orbitrap for simultaneous determination of AFs and ochratoxin A in snus [27]. The utilization of Heart-cutting 2D-LC enables to reduce matrix effect, leading to better precision of the AF contents. The mobile phase is normally a mixture of water and methanol (MeOH) or acetonitrile (ACN). Formic acid (FA), acetic acid (AA), ammonium formate or ammonium acetate are used as additives. The stationary phase was mainly $C_{18}$ although $C_8$ has been also proposed [28]. Slobodchikova et al. [22] also used a pentafluorophenyl (PFP) column whereas Qi et al. [27] combined both $C_{18}$ and PFP columns in the Heart-cutting 2D-LC system.

The analysis of biological samples focused on the monitoring of the four most important AFs (AFB1, AFB2, AFG1 and AFG2), although their adducts due to the interaction of AFB1 with proteins or DNA, AFB1-N7-guanine and AFB1-lys, respectively, as well as its hydrolysed derivative AFM1 have also been determined. In food samples, besides the four main AFs, some metabolites such as AFM1, AFM2, or AFL were also detected.

Both data dependent (dd-$MS^2$) and data independent (DIA) acquisition have been proposed. For the analysis of biological samples, Full MS combined with dd-$MS^2$ by inclusion of a list of accurate masses of target or suspect compounds was more frequent. Although, Ogawa et al. [29] also proposed a dd-$MS^2$ by fixing an ion intensity threshold. Regarding food analysis, authors normally prefer Full MS and DIA, specifically, all-ion fragmentation (AIF) mode, where no precursor ion isolation is carried out. Other modes such as simple Full MS, selected ion monitoring (SIM) or parallel reaction monitoring mode (PRM) have also been investigated. Renaud et al. [30] compared three acquisition modes: dd-$MS^2$ with inclusion list,

AIF and AIF using targeted high energy collision dissociation (HCD) events across a mass range for MS/MS. Good linearity was achieved by AIF with different HCD events at low concentrations, demonstrating that the limits of detection (LODs) are much higher without a Q mass filtering. The potential of AIF with different HCD events has also been studied for the determination of five AFs in nutraceutical obtained from green tea [31].

Most authors who carried out a non-targeted acquisition opted for target processing, in order to quantify and/or confirm AFs. Only Jia et al. [31] carried out a non-targeted processing consisting of: non-target fourier peak picking, (ii) spectra automated componentization, (iii) suspicion spectral library searching, and (iv) marked fragments filtering. Finally, compounds were confirmed with reference standard. In addition, Castaldo et al. [32] and Renaud et al. [30] carried out a non-targeted processing using spectral library for the tentative identification of other fungal metabolites, although they processed AFs following a targeted approach.

**Table 1** summarizes the separation and detection condition of HRMS methods for AF monitorization.

| AF studied | Matrix | Instrument | LC conditions | Acquisition | Ref. |
|---|---|---|---|---|---|
| AFB1, AFB2, AFG1, AFG2, AFM1 | Breast milk | UHPLC–Orbitrap HESI + | Hypersil GOLD $C_{18}$ (100 × 2.1 mm, 1.9 µm) $H_2O$/MeOH with FA and $HCOONH_4$ | Full MS (*m/z* 100-1000) | [33] |
| AFB1, AFB2, AFG1, AFG2 | Isoflavone supplements | UHPLC-Orbitrap HESI + | Hypersil Gold $C_{18}$ (100 × 2.1 mm, 1.9 µm) $H_2O$/MeOH with FA and $HCOONH_4$ | Full MS (*m/z* 100-1000) and AIF (*m/z* 65-700) | [34] |
| AFB1, AFB2, AFG1, AFG2 | Ginkgo biloba supplements | UHPLC-Orbitrap HESI + | Hypersil Gold $C_{18}$ (100 × 2.1 mm, 1.9 µm) $H_2O$/MeOH with FA and $HCOONH_4$ | Full MS and AIF (*m/z* 100-1000) | [35] |
| AFB1, AFB2, AFG1, AFG2 | Green tea and royal jelly supplements | UHPLC-Orbitrap HESI + | Hypersil Gold $C_{18}$ (100 × 2.1 mm, 1.9 µm) $H_2O$/MeOH with FA and $HCOONH_4$ | Full MS and AIF (*m/z* 100-1000) | [36] |
| AFB1, AFB2, AFG1, AFG2, AFM1, AFL | Coix seed | UHPLC-Orbitrap HESI + | $C_{18}$ (100 × 2.1 mm, 1.6 µm) $H_2O$/MeOH with FA and $CH_3COONH_4$ | Full MS (*m/z* 100-800) | [37] |
| AFB1, AFB2, AFG1, AFG2 | Feed | UHPLC-Orbitrap HESI + | Hypersil Gold $C_{18}$ (100 × 2.1mm,1.9 µm) $H_2O$/MeOH/ACN with AA | Full MS and AIF (*m/z* 55-1000) | [38] |
| AFB1, AFB1-lys | Human serum | UHPLC-Q-Orbitrap HESI + | $C_{18}$ (100 × 2.1 mm, 1.7 µm) $H_2O$/MeOH with FA and $HCOONH_4$ | Full MS (*m/z* 100-700) and dd-$MS^2$ (list dependent) | [39] |
| AFB1, AFM1, AFB1-N7-guanine | Human urine | UHPLC-Q-Orbitrap HESI + | Acquity BEH $C_{18}$ (100 × 2.1 mm, 1.7 µm) $H_2O$/MeOH with FA and $HCOONH_4$ | Full MS (no range) and dd-$MS^2$ (list dependent) | [40] |

| AF studied | Matrix | Instrument | LC conditions | Acquisition | Ref. |
|---|---|---|---|---|---|
| AFB1, AFM1 | Milk | UHPLC-Q-Orbitrap HESI + | Luna Omega $C_{18}$ (50 × 2.1 mm, 1.6 μm) $H_2O$/MeOH with FA and $HCOONH_4$ | Full MS and AIF (*m/z* 100-1000) | [41] |
| AFB1, AFB2, AFG1, AFG2, AFM1, AFM2 | Milk | UHPLC-Q-Orbitrap HESI + | Accucore $C_{18}$ (150 x 2.1 mm, 2.6 μm) $H_2O$/ACN with FA and $CH_3COONH_4$ | Full MS (*m/z* 50-1000) and dd-$MS^2$ (list dependent) | [42] |
| AFB1, AFG1, AFG2 | Maize | UHPLC-Q-Orbitrap HESI + | Zorbax Eclipse Plus RRHD $C_{18}$ column (50 × 2.1 mm, 1.8 μm) | Full MS, dd-$MS^2$ (list dependent), AIF and AIF with HCD events | [30] |
| AFB1, AFB2, AFG1, AFG2 | Cashew nut | UHPLC-Q-Orbitrap HESI + | HSS T3 (100 x 2.1 mm, 1.8 μm) $H_2O$/MeOH with FA and $HCOONH_4$ | PRM | [43] |
| AFB1, AFB2, AFG1, AFG2 | Cereals | UHPLC-Q-Orbitrap HESI + | Kinetex $C_{18}$ (50 × 3 mm, 1.7 μm $H_2O$/MeOH with AA and $CH_3COONH_4$ | Full MS and AIF (*m/z* 50-1000) | [44] |
| AFB1 | Durum wheat pasta and baby food pasta | UHPLC-Q-Orbitrap HESI + | Accucore $C_{18}$ (100 × 2.1 mm 2.6 μm) $H_2O$/MeOH with FA and $HCOONH_4$ | Full MS (*m/z* 90-1000) | [45] |
| AFB1, AFB2, AFG1, AFG2, AFM1 | Green tea supplements | UHPLC-Q-Orbitrap HESI + | Hypersil Gold $C_{18}$ (100 × 2.1 mm, 1.9 μm) $H_2O$/MeOH with FA and $HCOONH_4$ | Full MS (*m/z* 100-800), AIF, and AIF with HCD events | [31] |
| AFB1, AFB2, AFG1, AFG2 | Medicinal herbs | UHPLC-Q-Orbitrap HESI + | Kinetex $C_{18}$ column (100 × 2.1 mm, 1.7 μm) $H_2O$/MeOH with FA | SIM | [46] |
| AFB1, AFB2, AFG1, AFG2 | Pet foods | UHPLC-Q-Orbitrap HESI + | Luna Omega $C_{18}$ (50 × 2.1 mm, 1.6 μm) $H_2O$/MeOH with FA and $HCOONH_4$ | Full MS and AIF (*m/z* 100-1000) | [32] |
| AFB1, AFB2, AFG1, AFG2 | Waters | UHPLC-Q-Orbitrap HESI + | $C_{18}$ (125 × 2 mm, 5 μm) $H_2O$/ ACN with FA | Full MS (no data) and dd-$MS^2$ (list dependent) | [47] |
| AFB1-lys | Human plasma | NanoLC–Q-Orbitrap HESI + | Acclaim $C_{18}$ (15 cm, 75 μm) $H_2O$/ACN with FA | Full MS (*m/z* 50-900) and PRM | [26] |
| AFB1, AFB2, AFG1, AFG2 | Snus | Heart-cutting 2D-LC-Q-Orbitrap HESI + | Hypersil Gold $C_{18}$ (100 × 0.5 mm, 3 μm) and ACQUITY HSS PFP (100 × 2.1 mm, 1.7 μm) $H_2O$/MeOH/ACN with FA and $HCOONH_4$ | PRM | [27] |
| AFB1, AFB2, AFG1, AFG2 | Human plasma | UHPLC–IT-Orbitrap HESI + | PFP (50 × 2.1 mm, 2.6 μm) $H_2O$/MeOH with AA | Full MS (*m/z* 280-500) | [22] |

| AF studied | Matrix | Instrument | LC conditions | Acquisition | Ref. |
|---|---|---|---|---|---|
| AFB1, AFB2, AFG1, AFG2 | Beer | UHPLC-IT-Orbitrap HESI + | Gemini $C_{18}$ (150 × 2 mm, 5 μm) $H_2O$/MeOH with FA and $HCOONH_4$ | Full MS (*m/z* 90-900) and dd-$MS^2$ (list dependent) | [23] |
| AFB1 | Beer | HPLC-TOF ESI + | Kinetex $C_{18}$ (50 × 3 mm, 1.7 μm) $H_2O$/MeOH with FA and $CH_3COONH_4$ | Full MS (*m/z* 50-1000) | [24] |
| AFB1 | Beer | UHPLC-TOF ESI + | Kinetex $C_{18}$ (50 × 3 mm, 1.7 μm) $H_2O$/ACN with FA and $CH_3COONH_4$ | Full MS (*m/z* 50-1000) | [25] |
| AFB1, AFB2, AFG1, AFG2 | Human plasma | UHPLC–Q-TOF ESI + | ODS $C_{18}$ (150 × 1.5 mm, 5.0 μm) $H_2O$/MeOH with $HCOONH_4$ | Full MS (no data) and dd-$MS^2$ (Ion intensity-dependent) | [29] |
| AFB1-lys | Human serum | UHPLC-Q-TOF ESI + | Acquity BEH $C_{18}$ (50 × 2.1 mm, 1.7 μm) $H_2O$/ACN with FA | Full MS (*m/z* 280-650) and dd-$MS^2$ (list dependent) | [48] |
| AFB1, AFM1 | Plasma, urine, feces (pig, broiler) | UHPLC-Q-TOF ESI + | Acquity HSS T3 $C_{18}$ (100 × 2.1 mm, 1.8 μm) $H_2O$/MeOH with FA and $HCOONH_4$ | Full MS and AIF (mass range *m/z* 50-1200) | [49] |
| AFB1 | Seeds, milk, flour, beer | UHPLC-Q-TOF ESI + | Eclipse Plus $C_8$ RRHD (50 × 2.1 mm, 1.8 μm) $H_2O$/ACN with FA | No data | [28] |
| AFB1, AFB2, AFG1, AFG2 | Corn | UHPLC-Q-TOF ESI + | Hypersil Gold $C_{18}$ (100 × 2.1mm, 1.9 μm) $H_2O$/MeOH with FA and $CH_3COONH_4$ | Full MS (*m/z* 100-1000) | [50] |

**Table 1.**
*Summary of LC-HRMS condition for AF determination.*

## 3.2 HRMS applications for food analysis

AFs can grow on many foods, mainly peanuts, maize and cottonseed, although they have also been found in all types of nuts, copra, cereals, sunflower and soya beans, unrefined vegetable oils, spices, dried fruits, coffee, cocoa and animal feed [1, 16].

**Milk** is the most consumed beverage in the world, and it is the primary source of nourishment for the normal growth of infants and children. The maximum permissible level of AFM1 in milk is set at 0.5 μg $kg^{-1}$ in China and USA, and 0.05 μg $kg^{-1}$ in Europe. Zhao et al. [42] proposed the determination of AFB1, AFB2, AFG1, AFG2, AFM1, AFM2 and other mycotoxins in liquid milk using UHPLC-Q-Orbitrap. Limits of quantification (LOQs) were in the range of 0.015–0.150 μg $kg^{-1}$. AFM1 was detected in four samples in a range from 0.026 to 0.039 μg $kg^{-1}$. Rodríguez-Carrasco et al. [41] proposed to study the contamination of milk with AFM1 and its parent compound, AFB1, using also UHPLC-Q-Orbitrap. In this case, LOQs were 0.001 and 0.002 μg $L^{-1}$ for AFM1 and AFB1, respectively. The validated method was applied to 40 Italian milk samples and neither AFB1 nor AFM1 were found above the LOD in any of the analyzed samples.

Because occurrence of mycotoxins in **cereals** has been object of health concern worldwide for long time, numerous analytical methods for control of their presence have been developed. Vaclavik et al. proposed the use of direct analysis in real time (DART) with Orbitrap in positive mode for the control of different mycotoxins, including AFB1, AFB2, AFG1 and AFG2 in cereals, as wheat and maize [51]. Only ionization of some of tested AFs (AFB1, AFB2) was achieved by DART, being the sensitivity poor compared with triple quadrupole (QqQ). Lattanzio et al. [44] developed a LC-HRMS procedure for the simultaneous determination of AFs (B1, B2, G1, G2), and other mycotoxins in wheat flour, barley flour and crisp bread. Mycotoxin fragmentation patterns were obtained using Orbitrap. LODs in the 0.5–3.4 mg $kg^{-1}$ range were obtained for three cereal matrices and a critical comparison between the proposed method and a method based on QqQ showed similar performance. A comparison was also made by Renaud et al. [30] between a Q-Orbitrap and LC–MS/MS for AFB1, AFB2, AFG1 and AFG2 and other mycotoxins in maize. The linearity and LODs achieved were comparable by both methods. The technique TOF secondary ion mass spectrometry offers high sensitivity and identification of small molecules using the corresponding secondary molecular ions, which enabled a quantitative analysis of different aflatoxin analogues from corns with immunoaffinity columns (IACs) [52]. The detection sensitivity was estimated to be 10 μg $L^{-1}$ for the main four AFs. Tropical climate is a significantly favorable condition for fungus to develop as demonstrated by Giang et al. [43]. For this reason, mycotoxin contaminations are likely to occur on the cashew, especially aflatoxin. The toxins AFB1, AFB2, AFG1 and AFG2 were determined by UHPLC-HRMS in positive ion mode with LOQs ranged from 0.5 to 1.0 μg $kg^{-1}$. A method for the simultaneous determination of 9 mycotoxins, including the four main AFs in corn using UHPLC-Q-TOF was developed by Wang et al. [50]. LOQs ranged from 0.1 to 200 μg $kg^{-1}$. The developed method was applied to 130 corn samples, being AFB1 one of the most predominant mycotoxins, as it was found in 37 corn samples with concentrations between non-detected up to 593 μg $kg^{-1}$.

A simple and rapid multi-mycotoxin method for the determination of 17 mycotoxins simultaneously is described on **durum and soft wheat pasta baby food** samples [45] by UHPLC-Orbitrap in positive mode for AFB1. Twenty-nine samples were analyzed, 27 samples of durum wheat pasta, and two samples of baby food, and AFB1 was not detected in any sample (LOQ 0.11 μg $kg^{-1}$).

**Beer** is one of the most consumed cereal-based alcoholic beverages in the world, being usually obtained by fermenting certain starch-rich grains, such as malted barley and wheat, although other cereals like maize, oats, unmalted barley or rice, may be used. These raw materials can contain mycotoxins that are transferred to the final product. Bogdanova et al. [24] reports data on the occurrence of nine mycotoxins, including AFB1, in 100 beers using HPLC-TOF in positive mode. A LOQ of 0.150 μg $kg^{-1}$ was obtained for AFB1, being found contents between 0.1–0.19 μg $kg^{-1}$ for light beer samples. The low concentrations of AFB1 found in only a few samples could be related to its usually low prevalence in products manufactured and stored in the northern countries. AFB1 and other mycotoxins have also been determined in beer using LC-HRMS in positive mode by Rozentale et al. [25]. The LOD was 0.021 μg $L^{-1}$, and the toxin was not detected in any beer sample. Beer was also analyzed by Rubert et al. [23] using LC-ESI-IT-Orbitrap for the determination of 18 mycotoxins, including AFs (B1, B2, G1 and G2). The LOQs ranged from 9 to 30 μg $L^{-1}$. The method was applied to the analysis of 25 commercial beers, but no AFs were found.

**Nutraceutical products as dietary supplements and functional foods** contribute to a good nutrition, providing different alternatives for healthcare.

A multi-analytical strategy was proposed by Jia et al. [31] to screen mycotoxins and their transformation products in nutraceuticals from green tea. AFB1, AFB2, AFG1, AFG2 and AFM1 were determined using UHPLC-HRMS, obtaining entire spectrum of fragment ion peaks for each AF, which allows screening and quantitation of non-target mycotoxins. LOQs ranged between 0.02 and 0.40 μg $kg^{-1}$ and AFB1 was found in two samples (0.95 and 0.97 μg $kg^{-1}$). Among the plants that can be used for the preparation of nutraceuticals, *Ginkgo biloba* is widely used, obtaining the extract from ginkgo leaves. Martínez-Domínguez et al. [35] determined more than 250 toxic substances, including pesticides and mycotoxins, in *Ginkgo biloba* nutraceutical products using UHPLC-Orbitrap. LOD and LOQ below 5 and 10 μg $kg^{-1}$ were obtained, respectively. In the case of AFs, AFB1 (5–54 μg $kg^{-1}$) and AFB2 (4–300 μg $kg^{-1}$) were found in 6 samples. It should be noted that these levels are very high, especially the value obtained for AFB2 in one sample, considering the maximum contents allowed by the European legislation, and that AFB2 is one of the most toxic mycotoxins. The same authors [34] also applied the same approach for the analysis of isoflavone supplements obtained from soy, detecting AFB1 (8.2–17.1 μg $kg^{-1}$) and AFG2 (6.4 μg $kg^{-1}$), as well as to green tea and royal jelly supplements [36], quantifying AFB1 (5.4 μg $kg^{-1}$) in one of the green tea samples. Analysis of mycotoxins in functional and medicinal herbs is a challenge because herbs have complicated and diverse matrices from different parts of plants as well as different species. Thus, Cho et al. [46] developed a LC-tandem mass spectrometry (MS/MS) method for the determination of multi-class mycotoxins (including AFB1, AFB2, AFG1 and AFG2) in twenty different species of herbs that are used for both food and medicinal purposes. The results were further verified using Orbitrap in positive mode. AFB1 was found in six samples at levels around 5 ng $g^{-1}$. Coix seed is an important food and traditional Chinese medicine which is currently being used for the treatment of COVID-19 in China. Wu et al. [37] developed a method by UHPLC-HRMS for the simultaneous detection of 24 mycotoxins in coix seeds. The LOQs for AFB1, AFB2, AFG1, AFG2 and AFM1 were 0.5 μg $kg^{-1}$. More than 70 samples of coix seeds were collected from Chinese markets and were analyzed, being the results as follow: AFB1 positive ratio: 29.9%, range: 0.39–14.7 μg $kg^{-1}$; AFB2 positive ratio: 5.2%, range: 0.15–0.97 μg $kg^{-1}$; AFG1 positive ratio: 1.3%, range: 0.26–0.26 μg $kg^{-1}$; AFG2 positive ratio: 1.3%, range: 0.12–0.12 μg $kg^{-1}$; AFM1 positive ratio: 0%.

Mycotoxins are frequently present in **animal feed** due to their misuse, carry-over or environmental contamination. The consequence is the incorporation of these substances into the food chain and monitoring the presence of these hazardous chemicals remains one of the main tasks for ensuring feed safety and human health [1]. León et al. [38] developed a procedure for the quantitative target analysis of mycotoxins and other substances in feed using LC–HRMS using Orbitrap. For post-target screening a customized theoretical database including the exact mass, the polarity of acquisition and the expected adducts was built. Castaldo et al. [32] used a strategy combining a quantitative method for 28 mycotoxins, including AFB1, AFB2, AFG1 and AFG2, and a post-target screening for other 245 fungal and bacterial metabolites in dry **pet food** samples using UHPLC-Q-Orbitrap in positive mode. Results showed mycotoxin contamination in 99% of pet food samples at concentrations of up to hundreds μg $kg^{-1}$.

A **wide range of foods** such as peach seed, milk powder, corn flour and beer samples have been analyzed by Du et al. [28] for determining AFB1 and other fungi metabolites by UHPLC-Q-TOF with ESI in the positive mode. LODs were 0.0036–0.033 μg $kg^{-1}$ for solid samples and 0.0022–0.017 μg $L^{-1}$ for beer.

Modern MS detectors can be used not only as detectors, but also as a "separation" tool, due to significant advances in HRMS, achieving greater sensitivity and selectivity. Thus, **flow injection (FI)** can be used to introduce the sample into the MS instrument, saving time and solvent compared to UHPLC analysis. Using this approach, Sapozhnikova et al. [53] proposed the simultaneous detection of twelve pesticides and seven mycotoxins in food and feed samples by FI-MS, using QqQ and ion mobility HR-TOF. LODs in standard solutions were below maximum permitted content, except for AFB1 with the lowest maximum permitted content of 0.002 mg $kg^{-1}$.

Mycotoxins can be present in their parent forms and also in other forms, as **"modified mycotoxins"**, which are conjugated with glucoside, acetyl, sulphate, and/or glutathione or other substances. This term was first used for the hydroxylation product AFM1 of AFB1, which was present in mycotoxin-contaminated feed. Lu et al. [5] summarizes the target and non-target qualitative and quantitative analysis for modified mycotoxins using HRMS instruments, such as TOF and Orbitrap.

### 3.3 HRMS applications for biological sample analysis

The determination of mycotoxin exposure of human populations is difficult due to the heterogeneous distribution of mycotoxins in foods and the time lag between toxin intake and the development of chronic disease. Therefore, a more reliable and relevant indication of individual exposure could be provided by biomarkers measured in biological fluids.

Aflatoxins can bioaccumulate in the organs and tissues of animals and humans or be excreted by biological fluids or feces [39, 40]. Sensitive analytical procedures are required for the determination of AFs in biological samples due to the very low concentrations involved. Most of the analytical methods proposed are based on LC coupled to different detection systems such as spectrophotometry, fluorescence, MS or MS/MS. Recently, HRMS, including TOF and Orbitrap, resulted an excellent technique for target analysis of AFs as well as for identifying and screening of non-target compounds in metabolomic strategies for studies concerning bioaccumulation, toxicokinetics and excretion of AFs and their metabolites.

Most of the studies are related with **urine and blood** because sampling is non-invasive in the case of urine and minimally invasive in that of blood.

**Urine** is an easily accessible sample which can be easily collected in a large quantity and contains numerous metabolites. Urine samples were analyzed for the presence of AFB1 and AFM1 and AFB1-N7-guanine adduct by Debegnach et al. [40]. LODs obtained using LC–HRMS were 0.8 and 1.5 ng $L^{-1}$ urine for AFB1 and AFM1, respectively. No quantitative determination was possible for the adduct AFB1-N7-guanine. In the 120 urine samples analyzed, AFM1 was found in 14 samples in the range of 1.9–10.5 ng $L^{-1}$ urine, while AFB1 and its adduct were not detected. These results indicated that no workplace exposure was originated.

In addition, **blood** is a biofluid which incorporate the functions of different parts of the body into a single sample, being very useful for metabolomic studies. Human plasma samples were used for monitoring 17 mycotoxins, including AFB1, AFB2, AFG1 and AFG2, using HRMS on hybrid IT-Orbitrap in ESI positive mode by Slobodchikova et al. [22]. The LOQs of all the AFs were 0.2 μg $L^{-1}$. By using HRMS, the method can also be used for screening of the presence of different metabolites. Also, Slobodchikova et al. [54] performed human in vitro microsomal incubations of 17 mycotoxins and systematically characterize all resulting metabolites using LC–HRMS to build a library with screening of additional 188 metabolites, including 100 metabolites reported for the first time. NanoLC-Q-Orbitrap with isotope dilution MS was applied by McMillan et al. [26] to quantitate AFB1-lys in plasma samples from an extremely vulnerable population of Nigerian children suffering from severe acute malnutrition. The plasma levels of AFB1-lys in the population were between 0.2 and 59.2 μg $kg^{-1}$ albumin, with a median value of 2.6 μg $kg^{-1}$ albumin. AFB1-lys concentrations were significantly higher in children suffering with severe acute malnutrition. Identification of 56 natural toxic substances by LC–Q-TOF has been proposed by Ogawa et al. to create a forensic toxicological library [29]. The product ion spectra include the four main AFs, with positive ionization. The method was applied to post-mortem blood samples from a death resulting from the intake of aconite. The developed library permits the screening of natural toxic substances in routine forensic toxicological analysis. Serum samples were collected for the determination of AFB1 and AFB1-lys adduct [39]. For AFB1, a high number of non-detected samples was found (LOQ 5 μg $kg^{-1}$ serum) and none of the analyzed samples showed the presence of AFB1-lys adduct, thus the presence of AFB1 in serum cannot be attributable to occupational exposure. Serum AFB1-lys was also evaluated as an AFB1-specific biomarker for diagnostic purposes and for evaluating the efficacy of chemoprotective interventions in pigs [54]. The LOQ value was 10.3 μg $L^{-1}$ and results indicated that AFB1-lys has potential as an AFB1 specific biomarker for diagnostic purposes.

In comparison to other biological fluids such as blood, plasma and urine, the database on multi-mycotoxin levels in **human milk** is rather small. Breast milk is a relevant source of mycotoxins for neonates. Rubert et al. [33] proposed the use of LC–HRMS as excellent tool in the screening, quantitation and confirmation of targeted mycotoxins and their metabolites, including AFB1, AFB2, AFG1, AFG2 and AFM1. None of the AFs were detected in the breast milk samples.

Several studies propose to analyze **several biological samples** for metabolic studies. Thus, the correlation between exposure to AFB1 and early-stage renal damage was evaluated by Díaz de León-Martínez et al. [48] by analyzing urine and blood samples. The exposure to AFB1 was measured through the biomarker AFB1-lys. Plasma, urine and feces of pigs and plasma and urine of broiler chickens were used in a LC–HRMS procedure by Lauwers et al. [49] to determine mycotoxins, including AFs, and their metabolites with LOQ values of 1 μg $L^{-1}$. LC–HRMS was used on non-targeted qualitatively determination phase I and II metabolites, for which analytical standards are not always commercially available. The multi-method was successfully applied in a toxicokinetic study and a screening study to monitor the exposure of individual animals.

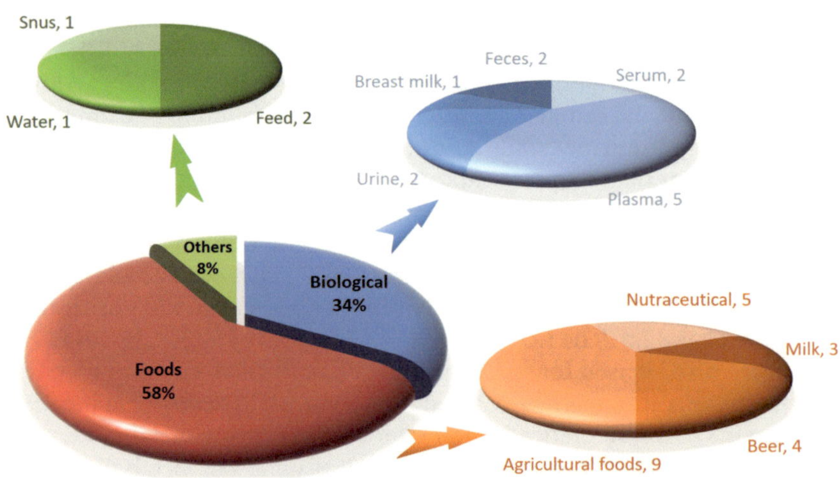


**Figure 3.**
*Type of samples more frequently analyzed. The number of published articles dealing with each matrix is indicated.*

**Figure 3** shows a distribution of the type of food and biological samples for which LC-HRMS methods have been applied in AF determination.

## 4. Sample treatments for determination of aflatoxins

Method accuracy and precision are strongly conditioned by the effectiveness and robustness of the sample treatment stage. Both physicochemical properties of the AFs and the sample matrix composition need to be considered in the extraction procedure selection, which should ideally isolate and concentrate the analytes, eliminate interferences, and provide extracts compatible with the analytical technique to be used. For example, AFB1 was extracted in acidified ethyl acetate (EtAc) from serum previously submitted to enzymatic digestion (ED) and lipid removing by liquid–liquid extraction (LLE) with hexane. Nevertheless, this extraction medium was unable to isolate the hydrophilic metabolite AFB1-lys from the same sample and, a salting-out step with a quick, easy, cheap, effective, rugged and safe (QuEChERS) mixture was applied [39]. The objective conditions the adoption of a more or less selective sample treatment. Thus, non-selective extractions are applied for non-targeted strategies, allowing retrospective analysis of any potential compound, whereas for targeted analysis, clean and concentrated extracts are required.

Solid samples are generally homogenized by grinding [37, 38, 43, 44, 46], in order to obtain representative sample aliquots before being submitted to a solid–liquid extraction (SLE) stage. Freeze-drying of feces has also been proposed for eliminating any variations due to different moisture contents [49]. For SLE, aqueous mixtures of polar organic solvents such as MeOH, acetone or ACN have been used for AFs isolation from biological [49] and food [37, 43, 44, 46, 52] samples, being the mixtures mechanically shaken. The application of external energy in SLE procedures is sometimes proposed in order to enhance analyte recoveries in low times. Ultrasound assisted extraction (UAE) [30, 32, 50, 55] and microwave assisted extraction (MAE) [28] have efficiently extract AFs from food matrices.

On the other hand, even though food and biological liquid samples could be directly analyzed HRMS or LC combined with HRMS, previous steps are generally applied to minimize matrix effects. Thus, the addition of organic solvents such as ACN or MeOH allowed deproteinization of plasma [26, 29, 49] and milk [42] samples. Enzymatic reactions have also proven to be effective for human serum deproteinization [39, 48].

The removing of non-polar sample components, such as phospholipids, has been proposed by LLE with hexane [39, 46], by solid-phase extraction (SPE) using SPE-phospholipid cartridges for pig feces [49] and well-plates for chicken plasma [49].

The isolation of AFB1, AFB2, AFG1, AFG2 and AFM1 by LLE using EtAc has been applied for urine [49] and serum [22, 39], being recommended though a three-step LLE by Slobodchikova et al. [22] which resulted in better recoveries than those provided by SPE or protein precipitation (PP) procedures in a multi-mycotoxin method.

The simultaneous sample matrix purification and AF isolation is accomplished by many of the applied treatments in a single step. Thus, an on-line SPE device allowed the simultaneous isolation of 12 mycotoxins, including AFB1, and matrix purification of beer samples. Although SPE is more commonly applied under off-line mode, as used by Rubert et al. for isolation of AFB1, AFB2, AFG1, AFG2 in a multi-mycotoxin method proposed for beer [23]. SLE extracts obtained from solid food matrices have also been submitted to SPE [43, 44]. Polymeric sorbents are used in SPE isolation of AFs in their free forms. Whereas mixed-mode SPE-sorbents are selected for the retention of AFB1-lys adduct. Thus, a modified extraction procedure involving a PP step before enzymatic digestion (ED) with Pronase® and

SPE-clean-up using strong ion mixed-mode-SPE has allowed both metabolic profiling and AFB1-lys adduct quantification in serum samples [26, 48].

Specific antibody-analyte binding is exploited as clean-up procedure in IACs, reporting interesting applications in AF analysis. Thus, gel suspensions of monoclonal antibody specific for AFs have allowed the purification of AFB1, AFB2, AFG1 and AFG2 from urine [40]. IAC have also been proposed for multi-mycotoxin studies, including AFs, for the analysis of functional and medicinal herbs [46]. In both articles reviewed dealing with IAC, AFs were eluted with MeOH after a washing step for impurities elimination using water [40] of aqueous buffer solutions [46].

QuEChERS methodology has been applied for AFs determination in both food [24, 32, 38, 41, 45, 50, 51, 53, 56] and biological samples [33, 39], using ACN as extractant solvent and a dispersive SPE (DSPE) step with the appropriate sorbents. When QuEChERS clean-up is applied omitting the use of sorbents, so that only implying organic solvent and salts, the procedure is named as simplified QuEChERS, and it has been proposed for isolation of AFB1, AFB2, AFG1, AFG2 and AFM1 from human breast milk [33] and AFB1 from durum wheat pasta [45]. The possibilities of different mixtures of solid sorbents for multi-class determinations of more than 250 compounds, pesticides and mycotoxins, including AFB1, AFB2, AFG1 and AFG2, applied to nutraceutical products have been studied by Martínez-Domínguez et al. [34–36] and compared with SLE, called in this case as "dilute and shoot" procedure. Best results have been reported by the latter procedure followed by a clean-up step using a mixture of sorbents in a DSPE mode [35, 36] or cartridge packed [34], this clean-up stage applied in order to enhance analyte recoveries and/or maintain the equipment performance for longer periods of times. When "dilute and shoot" procedure was compared to IAC for AFs in urine sample, lower LODs were achieved by the latter, because cleaner extracts with higher AF concentrations were obtained, being therefore selected [40]. An on-line automated sample preparation procedure is developed by Jia et al. [31] for multiple mycotoxin screening in nutraceutical products involving SLE, using aqueous acid solution and ACN, and the obtained supernatant being transferred to a disposable pipette extraction containing salt previously to the application of a clean-up step based on DSPE.

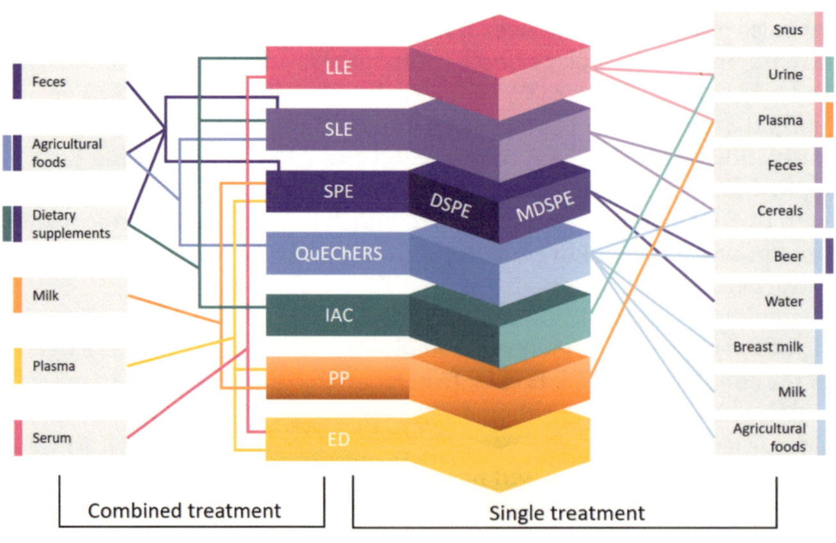


**Figure 4.**
*Sample treatments for AF determination by LC-HRMS.*

| Matrix | Sample treatment | Ref. |
|---|---|---|
| *Biological samples* | | |
| Human serum | ED of 0.5 mL sample with Pronase®, LLE degreasing with hexane and: LLE with acidified EtAc (for AFB1), QuEChERS (for FB1-lys) | [39] |
| Human serum | ED of 0.25 mL sample with Pronase® and mixed-mode SPE. Elution with acidified MeOH | [48] |
| Human plasma | PP of 0.23 mL sample with MeOH/water, supernatant ED with Pronase® and mixed-mode SPE. Elution with acidified MeOH | [26] |
| Human plasma | PP of 0.1 mL sample with EtOH/ACN | [29] |
| Human plasma | 3-step LLE of 0.1 mL sample with EtAc | [22] |
| Human urine | IAC for 2 mL sample. Elution with MeOH | [40] |
| Human breast milk | Simplified QuEChERS | [33] |
| Pig plasma, urine, and feces. Broiler chicken plasma and excreta | Pig plasma: PP of 0.25 mL sample with ACN. Pig urine: LLE of 0.5 mL sample with EtAc. Pig feces: SLE of 0.25 g sample with acetone and SPE for phospholipid removal.<br>Chicken plasma: PP of 0.15 mL sample with ACN and well-plates. Chicken excreta: SLE of 0.25 g sample with ACN | [49] |
| *Foods* | | |
| Beer | QuEChERS for 5 mL sample | [24] |
| Beer | On-line SPE for 0.5 mL sample. Elution with acidified ACN/$CH_3COONH_4$ | [25] |
| Beer | SPE for 10 mL sample. Elution with ACN/MeOH | [23] |
| Milk | PP of 4 g sample with ACN and MDSPE with 10 mg MNPs. Desorption with acidified EtAc | [42] |
| Milk | QuEChERS for 10 mL sample | [41] |
| Peach seed, milk powder, corn flour and beer | MAE of solid samples (0.2 g) in MeOH/water and DSPE with 2 mg zirconia NPs. Desorption with MeOH | [28] |
| Maize | UAE of 0.7 g sample in acidified MeOH/dichloromethane/EtAc | [55] |
| Maize | UAE of 0.5 g sample with acidified ACN | [30] |
| Corn | UAE of 2 g sample in ACN/water and QuEChERS | [50] |
| Cereal foods (flours and bread) | SLE of 10 g sample with ACN/water and SPE. Elution with MeOH | [44] |
| Durum wheat pasta and baby food pasta | Simplified QuEChERS for 4 g sample | [45] |
| Cashew nut | SLE of 1 g sample in MeOH/water and SPE. Elution with MeOH | [43] |
| Coix seed | SLE of 5 g sample with acidified ACN | [37] |
| Isoflavone supplements | SLE of 2.5 g sample with acidified ACN and clean-up by SPE | [34] |
| Ginkgo biloba nutraceuticals | SLE of 2.5 g sample with acidified ACN and clean-up by DSPE | [35] |
| Green tea and royal jelly supplements | SLE of 2.5 g sample with acidified ACN and clean-up by DSPE | [36] |
| Green tea nutraceuticals | SLE of 1 g sample with acidified ACN and clean-up by DSPE | [31] |
| Functional and medicinal herbs | SLE of 2 g sample with PBS, LLE degreasing with hexane and IAC. Elution with MeOH | [46] |

| Matrix | Sample treatment | Ref. |
|---|---|---|
| *Others* | | |
| Pet foods | UAE of 2 g sample in acidified ACN and QuEChERS | [32] |
| Feed | Simplified QuEChERS | [38] |
| Surface and drinking waters | SPE for 100 mL sample. Elution with MeOH/water/acetone | [47] |
| Snus | LLE with acidified EtAc | [27] |

**Table 2.**
*Summary of the sample treatments used in the AF determination by LC-HRMS.*

In the last years, nanoparticles (NPs) have received great attention in analytical chemistry due to the high surface area to volume ratio if compared to particles of higher dimensions, thus leading to very efficient extractions in lower times. A mass of 2 mg of zirconia NPs dispersed in the aqueous extract obtained by MAE from food samples allowed the DSPE isolation of AFB1 in 2 min, being then submitted to a desorption step in acidified chloroform [28]. When magnetized NPs are used, the collection of the enriched NPs is easily achieved by applying an external magnetic field, avoiding the centrifugation step. Under this named magnetic dispersive solid-phase extraction (MDSPE) methodology, AFB1, AFB2, AFG1, AFG2, AFM1 and AFM2, in a multiclass mycotoxin analysis method, have been preconcentrated with multi-walled carbon nanotubes (MWCNTs) modified with polyethylene glycol [42]. Although not implying HRMS detection for LC, it is noteworthy that AFB1 has also been preconcentrated with amino-modified magnetic MWCNTs [57].

With the aim to enhance sensitivity and clean-up purposes, the AF extracts finally obtained by applying the selected isolation procedure, are generally evaporated to dryness and reconstituted in low volumes of solvents compatible with the instrumental measurement step.

The data provided in this review demonstrate that most of the studies dealing with AF determination by LC-HRMS are focused on food, feed and biological samples analysis. In fact, only two manuscripts dealing with other matrices, waters [47] and snus [27], were found. A triple-stage SPE, consisting of a hand-made cartridge, packed with porous graphitized carbon and modified styrene-divinylbenzene polymer, coupled to a commercial HLB plus cartridge, allowed the isolation of natural toxins of different polarities. Thus, a screening method is proposed for the tentative identification of mycotoxins, cyanotoxins and plant toxins in surface waters [47]. The use of multiple Heart-cutting 2D-LC-Q-Orbitrap for AF separation and detection, respectively, has probably allowed to apply a very simple procedure in the treatment of snus samples. Thus, LLE in acidified EtAc provided similar analyte recoveries than QuEChERS method [27].

As can be appreciated in **Figure 4**, sample treatments for AF determination by LC-HRMS have been proposed both applying a unique methodology or through the combination of different procedures generally sequentially applied, for both food and biological samples.

A summary of the sample treatments involved in the reviewed LC-HRMS methods appearing in the literature for AF determination in different matrices is provided as well in **Table 2**.

## 5. LC-HRMS for AF biosynthesis and degradation studies

AFs are synthesized via multiple intermediates by a complex pathway in several species of the *Aspergillus* genus, including *Aspergillus flavus*. LC-HRMS combination has allowed the study of the biosynthesis pathway by monitoring the changes in metabolite profiles, as proposed Xie et al. [58] under different growth and environmental conditions and using Orbitrap. On the other hand, the role of quercetin as inhibitor of the AF biosynthesis has been studied by Tiwari and Shankar [59], using nano-LC-Q-TOF for protein identification and HPLC-UV for AFB1 levels monitorization. The results obtained showed the power of quercetin as anti-aflatogenic agent in *A. flavus*. A strategy based on UHPLC-Orbitrap has been proposed by Arroyo et al. [60] to study the function of certain genes of *A. flavus*, allowing to verify some steps of the biosynthesis pathway of AFs.

As regards mycotoxin degradation, decontamination techniques for AFs in food and feed attract continuous interest due to their adverse health effects and large economic losses for producers. In this sense, physical, chemical and biological strategies have been proposed. Thus, ABF1 degradation products by electron beam irradiation have been identified, as well as the possible pathway, using UHPLC-Q-TOF-MS [61, 62]. High-voltage atmospheric cold plasma (HVACP) is other physical strategy applied for AFB1 decontamination, providing a 76% efficiency when the non-thermal treatment was applied for 5 min in air containing 40% relative humidity. Thus, molecular formulas of six degradation products were elucidated by HPLC-TOF and their structures were further studied by Orbitrap MS. Two of the detected degradation compounds were ozonolysis products of AFB1, and the other four indicated the action of other reactive species besides ozone, generated during HVACP treatment [63]. The proven degradation power of ultrasounds for AFB1 aqueous solutions allows to perceive this physical detoxification technology as promising for food industry. An ultrasound exposure of 80 min degraded AFB1 by 85.1%, being eight main reaction products identified by UHPLC-Q-Orbitrap [64]. The study of degradation pathways and structural identification of photodegradation products of AFB1 in aqueous medium [65], ACN [66] and on peanut surface [67], has been carried out using UHPLC-Q-TOF after ultraviolet irradiation of different intensities.

Biological degradation, mainly caused by bacterial and fungal enzymes, appears as a strategy for AFB1 removal, with inherent advantages over physical and chemical strategies such as being friendly to the environment. LC-Q-TOF has been applied in the monitorization of AFB1 degradation products, and the obtained results lead the authors to propose bacterial strain *Bacillus licheniformis* BL010 for detoxification of AFB1 [68]. The degrading properties of *P. aeruginosa* towards AFB1 have been studied by Sangare et al. [69], and as no degradation products were identified by LC-Q-TOF, the decontamination route was proposed through the formation of products of chemical properties different from that of the parent AF. On the other hand, the enzymatic reaction based on the recombinant Rh_DypB peroxidase for the *in vitro* biotransformation of AFB1 has been studied by Loi et al. [70], proving an efficient detoxification at low enzyme and hydrogen peroxide concentrations. A 96% AFB1 hydroxylation yield to a less toxic AF, AFQ1, was observed after 96 h of reaction. The authors indicated the convenience to explore the translation of this strategy towards contaminated matrices. On the other hand, the salt tolerant yeast *Candida versatilis* CGMCC has also demonstrated its capacity to degrade AFB1, through the formation of four non-toxic products which have been identified by LC-Q-TOF [71].

## 6. Conclusion

AFs are secondary toxic metabolites which may be present mainly in contaminated food and biological samples at very low levels. Among them, AFB1 is considered the most toxic, being classified as a human carcinogen. The analysis of food and biological samples is very complex and includes different steps as extraction, clean-up, separation, and detection approaches. This chapter reports the main analytical procedures developed for the AF determination by LC-HRMS. Different sample preparation techniques have been proposed, being QuEChERS, SPE and SLE the more frequently used. New nanomaterials including magnetic nanoparticles have been recently applied as adsorbents, increasing extraction efficiency and specificity. Separation of AFs is usually performed using HPLC, which performance was improved when using UHPLC. Different detectors are proposed, being MS or MS/MS widely applied, ensuring a specific confirmation for targeted analysis. However, the toxicological pathway of AFs in biological samples leads to the appearance of modified or masked mycotoxins, whose structures must be accurately established, making their detection difficult using routine analytical methods. On the other hand, the lack of commercial analytical standards results a great challenge for accurate identification and quantitation of modified AFs. In this field, HRMS has proven to be a very effective tool to enable the rapid determination of both parent and modified AFs. The use of metabolomic platforms combined with HRMS is nowadays considered the most appropriate way to study the toxicokinetic behavior of AFs in order to establish, when possible, maximum tolerable intakes and to investigate whether they have any relationship with certain clinical pathologies and cancer processes.

## Acknowledgements

The authors acknowledge the financial support of the Comunidad Autónoma de la Región de Murcia (CARM, Fundación Séneca, Project 19888/GERM/15), the Spanish MICINN (PGC2018-098363-B-100), the University of Murcia (R-987/2020) and the European Commission (FEDER).

## Abbreviations

| | |
|---|---|
| AA | acetic acid |
| ACN | acetonitrile |
| AFAR | aflatoxin aldehyde reductase |
| AFL | Aflatoxicol |
| AFs | aflatoxins |
| AFB1 | aflatoxin B1 |
| AFB2 | aflatoxin B2 |
| AFBO | aflatoxin-8,9-epoxide |
| AFG1 | aflatoxin G1 |
| AFG1 | aflatoxin G2 |
| AFM1 | aflatoxin M1 |
| AFM2 | aflatoxin M2 |
| AFP1 | aflatoxin P1 |
| AFQ1 | aflatoxin Q1 |
| AIF | all-ion fragmentation |
| AP | aputinic |
| DART | direct analysis in real time |
| 2D | Two-dimensional |
| dd-$MS^2$ | data dependent |
| DIA | data independent |

| | |
|---|---|
| DMSPE | dispersive magnetic solid-phase extraction |
| DPEP | dipeptidase |
| DSPE | dispersive solid-phase extraction |
| ED | enzymatic digestion |
| ESI | electrospray ionization |
| EtAc | ethyl acetate |
| EtOH | ethanol |
| FA | formic acid |
| FAPy | formamidopyramidine |
| FI | flow injection |
| GGT | γ-glutamyltransferase |
| GSH | glutathione |
| GST | glutathione S-transferase |
| HCD | high energy collision dissociation |
| HESI | heated electrospray ionization |
| HRMS | high resolution mass spectrometry |
| HVACP | high-voltage atmospheric cold plasma |
| IACs | immunoaffinity columns |
| IARC | International Agency for Research on Cancer |
| IDMS | isotope dilution mass spectrometry |
| IT | ion trap |
| LC | liquid chromatography |
| LLE | liquid–liquid extraction |
| LOD | limit of detection |
| LOQ | limit of quantification |
| lys | lysine |
| MAE | microwave assisted extraction |
| MDSPE | magnetic dispersed solid-phase extraction |
| MeOH | methanol |
| MS | mass spectrometry |
| MS/MS | tandem mass spectrometry |
| MWCNT | multi-walled carbon nanotubes |
| NAT | N-acetyltransferase |
| NPs | nanoparticles |
| PBS | phosphate-buffered solution |
| PFP | pentafluorophenyl |
| PP | protein precipitation |
| PRM | parallel reaction monitoring mode |
| Q | quadrupole |
| QqQ | triple quadrupole |
| QuEChERS | quick easy cheap effective rugged and safe |
| SIM | selected ion monitoring |
| SLE | solid–liquid extraction |
| SPE | solid-phase extraction |
| TOF | time-of-flight |
| TOF-SIMS | time-of-flight secondary ion mass spectrometry |
| UAE | ultrasound assisted extraction |
| UHPLC | ultra-high performance liquid chromatography |
| WHO | World Health Organization. |

## Author details

Natalia Arroyo-Manzanares, Natalia Campillo, Ignacio López-García and Pilar Viñas*
Department of Analytical Chemistry, Faculty of Chemistry, Regional Campus of International Excellence "Campus Mare Nostrum", University of Murcia, Murcia, Spain

*Address all correspondence to: pilarvi@um.es

## References

[1] Marin S, Ramos AJ, Cano-Sancho G, Sanchis V. Mycotoxins: Occurrence, toxicology, and exposure assessment. Food and Chemical Toxicology. 2013;60:218-237. DOI: 10.1016/j.fct.2013.07.047.

[2] EFSA Panel on Contaminants in the Food Chain (CONTAM). Scientific opinion on ergot alkaloids in food and feed. EFSA Journal. 2012;10(7):2798. DOI: 10.2903/j.efsa.2012.2798.

[3] Singh C, Prakash C, Mishra P, Tiwari KN, Mishra SK, More RS, et al. Hepatoprotective efficacy of *Premna integrifolia* L. leaves against aflatoxin B1-induced toxicity in mice. Toxicon. 2019;166:88-100. DOI: 10.1016/j.toxicon.2019.05.014.

[4] Freire L, Sant'Ana AS. Modified mycotoxins: An updated review on their formation, detection, occurrence, and toxic effects. Food and Chemical Toxicology. 2018;111:189-205. DOI: 10.1016/j.fct.2017.11.021.

[5] Lu Q, Qin JA, Fu YW, Luo JY, Lu JH, Logrieco AF, et al. Modified mycotoxins in foodstuffs, animal feed, and herbal medicine: A systematic review on global occurrence, transformation mechanism and analysis methods. TrAC-Trends in Analytical Chemistry. 2020;133:28. DOI: 10.1016/j.trac.2020.116088.

[6] Benkerroum N. Chronic and acute toxicities of aflatoxins: Mechanisms of action. International Journal on Environmental Research and Public Health. 2020;17(2):423. DOI:10.3390/ijerph17020423

[7] Kelly JD, Eaton DL, Guengerich FP, Coulombe RA. Aflatoxin B1 activation in human lung. Toxicology and Applied Pharmacology. 1997;144(1):88-95. DOI: 10.1006/taap.1997.8117.

[8] Marchese S, Polo A, Ariano A, Velotto S, Costantini S, Severino L. Aflatoxin B1 and M1: Biological properties and their involvement in cancer development. Toxins. 2018;10(6):214. DOI:10.3390/toxins10060214.

[9] Fouad AM, Ruan D, El-Senousey HK, Chen W, Jiang S, Zheng C. Harmful effects and control strategies of aflatoxin B1 produced by *Aspergillus flavus* and *Aspergillus parasiticus* strains on poultry: Review. Toxins. 2019;11(3):176. DOI:10.3390/toxins11030176.

[10] Scientific Committee on Food. "Opinion on aflatoxins, ochratoxin A and patulin" expressed on 23 september 1994. Reports of the Scientific Committee on Food-35° Series (European Commission, DG Industry). 1996.

[11] Claeys L, Romano C, De Ruyck K, Wilson H, Fervers B, Korenjak M, et al. Mycotoxin exposure and human cancer risk: A systematic review of epidemiological studies. Comprehensive Reviews in Food Science and Food Safety. 2020;19(4):1449-1464. DOI: 10.1111/1541-4337.12567.

[12] IARC, Monographs on the evaluation of carcinogenic risks to humans. Lyon, 2012; Vol. 100F, Chemical agents and related occupations.

[13] IARC, Monographs on the evaluation of carcinogenic risks to humans. Lyon, 1993; Vol. 56, Some naturally occurring substances: Food items and constituents, heterocyclic aromatic amines and mycotoxins.

[14] IARC, Monographs on the evaluation of carcinogenic risks to humans. Lyon, 2002; Vol. 82, Some traditional herbal medicines, some mycotoxins, naphthalene and styrene.

[15] Marin DE, Taranu I. Overview on aflatoxins and oxidative stress. Toxin

Reviews. 2012;31(3-4):32-43. DOI: 10.3109/15569543.2012.730092.

[16] Rushing BR, Selim MI. Aflatoxin B1: A review on metabolism, toxicity, occurrence in food, occupational exposure, and detoxification methods. Food and Chemical Toxicology. 2019;124:81-100. DOI: 10.1016/j.fct.2018.11.047.

[17] Gross-Steinmeyer K, Eaton DL. Dietary modulation of the biotransformation and genotoxicity of aflatoxin B1. Toxicology. 2012;299(2):69-79. DOI: 10.1016/j.tox.2012.05.016.

[18] Bammler TK, Slone DH, Eaton DL. Effects of dietary oltipraz and ethoxyquin on aflatoxin B1 biotransformation in non-human primates. Toxicological Sciences. 2000;54(1):30-41. DOI: 10.1093/toxsci/54.1.30.

[19] Commission Regulation (EC) No 1881/2006 of 19 December 2006 setting maximum levels for certain contaminants in foodstuffs. Official Journal of the European Union 2006;L364:5-24.

[20] Directive 2002/32/EC of the European Parliament and of the council of 7 May 2002 on undesirable substances in animal feed. Official Journal of the European Communities 2002;L140:10-21.

[21] Sekera ER, Wood TD. Sequencing proteins from bottom to top: Combining techniques for full sequence analysis of glucokinase. In: Woods AG, Darie CC, editors. Advancements of mass spectrometry in biomedical research. Cham: Springer International Publishing; 2019, p.111-119. DOI: 10.1007/978-3-030-15950-4_6.

[22] Slobodchikova I, Vuckovic D. Liquid chromatography – high resolution mass spectrometry method for monitoring of 17 mycotoxins in human plasma for exposure studies. Journal of Chromatography A. 2018;1548:51-63. DOI: 10.1016/j.chroma.2018.03.030.

[23] Rubert J, Manes J, James KJ, Soler C. Application of hybrid linear ion trap-high resolution mass spectrometry to the analysis of mycotoxins in beer. Food Additives & Contaminants Part A. 2011;28(10):1438-1446. DOI: 10.1080/19440049.2011.595015.

[24] Bogdanova E, Rozentale I, Pugajeva I, Emecheta EE, Bartkevics V. Occurrence and risk assessment of mycotoxins, acrylamide, and furan in Latvian beer. Food Additives & Contaminants Part B. 2018;11(2):126-137. DOI: 10.1080/19393210.2018.1440636.

[25] Rozentale I, Bogdanova E, Bartkevics V. A rapid and sensitive method for the control of selected regulated and emerging mycotoxins in beer. World Mycotoxin Journal. 2018;11(4):503-517. DOI: 10.3920/wmj2017.2298.

[26] McMillanA,RenaudJB,BurgessKMN, Orimadegun AE, Akinyinka OO, Allen SJ, et al. Aflatoxin exposure in Nigerian children with severe acute malnutrition. Food and Chemical Toxicology. 2018;111:356-362. DOI: 10.1016/j.fct.2017.11.030.

[27] Qi DW, Fei T, Liu H, Yao HM, Wu D, Liu BZ. Development of multiple heart-cutting two-dimensional liquid chromatography coupled to quadrupole-Orbitrap high resolution mass spectrometry for simultaneous determination of aflatoxin $B_1$, $B_2$, $G_1$, $G_2$, and ochratoxin A in snus, a smokeless tobacco product. Journal of Agricultural and Food Chemistry. 2017;65(45):9923-9929. DOI: 10.1021/acs.jafc.7b04329.

[28] Du LJ, Chu C, Warner E, Wang QY, Hu YH, Chai KJ, et al. Rapid microwave-assisted dispersive micro-solid phase

extraction of mycotoxins in food using zirconia nanoparticles. Journal of Chromatography A. 2018;1561:1-12. DOI: 10.1016/j.chroma.2018.05.031.

[29] Ogawa T, Zaitsu K, Kokaji T, Suga K, Kondo F, Iwai M, et al. Development and application of a forensic toxicological library for identification of 56 natural toxic substances by liquid chromatography-quadrupole time-of-flight mass spectrometry. Forensic Toxicology. 2020;38(1):232-242. DOI: 10.1007/s11419-019-00506-w.

[30] Renaud JB, Sumarah MW. Data independent acquisition-digital archiving mass spectrometry: application to single kernel mycotoxin analysis of *Fusarium graminearum* infected maize. Analytical and Bioanalytical Chemistry. 2016;408(12):3083-3091. DOI: 10.1007/s00216-016-9391-5.

[31] Jia W, Shi L, Zhang F, Fan C, Chang J, Chu X. Multiplexing data independent untargeted workflows for mycotoxins screening on a quadrupole-Orbitrap high resolution mass spectrometry platform. Food Chemistry. 2019;278:67-76. DOI: 10.1016/j.foodchem.2018.11.056.

[32] Castaldo L, Graziani G, Gaspari A, Izzo L, Tolosa J, Rodríguez-Carrasco Y, et al. Target analysis and retrospective screening of multiple mycotoxins in pet food using UHPLC-Q-Orbitrap HRMS. Toxins. 2019;11(8):434. DOI: 10.3390/toxins11080434.

[33] Rubert J, León N, Sáez C, Martins CPB, Godula M, Yusà V, et al. Evaluation of mycotoxins and their metabolites in human breast milk using liquid chromatography coupled to high resolution mass spectrometry. Analytica Chimica Acta. 2014;820:39-46. DOI: 10.1016/j.aca.2014.02.009.

[34] Martínez-Domínguez G, Romero-González R, Arrebola FJ, Garrido Frenich A. Multi-class determination of pesticides and mycotoxins in isoflavones supplements obtained from soy by liquid chromatography coupled to Orbitrap high resolution mass spectrometry. Food Control. 2016;59:218-224. DOI: 10.1016/j.foodcont.2015.05.033.

[35] Martínez-Domínguez G, Romero-González R, Garrido Frenich A. Determination of toxic substances, pesticides and mycotoxins, in *Ginkgo biloba* nutraceutical products by liquid chromatography Orbitrap-mass spectrometry. Microchemical Journal. 2015;118:124-130. DOI: 10.1016/j.microc.2014.09.002.

[36] Martínez-Domínguez G, Romero-González R, Garrido Frenich A. Multi-class methodology to determine pesticides and mycotoxins in green tea and royal jelly supplements by liquid chromatography coupled to Orbitrap high resolution mass spectrometry. Food Chemistry. 2016;197:907-915. DOI: 10.1016/j.foodchem.2015.11.070.

[37] Wu Y, Ye J, Xuan Z, Li L, Wang H, Wang S, et al. Development and validation of a rapid and efficient method for simultaneous determination of mycotoxins in coix seed using one-step extraction and UHPLC-HRMS. Food Additives & Contaminants: Part A. 2021;38(1):148-159. DOI: 10.1080/19440049.2020.1833089.

[38] León N, Pastor A, Yusa V. Target analysis and retrospective screening of veterinary drugs, ergot alkaloids, plant toxins and other undesirable substances in feed using liquid chromatography-high resolution mass spectrometry. Talanta. 2016;149:43-52. DOI: 10.1016/j.talanta.2015.11.032.

[39] De Santis B, Debegnach F, Sonego E, Mazzilli G, Buiarelli F, Ferri F, et al. Biomonitoring data for assessing aflatoxins and ochratoxin A exposure by Italian feedstuffs workers. Toxins.

2019;11(6):351. DOI: 10.3390/toxins11060351.

[40] Debegnach F, Brera C, Mazzilli G, Sonego E, Buiarelli F, Ferri F, et al. Optimization and validation of a LC-HRMS method for aflatoxins determination in urine samples. Mycotoxin Research. 2020;36(2):257-266. DOI: 10.1007/s12550-020-00389-6.

[41] Rodríguez-Carrasco Y, Izzo L, Gaspari A, Graziani G, Manes J, Ritieni A. Simultaneous determination of AFB1 and AFM1 in milk samples by ultra high performance liquid chromatography coupled to quadrupole Orbitrap mass spectrometry. Beverages. 2018;4(2):43. DOI: 10.3390/beverages4020043.

[42] Zhao Y, Yuan YC, Bai XL, Liu YM, Wu GF, Yang FS, et al. Multi-mycotoxins analysis in liquid milk by UHPLC-Q-Exactive HRMS after magnetic solid-phase extraction based on PEGylated multi-walled carbon nanotubes. Food Chemistry. 2020;305:125429. DOI: 10.1016/j.foodchem.2019.125429.

[43] Giang L, Thien TLT. Determination of aflatoxin B1, B2, G1, G2 in cashew nut by UHPLC-HRMS. Vietnam Journal of Chemistry 2020;58(4):540-547. DOI: 10.1002/vjch.202000027.

[44] Lattanzio VM, Gatta SD, Godula M, Visconti A. Quantitative analysis of mycotoxins in cereal foods by collision cell fragmentation-high-resolution mass spectrometry: performance and comparison with triple-stage quadrupole detection. Food Additives & Contaminants: Part A. 2011;28(10):1424-1437. DOI: 10.1080/19440049.2011.593192.

[45] Tolosa J, Graziani G, Gaspari A, Chianese D, Ferrer E, Manes J, et al. Multi-mycotoxin analysis in durum wheat pasta by liquid chromatography coupled to quadrupole Orbitrap mass spectrometry. Toxins. 2017;9(2):59. DOI: 10.3390/toxins9020059.

[46] Cho HD, Suh JH, Feng S, Eom T, Kim J, Hyun SM, et al. Comprehensive analysis of multi-class mycotoxins in twenty different species of functional and medicinal herbs using liquid chromatography-tandem mass spectrometry. Food Control. 2019;96:517-526. DOI: 10.1016/j.foodcont.2018.10.007.

[47] Picardo M, Sanchís J, Núñez O, Farré M. Suspect screening of natural toxins in surface and drinking water by high performance liquid chromatography and high-resolution mass spectrometry. Chemosphere. 2020;261:127888. DOI: 10.1016/j.chemosphere.2020.127888.

[48] Díaz de León-Martínez L, Díaz-Barriga F, Barbier O, Ortíz DLG, Ortega-Romero M, Pérez-Vázquez F, et al. Evaluation of emerging biomarkers of renal damage and exposure to aflatoxin-$B_1$ in Mexican indigenous women: a pilot study. Environmental Science and Pollution Research. 2019;26:12205-12216. DOI: 10.1007/s11356-019-04634-z.

[49] Lauwers M, De Baere S, Letor B, Rychlik M, Croubels S, Devreese M. Multi LC-MS/MS and LC-HRMS methods for determination of 24 mycotoxins including major phase I and II biomarker metabolites in biological matrices from pigs and broiler chickens. Toxins. 2019;11:171. DOI: 10.3390/toxins11030171.

[50] Wang Y, Dong YJ, Li ZM, Deng LG, Guo CY, Zhang SQ, et al. Fast determination of multi-mycotoxins in corn by dispersive solid-phase extraction coupled with ultra-performance liquid chromatography with tandem quadrupole time-of-flight mass spectrometry. Journal of Integrative Agriculture. 2016;15(7):1656-1666. DOI: 10.1016/s2095-3119(15)61287-4.

[51] Vaclavik L, Zachariasova M, Hrbek V, Hajslova J. Analysis of multiple mycotoxins in cereals under ambient conditions using direct analysis in real time (DART) ionization coupled to high resolution mass spectrometry. Talanta. 2010;82(5):1950-7. DOI: 10.1016/j.talanta.2010.08.029.

[52] Ahn JH, Jeong YS, Lee TG, Kim YP, Kim HS. Sensitive and multiplexed analysis of aflatoxins using time-of-flight secondary ion mass spectrometry. BioChip Journal. 2012;6(1):34-40. DOI: 10.1007/s13206-012-6105-8.

[53] Sapozhnikova Y, Zomer P, Gerssen A, Nuñez A, Mol HGJ. Evaluation of flow injection mass spectrometry approach for rapid screening of selected pesticides and mycotoxins in grain and animal feed samples. Food Control. 2020;116:107323. DOI: 10.1016/j.foodcont.2020.107323.

[54] Di Gregorio MC, Jager AV, Souto PCMC, Costa AA, Rottinghaus GE, Passarelli D, et al. Determination of serum aflatoxin B1-lysine to evaluate the efficacy of an aflatoxin-adsorbing feed additive in pigs fed an aflatoxin B1-contaminated diet. Mycotoxin Research. 2017;33(2):93-102. DOI: 10.1007/s12550-016-0267-5.

[55] Mitema A, Feto NA, Rafudeen MS. Development and validation of TOF/Q-TOF MS/MS, HPLC method and in vitro bio-strategy for aflatoxin mitigation. Food Additives & Contaminants: Part A. 2020;37(12):2149-64. DOI: 10.1080/19440049.2020.1815861.

[56] Sirhan AY, Tan GH, Al-Shunnaq, A, Abdulra'uf L, Wong RCS. QuEChERS-HPLC method for aflatoxin detection of domestic and imported food in JORDAN. Journal of Liquid Chromatography & Related Technologies. 2014;37(3):321-42. DOI: 10.1080/10826076.2012.745138.

[57] Li W-k, Zhang H-x, Shi Y-p. Simultaneous determination of aflatoxin B1 and zearalenone by magnetic nanoparticle filled amino-modified multi-walled carbon nanotubes. Analytical Methods. 2018;10(27):3353-63. DOI: 10.1039/C8AY00815A.

[58] Xie HL, Wang XP, Zhang LX, Wang T, Zhang W, Jiang J, et al. Monitoring metabolite production of aflatoxin biosynthesis by Orbitrap Fusion mass spectrometry and a D-optimal mixture design method. Analytical Chemistry. 2018;90(24):14331-8. DOI: 10.1021/acs.analchem.8b03703.

[59] Tiwari S, Shankar J. Integrated proteome and HPLC analysis revealed quercetin-mediated inhibition of aflatoxin B1 biosynthesis in *Aspergillus flavus*. 3 Biotech. 2018;8:47. DOI: 10.1007/s13205-017-1067-0.

[60] Arroyo-Manzanares N, Diana Di Mavungu J, Uka V, Malysheva SV, Cary JW, Ehrlich KC, et al. Use of UHPLC high-resolution Orbitrap mass spectrometry to investigate the genes involved in the production of secondary metabolites in *Aspergillus flavus*. Food Additives & Contaminants: Part A. 2015;32(10):1656-73. DOI: 10.1080/19440049.2015.1071499.

[61] Wang RQ, Liu RJ, Chang M, Jin QZ, Huang JH, Liu YF, et al. Ultra-performance liquid chromatography quadrupole time-of-flight MS for identification of electron beam from accelerator degradation products of aflatoxin $B_1$. Applied Biochemistry and Biotechnology. 2015;175(3):1548-56. DOI: 10.1007/s12010-014-1377-1.

[62] Liu RJ, Wang RQ, Lu J, Chang M, Jin QZ, Du ZB, et al. Degradation of $AFB_1$ in aqueous medium by electron beam irradiation: Kinetics, pathway and toxicology. Food Control. 2016;66:151-7. DOI: 10.1016/j.foodcont.2016.02.002.

[63] Shi H, Cooper B, Stroshine RL, Ileleji KE, Keener KM. Structures of

degradation products and degradation pathways of aflatoxin $B_1$ by high-voltage atmospheric cold plasma (HVACP) treatment. Journal of Agricultural and Food Chemistry. 2017;65(30):6222-6230. DOI: 10.1021/acs.jafc.7b01604.

[64] Liu YF, Li MM, Liu YX, Bian K. Structures of reaction products and degradation pathways of aflatoxin $B_1$ by ultrasound treatment. Toxins. 2019;11(9):526. DOI: 10.3390/toxins11090526.

[65] Liu RJ, Jin QZ, Tao GJ, Shan L, Huang JH, Liu YF, et al. Photodegradation kinetics and byproducts identification of the aflatoxin $B_1$ in aqueous medium by ultra-performance liquid chromatography-quadrupole time-of-flight mass spectrometry. Journal of Mass Spectrometry. 2010;45(5):553-559. DOI: 10.1002/jms.1741.

[66] Liu RJ, Jin QZ, Tao GJ, Shan L, Liu YF, Wang XG. LC-MS and UPLC-quadrupole time-of-flight MS for identification of photodegradation products of aflatoxin $B_1$. Chromatographia. 2010;71(1-2):107-112. DOI: 10.1365/s10337-009-1354-y.

[67] Chang M, Jin QZ, Liu YF, Liu RJ, Wang XG. Efficiency and safety evaluation of photodegradation of aflatoxin $B_1$ on peanut surface. International Journal of Food Science & Technology. 2013;48(12):2474-2479. DOI: 10.1111/ijfs.12238.

[68] Wang Y, Zhang HY, Yan H, Yin CH, Liu Y, Xu QQ, et al. Effective biodegradation of aflatoxin B1 using the *Bacillus licheniformis* (BL010) strain. Toxins. 2018;10(12):497. DOI: 10.3390/toxins10120497.

[69] Sangare L, Zhao YJ, Folly YME, Chang JH, Li JH, Selvaraj JN, et al. Aflatoxin $B_1$ degradation by a Pseudomonas strain. Toxins. 2014;6(10):3028-3040. DOI: 10.3390/toxins6103028.

[70] Loi M, Renaud JB, Rosini E, Pollegioni L, Vignali E, Haidukowski M, et al. Enzymatic transformation of aflatoxin $B_1$ by Rh_DypB peroxidase and characterization of the reaction products. Chemosphere. 2020;250:126296. DOI: 10.1016/j.chemosphere.2020.126296.

[71] Li JL, Huang J, Jin Y, Wu CD, Shen DZ, Zhang SY, et al. Mechanism and kinetics of degrading aflatoxin $B_1$ by salt tolerant *Candida versatilis* CGMCC 3790. Journal of Hazardous Materials. 2018;359:382-387. DOI: 10.1016/j.jhazmat.2018.05.053.